THE FAMILY
Naturopathic
ENCYCLOPEDIA

D0557854

THE FAMILY
Naturopathic
ENCYCLOPEDIA

*Your comprehensive, user-friendly guide to naturally
treating medical conditions for the whole family*

LINDA WOOLVEN M.H., C.A.c. & TED SNIDER
With Foreword By Michael T. Murray, N.D.

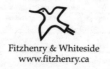

Fitzhenry & Whiteside
www.fitzhenry.ca

Published in Canada by Fitzhenry & Whiteside, 195 Allstate Parkway, Markham, Ontario L3R 4T8

Published in the United States by Fitzhenry & Whiteside, 311 Washington Street, Brighton, Massachusetts 02135

www.fitzhenry.ca godwit@fitzhenry.ca

10 9 8 7 6 5 4 3 2 1

Library and Archives Canada Cataloguing in Publication
Woolven, Linda
The family naturopathic encyclopedia / Linda Woolven and Ted Snider.
ISBN 978-1-55455-077-7
1. Naturopathy--Encyclopedias. I. Snider, Ted II. Title.
RZ440.W66 2011   615.5'3503   C2010-905750-3

Publisher Cataloging-in-Publication Data (U.S)
Woolven, Linda
The family naturopathic encyclopedia / Linda Woolven, and Ted Snider.
[256] p. :   cm.
Includes bibliographical references and index.
ISBN-13: 978-1-55455-077-7 (pbk.)
1. Naturopathy. I. Snider, Ted. II. Title.
615.5/35dc22   RZ440.W675 2011

Fitzhenry & Whiteside acknowledges with thanks the Canada Council for the Arts, and the Ontario Arts Council for their support of our publishing program. We acknowledge the financial support of the Government of Canada through the Book Publishing Industry Development Program (BPIDP) for our publishing activities.

 Canada Council
for the Arts
Conseil des Arts
du Canada

 ONTARIO ARTS COUNCIL
CONSEIL DES ARTS DE L'ONTARIO

Design by Kerry Designs
Cover image courtesy Photos.com
All images © 2011 Photos.com, a division of Getty Images
Printed in Canada

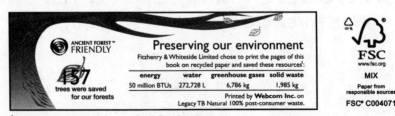

ANCIENT FOREST™
FRIENDLY

57

trees were saved
for our forests

Preserving our environment
Fitzhenry & Whiteside Limited chose to print the pages of this
book on recycled paper and saved these resources[1]:

energy	water	greenhouse gases	solid waste
50 million BTUs	272,728 L	6,786 kg	1,985 kg

Printed by **Webcom Inc.** on
Legacy TB Natural 100% post-consumer waste.

FSC
www.fsc.org
MIX
Paper from
responsible sources
FSC® C004071

[1]Estimates were made using the Environmental Defense Paper Calculator.

The Family Naturopathic Encyclopedia is dedicated to
the memory of our two mothers,
Helen Woolven and Dorothy Snider

ABOUT THE AUTHORS

Linda Woolven is a master herbalist, acupuncturist and solution-focused counselor with a practice in Toronto. She is the author of *Smart Guide to PMS and Pain-free Periods*, *The Vegetarian Passport Cookbook: Simple Vegetarian Dishes from around the World*, and hundreds of articles on natural health.

Together, Linda Woolven and Ted Snider are the authors of *Healthy Herbs: Your Everyday Guide to Medicinal Herbs and Their Use* and of *The Natural Path*, a monthly natural health newsletter.

CONTENTS

WOMEN'S HEALTH

MEN'S HEALTH

SENIORS' HEALTH

FOREWORD

by Michael T. Murray, N.D.

*"Nature is doing her best each moment to make us well.
She exists for no other end. Do not resist. With the least inclination
to be well, we should not be sick."*

Henry David Thoreau

A revolution is occurring in health care. As our understanding of the environment and human body evolves, new paradigms are developing. Science and medicine now have in their possession the technology and understanding necessary to develop new frameworks. This situation is most evident in physics. The classical cause-and-effect views of Descartes and Newton have been replaced by quantum mechanics, Einstein's theory of relativity, and the theoretical physics of Stephen Hawking.

In physics, the major shift has been away from the view that for every action there is an equal and opposite reaction. Today's contemporary view incorporates possibilities instead of certainties, taking into consideration the tremendous "interconnectedness" of the universe—a more wholistic rather than reductionist view.

Modern medicine also focuses on interconnectedness, the interconnectedness of body, mind, emotions, social factors, and the environment in determining the status of health within an individual. Earlier, health care professionals and healers viewed the body basically as a machine, one that could best be fixed with drugs and surgery. Our new model suggests that these practices should be secondary to natural, non-invasive, techniques which work to promote wholistic health and healing. Similarly, the relationship between physician and patient has evolved: the era of physician as a demigod is over; the era of self-empowerment is beginning.

OLD PARADIGM

Bio-mechanical view that the body is a machine
The body and mind are separate
Emphasis on eliminating disease
Treatment of symptoms
Specialization at the expense of tunnel vision
High technology, heroic measures
Physician should be emotional-neutral, detached
Physician is the all-knowing authority
Physician is in control of patient's health decisions
Focus on objective information (how the patient is doing based on charts, statistics, tests results, etc.)

NEW PARADIGM

Wholistic view concerned with the whole patient
The body and mind are interconnected
Emphasis on achieving health
Treatment is designed to address underlying causes
An integrated approach
Focus on diet, lifestyle and preventive measures
Physician's caring and empathy is critical to healing
The physician is a partner in the healing process
Each patient is in charge of his or her health care choices
Focus on subjective information (how the patient is feeling)

How to Be Well – 7 Steps

The achievement of wellness requires a systems approach. Attention must be given to all areas in an individual's life as every component of life affects another. Wellness requires a "whole person" perspective that revolves around the myriad choices we make with attitude, habits, diet, lifestyle, etc. People need to realize that getting and staying well is achieved by assuming personal responsibility for one's life: one's current situation, and one's health. Every aspect of your life must be utilized to propel you towards the goal of wellness. The question of health or disease often comes down to individual responsibility. In this context, responsibility means choosing a healthy alternative over a less healthy one. If you want to be healthy, make healthy choices on a consistent basis.

No matter what your current state of wellness might be, you **can** take steps to improve. The human body is constantly regenerating. Every three to four days, each of us gains a whole new lining in our gastrointestinal tract as new cells are formed to replace damaged old ones. We renew our entire skin in just thirty days, and every six weeks we make an entirely new liver. We live within an incredible vessel of complexity designed to propel us through life. Although we may abuse it, our body is very forgiving when we give it the right support and time to heal. Here are my seven steps to wellness to help you get the right support.

STEP #1

Incorporate spirituality in your life

Spirituality means different things to different people. For me, it means recognizing that there is a power greater than myself that connects us all. I believe it is critically important to make the connection with that inner presence at the core of our being that connects us to that higher power. I know many people try to live without faith, religion, or God, but quite frankly I don't see how life would have much meaning without these supports. And I believe that incorporating spirituality in our lives can have a profound effect on our

STEP #2

Develop a positive mental attitude

It is not the challenges in our lives that determine our direction; it is our response to these obstacles that shapes the quality of life and determines to a very large degree our level of health. It is often true that hardship, heartbreak, disappointment, and failure may serve as the sparks for joy, ecstasy, compassion, and success. The determining factor is how we view these challenges either as stepping stones or as stumbling blocks. Optimism is not only a necessary step toward achieving optimal health, it is critical to happiness and a higher quality of life.

STEP #3

Focus on establishing positive relationships

Human beings need each other, and human relationships. We need to work with others, exchange services, share information, and provide emotional comfort. Positive human relationships sustain us and nourish us—body and soul. Scientific evidence suggests that positive relationships can prevent disease and extend life: negative close relationships or the lack of close confidants can be very harmful to our health. Poor marital quality is linked to heart attacks, heart failure, metabolic syndrome, and type 2 diabetes. In one very detailed study, 9,011 British civil servants (6,114 men and 2,897 women) answered a questionnaire which assessed their relationship status. Of the 8,499 individuals who did not have coronary heart disease (CHD) at the beginning of the study and who provided sufficient information for analysis, 589 reported a CHD event (e.g., heart attack). After adjusting for factors like obesity, hypertension, diabetes, and cholesterol levels, smoking, alcohol intake, exercise, and fruit and vegetable consumption, researchers found that people who experienced negative aspects of a close relationship had a 34 per cent higher risk of incident coronary events than those who did not. Their conclusion: if people wish to avoid CHD and live longer, they should "be nicer to each other."

STEP #4

Follow a healthy lifestyle

Lifestyle reflects daily habits. In many ways, these habits define our health. By avoiding harmful habits and embracing health-promoting habits we can transform our lives toward wellness. Here are the seven key components of a healthy lifestyle (NOTE: exercise is so important it is dealt with separately):

- **Key 1.** Do not smoke.
- **Key 2.** Drink alcohol only in moderation.
- **Key 3.** Get adequate rest.
- **Key 4.** Develop a positive way to manage stress.
- **Key 5.** Practise effective time management.
- **Key 6.** Connect with nature.
- **Key 7.** Laugh long and often.

STEP #5

Be active and get regular physical exercise

While the immediate effect of exercise is stress on the body, the body will adapt to regular exercise; it becomes stronger, functions more efficiently, and has greater endurance. The whole body benefits from regular exercise, largely as a result of improved cardiovascular and respiratory function. Exercise enhances the transport of oxygen and nutrients into cells. At the same time, exercise enhances the transport of carbon dioxide and waste products from the tissues of the body to the bloodstream and ultimately to the eliminative organs. As a result, regular exercise increases stamina and energy levels.

Regular exercise is also a powerful prescription for a positive mood. Tensions, depressions, feelings of inadequacy, and worries diminish greatly with regular exercise. Exercise alone has been demonstrated to have a tremendous impact on improving mood and the ability to handle stressful life situations.

STEP #6

Eat a health-promoting diet

Diet is fundamental to good health, yet few of us really spend much thought or time on designing a diet that will promote health. Far too many people have fallen prey to the comforts of modern life, leading to physical inactivity and the reliance on foods that provide temporary sensory gratification at the expense of true nourishment. It is easy to give your body its best chance of maintaining or achieving health. Following are some important keys to eating a health-promoting diet:

• **Key 1.** Eat to control blood-sugar levels—refined sugars, white flour products, and other sources of simple sugars are quickly absorbed into the bloodstream, causing a rapid rise in blood sugar leading to poor blood-sugar regulation, obesity, and ultimately type 2 diabetes. The stress on the body that these sugars cause, including secreting too much insulin, can also promote the growth of cancer and increase the risk of heart disease. So, let me make this simple recommendation: Don't eat "junk foods" and high-sugar foods.

• **Key 2.** Eat five or more servings daily of vegetables and two servings of fruit—a diet rich in fruits and vegetables is your best bet for preventing virtually every chronic disease.

• **Key 4.** Eat organic foods (in the United States alone, more than 1.2 billion pounds of pesticides and herbicides are sprayed or added to food crops each year—roughly five pounds of pesticides for each American man, woman, and child). There is a growing concern that in addition to pesticides directly causing a significant number of cancers, exposure to these chemicals through food consumption damages the body's detoxification mechanisms, thereby increasing the risk of cancer and other diseases.

- **Key 5.** Reduce the intake of meat and other animal products—study after study confirms one basic truth: the higher the intake of meat and other animal products, the higher the risk of heart disease and cancer, especially for major cancers like colon, breast, prostate, and lung cancer. There are many reasons for this association. If you choose to cat red meat:
    - Limit your intake to no more than three or four ounces daily—about the size of a deck of playing cards. And choose the leanest cuts available, keeping in mind that in the U. S. the USDA allows the meat and dairy industry to label fat content by weight rather than by per cent of calories.
    - Avoid consuming well-done, charbroiled, and fat-laden meats.
    - Consider buying free-range meats or wild game.

- **Key 6.** Eat the right type of fats. It is important to consume less than 30 to 40 per cent of calories as fat. However, just as important as the amount of fat is the type of fat you consume. The goal is to decrease your intake of saturated fats and the omega-6 fats found in most vegetable oils, including soy, sunflower, safflower, and corn; while increasing the intake of monounsaturated fats from nuts, seeds, olive oil, and canola oil, in addition to insuring an adequate intake of omega-3 fatty acids found in fish and flaxseed oil.

- **Key 7.** Keep salt intake low. Too much sodium in the diet from salt (sodium chloride) can not only raise blood pressure in some people, it also increases the risk of cancer. In North America, prepared foods contribute 45 per cent of our sodium intake, 45 per cent is added in cooking, and another 5 per cent is added as a condiment. Only 5 per cent of sodium intake comes from the natural ingredients in food.

STEP #7

Support your body through proper nutritional supplementation and body work

The physical care of the human body involves making sure that it has all of the necessary nutritional blocks to build good health. Pay attention to four other key areas: exercise, breathing, and posture. I believe there are three key supplements to take every day:

- A high potency multiple vitamin and mineral formula.

- A pharmaceutical-grade fish oil supplement. The health benefits of the long-chain omega-3 oils from fish oils are now well known. Using a high-quality fish oil supplement is the perfect solution to people wanting the health benefits of fish oils without the mercury, PCBs, dioxins, and other contaminants often found in fish. All told, fish oil supplementation can reduce the effects of about sixty different health conditions, including, diabetes, cancer, heart disease, rheumatoid arthritis and other autoimmune diseases, psoriasis, eczema, asthma, attention deficit disorder, and depression. It is estimated that the use of fish oil supplements may reduce overall cardiovascular mortality by as much as 45 per cent. For optimum benefit, take a dosage of fish oil sufficient to provide a combined total of 1000 mg of EPA and DHA daily.

- A "greens drink" or supplement containing concentrated sources of phyto-chemicals. The term "green drinks" refers to green tea and a number of commercially available products containing dehydrated barley grass, wheat grass, or algae sources such as chlorella or spirulina. Such formulas are rehydrated by mixing with water or juice. These products—packed full of phytochemicals, especially carotenes and chlorophyll—are more convenient than trying to sprout and grow your own source of greens. An added advantage is that they tend to taste better than, for example, straight wheatgrass juice.

Finally, I recommend engaging in yoga, tai chi, or stretching. These activities are very important as they not only increase flexibility and reduce tension in our musculoskeletal system, but also once again bring an awareness to posture and breathing. It is also a great thing for your health if you can see a body worker on a regular basis. Bodywork is a general term referring to therapies involving touch, including various massage techniques, chiropractic spinal adjustment and manipulation, reflexology, shiatsu, and many more.

My hope

It is my sincere hope that you—or someone you care about—will use the information provided in the following pages to achieve greater health and happiness. *The Family Naturopathic Encyclopedia* is an excellent resource that provides clear recommendations to better your health.

Live in good health with passion and joy!

Michael T. Murray, N.D.
July 2010

INTRODUCTION

Finally, a book that you can use to help the whole family stay healthy and prevent disease; a book that uses natural, safe and effective, well-researched methods. A book that is a must in every house.

People who live long, healthy lives, have certain things in common: they don't smoke, they maintain a healthy weight, they stay in shape, they eat lots of plant foods, they keep their blood pressure and blood-sugar under control and they do not drink alcohol excessively.

None of these habits is a surprise. Research also finds that the more informed or educated a person is, the more likely he or she will to live a longer, healthier life[1]. The greatest gap in public education about health care, and the greatest crime in the modern chemical and pharmaceutical approach to health, is that people do not have to wait until they are sick to get rid of the disease, and they do not always have to treat disease with drugs with all of their potentially harmful side effects.

The natural approach to a long, happy, healthy life offers a different path. This approach aims not at the removal of diseases we have come to see as almost inevitable, but at the preservation of a flourishing state of health. Did you know that we know how not to get most illnesses? And when we do succumb to one of them, most are manageable or treatable with safe, natural herbs, vitamins, dietary and lifestyle changes that can be as or more effective than the chemical pharmaceuticals, and without the dangerous and often terrible side effects?

At this point, critics of natural medicine used to say—and some who clearly don't look at the literature still do—that there was no scientific research behind such a claim. Not so. The explosion of studies in the past several years refutes the naysayers, as you will see in this book. Other critics suggest that the research into natural medicine was not properly documented scientifically, and was of a lower quality than research on pharmaceutical drugs. But now that objection is no longer available either. Not so. When researchers actually compared herb studies with drug studies for the same conditions, they found that " . . . the quality of trials of . . . herbal medicine is on average superior to trials of conventional medicine"[2].

Often the information the public is receiving—or not receiving—about our health, is that there are many safe, natural alternatives out there, alternatives we are not being told about that could be alleviating much suffering and making us feel whole lot healthier and happier.

Herewith is the purpose of this book.

And just as some of the best moments in life happen when all of your family and friends are together, a wealth of natural health information you need for your whole family and friends has been collected together in this volume. You will find information on how to prevent and treat naturally the most common conditions that afflict the whole family, conveniently divided into sections on children's health, health for everyone in the family, women's health, men's health and health for seniors: the complete family guide to natural health.

We hope that this book helps your whole family have long, flourishing, happy and healthy lives!

Chapter Endnotes

1. Vaillant, G.E., Mukamal K., Successful Aging. *Am J Psychiatry* 2001;158:839-47; Bradley, J., *et al*. Midlife Risk Factors and Healthy Survival in Men. *JAMA* 2006; 296:2343-50.

2. Nartey, L., *et al*. Matched-pair study showed higher quality of placebo-controlled trials in Western phytotherapy than conventional medicine. *Journal of Clinical Epidemiology*. 2007; 60:787-94.

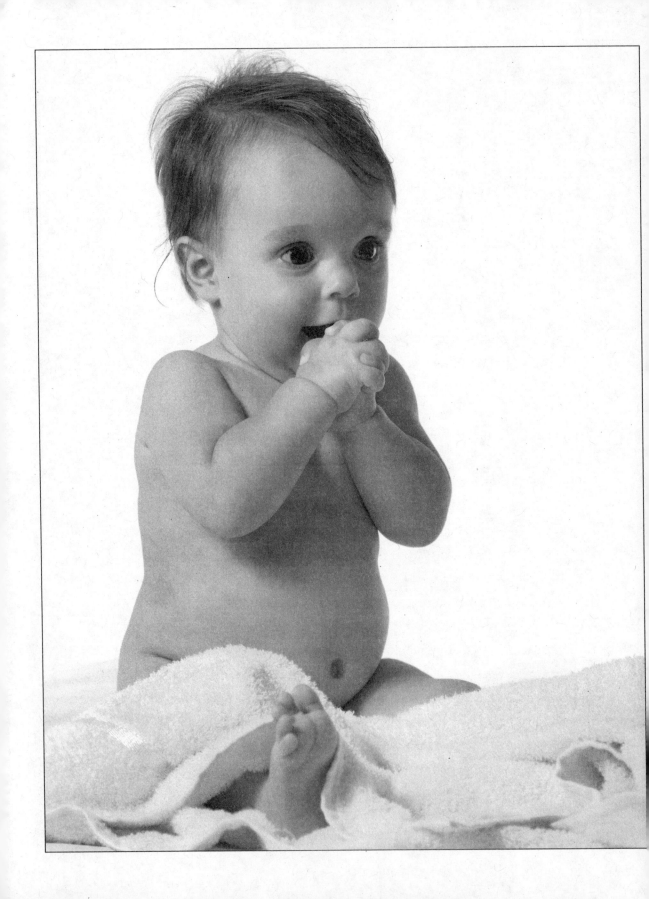

CHILDREN'S HEALTH

Children are still forming, their bodies making cells that will make them into who they are and will grow up to be. With this kind of important changing and growing going on, it is important to give their bodies what they need and to avoid harmful substances, like drugs and chemicals, drugs that may have bad side effects and affect the child's health. Some drugs that are prescribed widely to children, like Ritalin, have not even been approved as safe for children; yet, children continue to be on them.

So, when treating health conditions that may arise in children, it becomes even more important to use a natural approach, using nutrition, vitamins, herbs and other supplements. This approach is gentler, safer and effective and will help to heal the underlying health problems that children can get. It's the old "We are what we eat," and herbs, vitamins, and other supplements are healthy nutrients to eat, nutrients you can feel good about your child ingesting.

This section of the encyclopedia will focus on some of the more common health concerns that frequently affect children. It will look at colic, thrush, diaper rash, teething, bedwetting, childhood constipation, ear infection, childhood colds and flus, head lice, autism, attention deficit hyperactivity disorder and acne.

ACNE

Breakouts affect not only teenagers, but adults as well. While conventional medicine may help to get rid of the problem, it does so by using antibiotics that can wipe out friendly flora, leading to a host of possible problems down the road, such as candida. The natural approach to clearing up pimples corrects dietary problems and uses skin-, blood-, liver-, and bowel-purifying herbs and other nutrients.

Causes of Acne

Acne can be caused by hormone imbalances, poor diet, nutritional deficiencies, genetics, stress, thyroid problems, and toxins. One study showed that 50 per cent of patients with severe acne had increased blood levels of toxins that had been absorbed from the intestines[1]. In other words, bowel toxemia is a key factor. So is hormone imbalance. According to Michael T. Murray, N.D., patients with acne have more activity of 5-alpha-reductase, an enzyme in their skins, which converts testosterone to a more potent form know as dihydrotestosterone (DHT), which causes acne[2].

Diet for Acne

To avoid acne, the diet should be free of sugar, trans-fatty acids, milk and milk products, fried foods, and excess iodine. All refined sugar should be avoided since it can lead to poor nutritional health and cause an overgrowth of candida that could cause skin breakouts. High-fat foods and foods containing trans-fatty acids, such as milk and milk products, margarine, and hydrogenated vegetable oils, should also be avoided since they are linked with skin breakouts. Animal-fat and milk products cause the body to produce arachidonic acid, which produces inflammation that can cause pimples. In general, the more fibre you eat to help keep the colon clean, the less likely you are to get skin breakouts. Food allergies should be determined and then these foods avoided since they are linked to acne. Parasites such as candida should also be eliminated, since they, too, cause skin problems.

Important Supplements for Acne

Key nutrients that are used to treat acne include chromium, vitamins A and E, selenium and zinc.

Chromium

Chromium has been shown in a study to help eliminate acne[3]. The reason chromium works seems to be because people with acne seem not to metabolize sugar properly. Some even refer to acne as *skin diabetes*. Chromium improves glucose tolerance and enhances insulin sensitivity.

Vitamin A

Vitamin A is used topically by dermatologists in the treatment of acne. Although it can be effective in this form, it can cause excessive dryness and redness that many people find very painful. But taken internally, vitamin A has been shown in many studies to reduce sebum production and the build-up of keratin in the follicle, helping to prevent skin breakouts[4]. So far, only high dosages of vitamin A have been used in the studies, and these high dosages should not be undertaken without supervision.

Zinc

Zinc is, we believe, the most important nutrient for skin health. In her clinic, Linda has seen acne cleared up with supplementation with this nutrient alone. Zinc is involved in regulating testosterone levels, a hormone that, when it is imbalanced, can cause acne. Zinc also helps in wound-healing, immune-system function, inflammation control, and tissue regrowth. Several double-blind studies have shown results using zinc in the treatment of acne[5]. One study found that 75 per cent of people with acne who used zinc gluconate improved, compared to only 23.5 per cent of those using a placebo[6]. Thirty mg of zinc were used in this study. Those using zinc for acne should allow twelve weeks to see results. Even better results may be seen with better forms of zinc. Clinically, Linda uses the better forms of zinc such as zinc citrate, acetate, picolinate or mononethionine to clear up acne.

Vitamin E and Selenium

Vitamin E and selenium not only are useful on their own for aiding acne, but also help with the functioning of vitamin A. Vitamin A blood levels will stay low no matter how much vitamin A is supplemented if vitamin E is low. Vitamin E also interacts with selenium, which is important for preventing inflammation. After treatment with vitamin E and selenium, acne has been shown to be reduced[7].

B Vitamins

It is also useful to take a B-complex when treating skin breakouts. Pantothenic acid, also known as B5, has been shown to reduce sebum production relatively quickly[8]. Excess sebum production can cause acne. Pantothenic acid also stopped new pimples from forming and healed existing ones. High dosages were used in the study with no side effects. B6 can aid women with PMS-related acne[9], as can a herb called chastetree berry[10], which helps to balance hormone levels.

Topical Tea Tree

One of the most effective topical preparations that can be used is tea tree oil. Tea tree oil is antiseptic and has been shown to be effective against a wide range of organisms, including twenty-seven strains of acne. It is absorbed well and does not cause great irritation to the skin. A study done in Australia showed a 5 per cent tea tree oil solution to be as beneficial as benzoyl peroxide in treating acne, with fewer side effects[11]. For severe acne, stronger tea tree solutions of up to 15 per cent should be used. Numerous studies have shown tea tree oil to be extremely safe.

Cleaning the Skin from the Inside Out

If you have acne, it is crucial to cleanse the body and get rid of the toxemia. To help cleanse the blood, bowels, liver, and skin and to support immune function, it is a good idea to take a combination of herbs such as milk thistle, buckthorn, sarsaparilla, sassafras, burdock, red clover, yellow dock, echinacea, goldenseal, and dandelion. Cleansing the body can aid in clearing acne, as can supporting the immune function. You can get many of these herbs already combined in health food stores. Linda has found grapefruit seed extract valuable for treating acne as well, and it has been shown to kill off bacteria, viruses, and fungi, including candida. Cleansing the urinary tract system can also be of benefit. Use herbs like buchu, *uva ursi*, corn silk, and dandelion.

Acidophilus and bifidus can also be of help, since these probiotics aid in correcting an improperly balanced colon, helping the body to excrete toxins. And green foods, such as chlorella, alfalfa, barley grass, wheat grass, and spirulina, can also be of aid, since they help to detoxify the body and provide nutrients.

Castor-oil packs can also be a huge benefit for acne, as they help to clear the body of toxins.

More Help

Several studies have shown that acupuncture is very helpful for acne[12].

For cystic acne and rosacea, take guggulipids[13], which help to get rid of excess oil build-up on the skin. It is also useful to take a fat- and protein-digesting enzyme.

It is helpful to change pillowcases often, to avoid heavy creams and oils on the skin, and to avoid over-washing of the skin. Keep the skin clean, keep hands away from the face, and avoid make-up that blocks pores. Oral contraceptives, progesterone, steroids, corticosteroids, and drugs that contain bromides or iodides should also be avoided, since they can contribute to the problem.

Sunlight or ultraviolet light decrease acne, but avoid overexposure to the sun.

Chapter Endnotes

1. Juhlin, L., G. Michaelson. "Fibrin microclot formation in patients with acne." *Acta Derm Venerol*, 1983; 63:538'40.

2. Takayasu, S., *et al.* "Activity of testosterone 5-alpha-reductase in various tissues of human skin." *J Invest Dermatol*, 1980; 74:187'91.

3. McCarthy, M. "High chromium yeast for acne?" *Med Hypoth*, 1984; 14:307'10.

4. Kugman, A., et al. "Oral vitamin A in acne vulgaris." *Int J Dermatol*, 1981; 20:278'85.

5. Michaelson, G., L. Juhlin, K. Ljunghall. "A double-blind study of the effect of zinc and oxytetracycline in acne vulgaris." *Br J Dermantol*, 1977; 97:561'65; Weimer, V., et al. "Zinc sulphate in acne vulgaris." *Arch Dermatol*, 1978; 114:1776'78; Michaelsson, G., A. Vahlquist, L. Juhlin. "Effects of oral zinc and vitamin A on acne." *Arch Dermatol*, 1977; 113:31'36; Hillström, *et al.* "Comparison of oral treatment with zinc sulfate and placebo in acne vulgaris." *Br J Dermatol*, 1977; 97:681-84; Verma, K. C., A. S. Saini, S. K. Dhamija. "Oral zinc sulphate therapy in acne vulgaris: a double-blind trial." *Acta Dermatovener (Stockholm)*, 1980; 60:337-40; Dreno, B., et al. "Low doses of zinc gluconate for inflammatory acne. *Acta Dermatovener (Stockholm)*, 1989; 69:541-43; Michaelsson, G. "Oral zinc in acne." *Acta Dermatovener (Stockholm)*, 1980; Suppl 89:87-93 [review].

6. Dreno, B., et al. "Low doses of zinc gluconate for inflammatory acne." *Acta Derma Venerol*, 1989; 69:541'43.

7. Michaelsson, G. and L. Edqvist. "Erythrocyte glutathione peroxidase activity in acne vulgaris and the effect of selenium and vitamin E treatment." *Acta Derm Venerol*, 1984; 64:9'14.

8. Leung, L. H. "Pantothenic acid deficiency as the pathogenesis of acne vulagris." *Med Hypoth*, 1995; 44:490'92.

9. Snider, B., D. Dieteman. "Pyridoxine therapy for premenstrual acne flare." *Arch Dermatol*, 1974; 110:103'01.

10. Giss, G., W. Rothenburg. Z Haut Geschlechtskr, 1968; 43:645'47; Amann, W. "Acne vulgaris and *Agnus castus* (Agnolyt (tm))." *Z Allgemeinmed,* 1975; 51:1645-58.

11. Bassett, I. B., D. L. Pannowitz, R. S. Barnetson. "A comparative study of tea-tree oil versus benzoyl peroxide in the treatment of acne." *Med J Austral*, 1990; 53:455-58.

12. Xu, Y. "Treatment of facial skin diseases with acupuncture-a report of 129 cases." *J Tradit Chin Med*, 1990; 10:22-25; Liu, J. "Treatment of adolescent acne with acupuncture." *J Tradit Chin Med*, 1993; 13:187-88.

13. Thappa, D. M., J. Dogra. "Nodulocystic acne: oral guggulipid versus tetracycline." *J Dermatol*, 1994; 21:729-31.

ATTENTION DEFICIT HYPERACTIVITY DISORDER

We desperately need a safe, effective treatment for Attention Deficit and Hyperactivity Disorder (ADHD). An astounding 3 to 6 per cent of children suffer from this disorder. That means that, on average, in every classroom in your child's school, at least one and probably two children are struggling through ADHD. And the rate is likely higher, as not everyone gets diagnosed. And aside from being addictive, the very common drug treatments such as Ritalin can cause a host of serious side effects, including abnormal heart rate and blood-pressure changes, anaemia, insomnia, depression, headaches, liver damage, appetite loss, and stunted growth. The safety of Ritalin for children under six has never been established. An effective and safe treatment is badly needed.

Correcting Nutritional Deficiencies

Children with ADHD are deficient in a number of nutrients. When those nutrients are supplemented, the children improve.

Essential fatty Acids

Deficiencies in omega-3 fatty acids have been linked to ADHD. Several studies have found that levels of essential fatty acids are significantly lower in affected children[1]. When kids with ADHD were given either a fatty acid supplement or a placebo for twelve weeks in a double-blind study, the fatty acid supplement produced significant improvement in cognitive function and behaviour, compared to the placebo[2].

Magnesium and B6

Magnesium deficiencies are far more common in children who have ADHD than in children who don't. When children with ADHD and low magnesium levels were given 200 mg a day of magnesium for six months, they had significantly less hyperactivity than before they were on the magnesium, and also significantly less than the control group who were not given magnesium[3].

Some children with ADHD are also deficient in B6[4]. So researchers tried giving both magne-

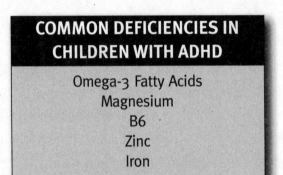

COMMON DEFICIENCIES IN CHILDREN WITH ADHD

Omega-3 Fatty Acids
Magnesium
B6
Zinc
Iron

sium and B6 to fifty-two children with ADHD. There was a significant improvement in their hyperexcitability[5].

Zinc

Zinc is another promising nutrient. Many studies have found that children with ADHD are more likely to be zinc-deficient than others. And once again, when the missing nutrient is provided, the ADHD improves. Average ADHD scores improved significantly more in a group of kids given 40 mg of zinc than in the group given a placebo in a large study of four hundred children with ADHD. They had significantly better improvement in hyperactivity, impulsiveness, and socialization[6]. A second study found that a lower dose of 15 mg of zinc a day led to significantly greater improvement in behaviour than a placebo[7].

Iron

Another recent study has found significantly lower levels of iron in children with ADHD. It also found that the lower the iron levels, the worse the distractibility, inattention and learning disorders[8].

So, topping up essential fatty acids, magnesium, B6, zinc and iron may be important. Supplementing L-carnitine might also help. Parents found a 54 per cent improvement in behaviour when their kids were given L-carnitine versus only a 13 per cent improvement when they were given a placebo. Teachers found similar but slightly less improvement. The dose was 100 mg per kilogram of body weight, up to 4 gms a day[9].

Supporting the idea that nutritional supplements help, a study has found that a supplement containing vitamins, minerals, essential fatty acids, probiotics, amino acids, and herbs was as effective as Ritalin in treating ADHD[10].

Other Supplements that Help

Probiotics are crucial, as they improve digestion, get rid of fungi and other parasites that may be present and causing a problem, and help improve the absorption of nutrients.

Also key are herbs such as ginkgo biloba, huperzene A, ginseng and gotu kola, as they can help to improve memory and concentration.

Herbs that help to relax the body, such as skullcap, hops, valerian, passionflower, linden, lemon vervain, chamomile, and other nervines, are also used to help calm the brain and nervous system.

Eliminate Allergens

And, perhaps most importantly, allergens in the diet are culprits. So getting rid of offending food allergies is key. Common culprits are dairy, wheat, gluten, corn, soy, eggs, peanuts, MSG, dyes and food additives, fish, oranges, and tomatoes. Food additives, sugar, caffeine, alcohol, and refined grains are also linked to this problem and people do better when these are eliminated.

Chapter Endnotes

1. Mitchell, E. A., M. G. Aman, S. H. Turbott, M. Manku. "Clinical characteristics and serum essential fatty acid levels in hyperactive children." *Clin Pediatr*, 1987; 26:406'11; Stevens, J. L., S. S. Zentall, J. L. Deck, et al. "Essential fatty acid metabolism in boys with attention-deficit hyperactivity disorder." *Am J Clin Nutr*, 1995; 62:761'68.

2. *Prog Neuropsychopharmacol Biol Psychiatry*, 2002.

3. Starobrat'Hermelin, B., T. Kozielec. "The effects of magnesium physiological supplementation on hyperactivity in children with attention deficit hyperactivity disorder (ADHD). Positive response to magnesium oral loading test." *Magnes Res*, 1997; 10:149'56.

4. Bhagavan, H. N., M. Coleman, D. B. Coursin. "The effect of pyridoxine hydrochloride on blood serotonin and pyridoxal phosphate contents in hyperactive children." *Pediatrics*, 1975; 55:437'41.

5. *Journal of the American College of Nutrition*, 2004; 23:545S-48S.

6. *Progress in Neuro-Psychopharmacology and Biological Psychiatry*, 2004; 28:181-90.

7. Akhondzadeh, S., M. R. Mohammadi and M. Khademi. "Zinc sulfate as an adjunct to methylphenidate for the treatment of attention deficit hyperactivity disorder in children: A double-blind and randomized trial." *BMC Psychiatry*, 2004; 4:9.

8. Konofal, E., M. Lecendreux, I. Arnulf, M-C. Mouren. "Iron Deficiency in Children With Attention-Deficit/Hyperactivity Disorder." *Archives of Pediatrics and Adolescent Medicine*, 2004; 158:1113'15.

9. *Prostaglandins Leukotrienes and Essential Fatty Acids*, 2002; 67:33-38.

10. Harding, K., R. Judah, C. Gant. "Outcome-based comparison of ritalin versus food-supplement treated children with AD/HD." *Alternative Medicine Review*, 2003; vol.8, no. 3:319'30.

AUTISM

The number of children suffering from autism is rising dramatically. The number of cases has risen up to five times since the early 1990s.

Autism is a serious condition that often shows up in the first thirty months of life. Autistic children are abnormally withdrawn and unable to develop social relationships or to use language to communicate. They are out of touch with reality and unable to learn from experience or to change their behaviour to fit changes in their environment. Their behaviour is marked by repetitive rituals. There is a huge range of degrees of autism, and conventional medicine has offered little hope.

The natural approach to autism seems to fare better. Treatment effectiveness ratings collected from 23,700 parents by the Autism Research Institute (ARI), consistently show greater benefit from nutrients than from drugs.

Important Dietary Changes for Autism

The natural approach should start with diet. First, food additives can be a problem. Second, sugar should be gradually eliminated or reduced. And third, autistic children can have intolerances to a number of foods, including egg, tomato, eggplant, avocado, red pepper, soy, and corn. But the biggest problem—and the biggest promise—comes from the milk protein casein and the grain protein gluten. According to an excellent article on autism by Paris Kidd, PH.D,[1], studies show that as many as 80 per cent of people with autism improve when casein and gluten are eliminated from their diet. A 1995 study found that 66 per cent improve with the removal of dairy alone[2]. That's incredible! Clinically, I have seen this to be true. Children who get off the offending foods seem to be much higher-functioning.

FOODS TO ELIMINATE

milk protein
gluten
food additives
sugar
eggs
tomato
eggplant
avocado
red pepper
soy
corn

Important Supplements for Autism

In addition to eliminating things from the diet, autistic people can benefit by supplementing the diet with nutrients. Most people with autism suffer from gastrointestinal problems. Because of these digestive problems, almost all people with autism have nutritional deficiencies. So taking a multivitamin/mineral and digestive enzymes is a good idea. The multi, however, should not have copper in it, as copper is the one nutrient that autistic people often have too much of. Bromelain and papain will not only help with the digestive problems, but also with the inflammatory problems of autism.

The most exciting nutrients for autism, though, are vitamin B6 and magnesium. In 2002, autism expert Bernard Rimland conducted a review of eighteen studies on autism and either B6 or a B6/magnesium combination. He found that every one of them was positive[3]. Though not a cure for autism, the combination of B6 and magnesium can bring about fantastic improvements. Rimland says that B6 is better supported by the scientific research than are drugs for autism[4]. Researchers have found, based on several studies, that the combination of B6 and magnesium is a "breakthrough autism treatment" for about half of all cases[5]. The ARI ratio for whether these nutrients make autistic people better or worse (B:W) is 4.3:1 for B6, 4.6:1 for magnesium, and an impressive 11:1 for the B6/magnesium combination.

Though B6 and magnesium are the stars, other nutrients can help also. Folic acid receives a 10:1. Calcium, which, along with magnesium, is a com-

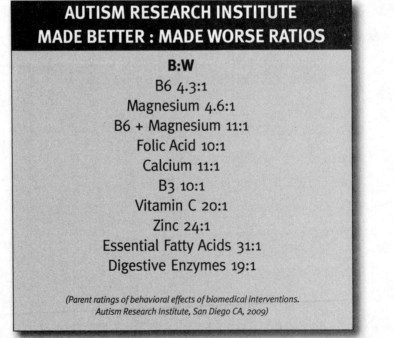

AUTISM RESEARCH INSTITUTE
MADE BETTER : MADE WORSE RATIOS

B:W
B6 4.3:1
Magnesium 4.6:1
B6 + Magnesium 11:1
Folic Acid 10:1
Calcium 11:1
B3 10:1
Vitamin C 20:1
Zinc 24:1
Essential Fatty Acids 31:1
Digestive Enzymes 19:1

(Parent ratings of behavioral effects of biomedical interventions.
Autism Research Institute, San Diego CA, 2009)

mon deficiency in people with autism, gets a whopping B:W rating of 11:1. Melvyn Werbach, M.D., discusses a case report in which three out of four autistic people reduced or stopped their self-injuring behaviour when they were supplemented with calcium[6].

Vitamin C can also help. A double-blind study found that vitamin C lessened the severity of symptoms[7]. An earlier study also demonstrated improvement with vitamin C[8]. Vitamin C's B:W rating is an impressive 20:1. One way vitamin C may work is by detoxifying the liver, getting offending built-up toxins, including heavy metals, out of the system. It would be worthwhile to do a full detox program with autistic people to get the offending toxins out of their systems. Work with a natural healer to do the detox, as, initially ,detoxes can spill toxins into the system, and there could be some side effects. So detoxes should be done gently and slowly.

Zinc is too low in people with autism, while copper is too high. So zinc should be supplemented, but copper should be left out of multivitamin/minerals. Zinc's B:W is 24:1.

And finally, nearly every person with autism is deficient in omega-3 fatty acids. Supplementing essential fatty acids gets a B:W rating of 31:1.

Heavy-metal detoxification and healing a leaky gut can also help. Forty-three per cent of children with autism have leaky-gut syndrome[9]. In cases of leaky-gut, L-glutamine, licorice, and probiotics will greatly help. These nutrients should be considered with all autistics as they help to improve digestion and absorption of nutrients, two key problems of people with autism. Antiparasitic and antifungal herbs, such as grapefruit seed extract, black walnut, pau d'arco, and wormwood, which address possible causes of leaky-gut syndrome, should also be considered.

Chapter Endnotes

1. Kidd, Paris M., Ph.D., "Autism, An Extreme Challenge to Integrative Medicine. Part II: Medical Management." *Alternative Medicine Review: A Journal of Clinical Therapeutics*, Vol. 7, No. 6, 2002, pp. 472'99.

2. Lucarelli, S, T. Frediani, A. M. Zingoni, *et al.* "Food allergy and infantile autism." *Panminerva Med*, 1995; 37:137'41.

3. Rimland, B. "The use of vitamin B6, magnesium, and DMG in the treatment of autistic children and adults." In Shaw, W., ed., *Biological Treatment for Autism and PDD*. Lenexa, K.S.: The Great Plains Laboratory, Inc., 2002.

4. Rimland. B. "Vitamin B6 versus Fenfluramine: a case study in medical bias." *J Nutr Med*, 1991; 2:321'322.

5. Lelord, G., J.P. Muh, C. Barthelemy, *et al.* "Effects of pyridoxine and magnesium on autistic symptoms-initial observations." *J Autism Dev Disord*, 1981; 11:219'30; Lelord, G., E. Callaway, J.P. Muh. "Clinical and biological effects of high doses of vitamin B6 and magnesium on autistic children." *Acta Vitaminol Enzymol*, 1982; 4:27'44.

6. Coleman, M. "Clinical presentations of patients with autism and hypocalciuria." *Developmental Brain Dysfunction*, 1994; 7:63'70.

7. Dolske, M. C., J. Spollen, S. McKay, *et al.* "A preliminary trial of ascorbic acid as supplemental therapy for autism." *Prog Neuropsychopharmacol Biol Psychiatry*, 1993; 17:765'74.

8. Tollbert, L. C. "Ascorbic Acid: Therapeutic Trial in Autism." Presentation at the Autism Society of America Annual Conference, Indianapolis, IN, July 1991.

9. D'Eufemia, P., M. Celli, R. Finocchiaro, et al. "Abnormal intestinal permeability in children with autism." *Acta Pediatr*, 1996; 85:1076'79.

BED-WETTING

Bed-wetting is one of the most difficult and embarrassing problems for children to overcome. The child goes to bed dry and wakes up wet, and this can go on for years.

What Are Some of the Causes of Bed-Wetting?

Sometimes children grow faster than their bladders, and the bladder simply cannot hold all of the liquid. Sometimes the child has parasites or an infection; sometimes he is simply a very deep sleeper; sometimes it's stress-related. It could be jealousy over a new sibling or favouritism, anxiety over a new school, moving, family arguments, friends, teachers, work at school, neglect, unhappiness, insecurity, fear, or overexcitement. Most children stop wetting the bed when they are two or three years old. Children who continue to wet the bed may also have nerves and muscles that are not governing the bladder well enough yet. Other causes include diabetes, structural abnormalities, hypoglycemia, family history of bed-wetting, constipation, dietary deficiencies—especially of nutrients such as calcium and magnesium—too much sugar or refined foods, chemicals, food allergies, and, for some children, getting too cold can cause bed-wetting. Even strong electromagnetic fields can cause a problem, perhaps from a computer too close to the bed.

What Can You Do to Help a Bed Wetter?

First of all, never blame the child. It is not the child's fault, and it will take all of your love and support to make the child feel secure, which can help to stop bed-wetting.

Also, you can try leaving the child in children's pull-up underwear overnight until he consistently wakes up dry. This will help the child and the bedclothes to stay dry and will make the child feel more confident. The pull-ups look and feel a lot like underwear so the child will feel less embarrassed about going to bed than if he was in diapers.

Although some sources do not agree with restricting liquids at all, most suggest restricting them one hour before bed.

Make sure the child goes to the bathroom right before bed and fully empties the bladder. Encourage the child to partially stand after he is finished urinating, at about a 45-degree-angle squat position, over the toilet, as this position forces any leftover urine out of the bladder.

Teach the child the bladder-clenching method known as the kegal method that pregnant and older women use to stop loss of bladder control.

Herbal Help for Bed-Wetting

Anne McIntyre, author of *The Herbal for Mother and Child,* uses teas made of horsetail, St. John's wort, and corn silk throughout the day to soothe the bladder and encourage normal nervous control of the bladder. Give small frequent doses and stop one hour before bedtime. Herbalist Rosemary Gladstar says that corn silk is the best herb to give for this problem.

You can use 1 tsp of the herbs per cup of boiling water and make an infusion. Or you can use tinctures of herbs, and give one drop of herb per 4 lbs of the child's weight.

Other useful herbal teas are made from cranesbill, oakbark, yarrow, and agrimony, which are astringents and can stop excess liquid. McIntyre also suggests parsley.

Or you could try uva ursi throughout the day, or dandelion root or garlic or goldenseal to

CAUSES OF BEDWETTING

small bladder
parasites
infection
deep sleeper
stress
jealousy
anxiety
neglect
unhappiness
insecurity
fear
over excitement
poor nerves or muscles that govern the bladder
diabetes
structural abnormalities
hypoglycemia
family history of bed wetting
constipation
dietary deficiencies
too much sugar or refined foods
chemicals
food allergies
cold
strong electromagnetic fields

strengthen the bladder and to stop irritation and infections that can cause bladder problems. A good kidney-strengthening formula is dandelion root, ginger, and parsley root. Give teas or tincture throughout the day. Be sure not to give diuretic herbs like uva ursi too close to bedtime.

An old-time herbal remedy for bed-wetting is poplar bark. This herb strengthens the bladder and reduces bed-wetting.

If the child's bed-wetting seems to be from stress or other emotional concerns, try using catnip, lemon balm, vervain, chamomile, hops, skullcap, passion flower, oats, lady's slipper, or valerian root.

You might want to try Anne McIntyre's suggestion: rubbing the child's lower spine and abdomen with oil of chamomile or St. John's wort while settling the child down for bed.

More Help

You can also try acupuncture or acupressure to strengthen weak kidneys and bladder and to relieve stress.

Give your child calcium and magnesium, which can help to relax the nervous system, and which are vital for control of bladder nerves and muscles. Also, silica helps to strengthen the bladder, so give horsetail or silica supplements. Give a multivitamin/mineral to make sure the child is not low on any nutrients that could be causing the problem.

If constipation is a problem, give stewed prunes, dandelion root, psyllium, or flaxseed or increase fibre in the diet from fruits, vegetables, seeds, nuts, and whole grains, and cut the dairy and the sugar, which can cause constipation. If constipation is severe, try aloe juice, or senna with fennel or ginger, or cascara sagrada and buckthorn for short periods of time.

And look to your child's diet. Many times, bed-wetting is caused by a food allergy that causes the bladder to spasm. The most likely culprits are dairy, fruit juice, corn, wheat, soy, eggs, tomatoes, and some fruits.

If hypoglycaemia is a problem, treat it. Use nutrients and herbs such as chromium and devil's club, and control the diet by removing any refined products and sugar. (See blood-sugar section).

If parasites are a problem, treat them. Use herbs such as wormwood, black walnut, cloves, male fern, grapefruit seed extract, psyllium, pomegranate seeds, pumpkin seeds, etc.

Clear electromagnetic fields from the child's bedroom if you feel they may be a factor.

Although it is a less likely cause, be sure to get the child checked out by a health care professional to ensure that the problem is not structural, an infection, or other health concern.

CHILDHOOD COLDS AND FLUS

All parents want their children to be healthy and strong and to live full and happy lives. Children are carefully watched over, loved, and nurtured, in hopes of them growing up to be healthy and happy adults. Sometimes the task of protecting your child from illness can seem overwhelming, but there is help for parents: Nature just happens to provide numerous valuable gifts that can be used to help children stay healthy and avoid illness, or aid them when they do succumb.

Make Their Immune Systems Stronger than the Virus

Day cares, music groups, and schools are great learning places for children, but they are also breeding grounds for viruses, bacteria, and parasites. Studies have shown that plastic toys carry common parasites on them that can easily be spread amongst children, especially if a child places the toy in his mouth. But if your child has a strong immune system, she will likely fight off most infectious agents and remain healthy. Why not give your child a head start on health and minimize her chances of becoming ill?

This head start is easily accomplished by feeding your child healthy food that is free of sugar, chemicals, and empty calories. A simple step is to replace white bread and white rice with whole grains, fresh vegetables, legumes, and fruit.

If your child likes milk shakes, but seems to get earaches or other problems when he drinks milk, try using milk substitutes such as rice, soy, or almond milk. Even Dr. Benjamin Spock, the man who first told parents that all children should drink milk, has since retracted that statement.

Try mixing up this healthy and pleasant-tasting drink in the morning, adjusting it to the age and size of the child. Blend one small banana with 1 to 2 cups of milk substitute, fresh fruit, such as strawberries, or carob powder, with 1/4

NUTRIENT RICH IMMUNITY DRINK

1 small banana
1-2 cups soy, rice or almond milk
fresh fruit like strawberry or other berry
carob powder (optional)
spirulina or other green food powder
echinacea
elderberry (optional)
soy protein powder (optional)

to 1tsp of spirulina or other green powder, and echinacea drops. Herbalist Anne Mcinture says that the standard dosage for tinctures for children is anywhere from 10 drops to 1/2 tsp. The standard dosage is often given at one drop of tincture or extract per 4 lbs body weight. You can use tinctures made of glycerine, as most children like the taste and will take it. You can also add soy protein for extra nutrition, or immune herbs such as elderberry, or just about anything else with a taste that your child likes.

The drink is an excellent way to get your child to take in nutrients, since it hides the taste that he may not like. This drink is fast and can also be adjusted to fit individual children's needs and tastes. Even very young children can take it in small doses. The drink is full of vitamins, minerals, proteins, and nutrients that will strengthen the child's immunity. Echinacea is an immune enhancer that is strongly recommended for anyone in an increased health-risk situation, such as children in day care or school. It is safe to use every day. A review of the research has concluded that long-term use of echinacea whole root powder is safe for all ages from infant to adult.

If your child is ever on antibiotics, be sure to supply acidophilus and bifidus to replenish friendly flora—otherwise the child may suffer from poor immunity and develop recurrent infections.

Anne McIntyre, author of *Herbal Healing for Mother and Child*, suggests giving children oils such as flaxseed oil, especially if they are prone to infections. Essential fatty acids are crucial for all children to maintain a strong immune system and must be taken into the body, as the body cannot produce them on its own.

Nutrients needed to boost immunity can be taken in a supplement form and crushed into a drink, or in a liquid form, and also can be increased in the diet.

Calcium can be found in tahini, seeds, nuts, legumes, deep leafy greens, and whole grains. Other nutrients can also be found in foods: magnesium in beans and nuts and deep leafy greens; B vitamins in yeast; iron in legumes, deep leafy greens and sea vegetables, zinc in eggs, pumpkin seeds, and nuts; beta-carotene in green leafy vegetables; vitamin C in fruits and vegetables; and proteins in legumes, whole grains, fruits, and vegetables, especially deep leafy greens.

The antioxidants beta-carotene, vitamin C, and zinc are especially important for keeping up a strong immune system and protecting against disease.

Iron can prevent anaemia, but should not be taken when bacteria are present as the bacteria feed on the iron.

The B vitamins are involved in almost everything that the body does and help ward off stress and fatigue, and calcium and magnesium are especially helpful for the nervous system, to build bones, and to promote healthy sleep.

Try using a green food like spirulina hidden in a drink, or a flavoured multivitamin/mineral formula, or both, to ensure that your child is not missing anything in his diet.

Extra vitamins and minerals should be supplied at age-specific dosages for preventing and treating colds and flus. And be sure that your child is getting plenty of fibre to help flush out toxins. These supplements will help to keep your child strong and healthy to help prevent colds and flus.

Some wonderful herbs that can be used safely to increase immunity in children are, amongst others, licorice, astragalus, garlic, myrrh, red raspberry, ginseng, echinacea, chamomile, elderberry, thyme, andrographis, and goldenseal. Give children weak teas, by the dropper if they are still nursing, or in a bottle use 1/4 tsp per 1 cup infusion, or give tinctures in a diluted form. Or for tinctures or extracts use 1 drop per 4 lbs of body weight. Older children should go by their weight divided by the standard adult weight 150 lbs to give you their dosage. For a 50 lb child, for example, 50/150 lbs = 1/3 the adult dosage.

Licorice: This herb is useful during or after an illness to help fight off viral infections, cleanse the lungs of mucous, and cleanse and soothe the bowels. It enhances the immune system, aids white blood cells, and supports the adrenal glands, aiding in times of stress.

Astragalus: A wonderful herb that can be used to increase immunity. Astragalus is used to treat all immune-system breakdowns, colds, flus, fevers, and infections. Astragalus produces interferon, which prevents viruses from gaining a hold on the respiratory system. Interferon binds to cell surfaces and stimulates the synthesis of proteins that prevent viral infections. Astragalus both prevents infections such as colds and treats them.

Garlic: This food can be used daily to ward off parasites, viruses, fungi, and bacteria, or it can be used as needed. It can be made into drops and used to fight off ear infections and is especially useful for strains of bacteria that have become antibiotic-resistant. Again, it is great for colds and flus.

Myrrh: Herbalist Michael Tierra calls myrrh one of the best antiseptic herbs that we have. It is wonderful for coughs, bronchitis, thrush, mouth infections, infected wounds, indigestion, and many other problems.

Red Raspberry: Raspberry leaf makes a wonderful tea that most children like. It can be used to clear up thrush, sore throats, stomach problems, and intestinal complaints. It is useful for clearing out decaying matter from the digestive system.

Ginseng: Ginseng can be very useful for children who are convalescing after an illness. It should not be used for acute illnesses, but is wonderful for pale, lethargic children to help increase their white blood count and to help the liver and spleen. Ginseng is known for its ability to increase energy and to help the body deal with stress. It can also be used to strengthen the body and to prevent colds and flus.

Echinacea: A wonderful herb that is useful for all viral and bacterial infections. It aids white blood cells. Echinacea can not only treat a cold, it can also prevent a cold. A meta-analysis of studies that looked only at high-quality, double-blind, placebo-controlled studies proved that echinacea is effective at preventing colds[1]. It stimulates the production of immune cells and then increases their ability to devour invading pathogens. It then turns on a secondary immune system in your body that is triggered when antibodies start to destroy invaders. And it also has the amazing ability to disable a virus's mechanism for spreading throughout the body.

Elderberry: Elderberry is one of our favourite herbs for preventing and treating cold and flus. In one double-blind, placebo-controlled study, sixty people with the flu were given either 15 ml of standardized black elderberry syrup or a placebo four times per day for five days. There was a significant difference on a scale that ranked improvement from 0 to 10. By the third or fourth day, most of the elderberry group had improved to near 10, while the placebo group did not achieve that level until after seven or eight days. By the fourth day, scores for aches and pains, sleep quality, respiratory-tract mucous, and nasal congestion had all climbed to over 9 in the elderberry group, but were still at or below 1 in the placebo group[2].

Research has found that while the placebo group took six days to get over the flu, 90 per cent of the elderberry group was better in two to three days.

Elderberry is effective against ten strains of flu viruses and has the incredible ability to stop viruses from penetrating into your cells, rendering them incapable of replication[3].

Herbal expert Paul Berger has suggested that elderberry could even outperform the flu shot. The flu shot is only effective against the few strains it recognizes.

Chamomile: This herb makes a mild-tasting tea that most children will drink. It is great for upset stomachs, insomnia, colds, flus, and, according to the Greeks, as we have found on our travels, just about everything.

Thyme: A common kitchen herb that is wonderful for thrush, whooping cough, asthma, coughs, flu, and fever.

Goldenseal: An excellent herb for immunity, colds, flus, food poisoning, allergies, diarrhea, hepatitis, gastritis, stomach problems, eczema, and many other ailments. It dries and cleanses mucous membranes. It has antibiotic, antiviral, and antifungal properties.

Andrographis: Andrographis is used for preventing and treating colds and is a good one for your child to take during the cold season. In a double-blind study, children were given andrographis during the winter months in dosages of 200 mg a day for three months. The children on andrographis had 2.1 times less risk of catching a cold than the children on the placebo[4].

More Help

There are many other herbs that can be used to strengthen immunity and treat illnesses. Mary Bove, N.D., suggests the following additional antiviral herbs to aid children: usnea, which is great for strep throat, linden flowers, yarrow flowers, catnip, meadowsweet, and lemon balm. She suggests using herbs as teas and in herbal popsicles to help soothe throats. These herbs are great for increasing the body's own immune system's ability to fight off infections, to induce sleep, to calm, and to reduce pain.

Another possible choice is to put herbs such as eucalyptus in infusers and vaporizers to reduce viruses and bacteria in the air and to clear sinuses. Lavender can also be used to induce calmness and sleep.

Try to encourage children to wash their hands frequently, as this can help prevent the spread of many infections.

Chapter Endnotes

1. Schoop, R., *et al.* "echinacea in the prevention of induced rhinovirus colds: a meta-analysis." *Clin Ther*, 2006; 28:174'83.

2. Zakay-Rones, Z., et al. "Randomized study of the efficacy and safety of oral elderberry extract in the treatment of influenza A and B virus infections." *J International Med Res*, 2004; 32:132-40.

3. Zakay-Rones, Z., *et al.* "Inhibition of several strains of influenza virus in vitro and reduction of symptoms by an elderberry extract (*Sambucus nigra L.*) during an outbreak of influenza B Panama." *J Altern Complement Med*, 1995; 1:361-69.

4. Caceres, D.D., *et al.* "Prevention of common colds with *Andrographis paniculata* dried extract. A pilot double-blind trial." *Phytomedicine*, 1997; Vol. 4:101'04.

COLIC

It's late at night, dark, cold and your child is up, crying, miserable and holding his tummy. You walk with him, try to soothe him, but this offers only some small comfort; he's still got his legs pulled right up against his belly. What's wrong with him? Well, in this case, it is childhood colic, one of the most common reasons for children's stomachaches. You ask yourself what you can do. It's been going on for several nights now, and both you and your child are exhausted.

Perhaps you have noticed that certain foods seem to make your child worse. You're right. Dietary changes are crucial in treating and preventing colic. A few herbs have been used around the world for centuries for treating colic that bring speedy relief. Incidentally, these herbs work very well on adult stomachaches as well.

And, although colic mainly affects young children and babies, it can affect adults as well. Colic causes cramp-like abdominal pain that occurs intermittently. Children suffering from colic will pull up their legs, cry and clench their fists. They may nurse or eat briefly, but will often stop eating to cry again. Usually the child gains weight normally and the stools are normal.

Causes of Colic

Because it is believed that emotional upset can contribute to, or even cause, colic, it is crucial that the baby's atmosphere is kept as calm and stress free as possible. Breast-feeding should be done calmly and not rushed.

Colic may be related to feeding problems. Mothers should check that their babies are latched on correctly. If you are unsure, there are breast-feeding clinics that can help, or you can consult a midwife.

Food, too, is a major contributing cause of colic. Often it is what the mother eats that causes problems for the child, since she is passing what she has eaten along in the breast milk. Often the foods that are causing problems are those that are allergens or irritants to the child, although they may not be bothering the mother. According to Mary Bove, N.D., author of *An Encyclopedia of Natural Healing for Children and Infants*, common foods that cause problems include all forms of dairy, alcohol, coffee, spicy foods, garlic, onions, legumes, too much fruit, cabbage, broccoli, cauliflower, and Brussels sprouts. The most troublesome ones of all are dairy, citrus, wheat, and corn. Anne McIntyre, author of *The Herbal for Mother and Child*, adds that green peppers, eggplants, cucumbers, zucchini, chocolate, tomatoes, eggs, and sugar can also be problems. Bove specifically recommends that breast-feeding women avoid dairy products in their diet for at least three months. A recent study looked at the allergy connection. Breast-feeding mothers of colicky babies were put either on a control diet or on a low-allergy diet that eliminated soy, wheat, eggs, peanuts, nuts, and fish. And the results were truly impressive: 74 per cent of the babies in the low-allergen group responded favourably, compared to only 37 per cent in the control group[1].

The best way to determine which foods are causing problems for the child is for the mother to eliminate all of the foods that commonly cause problems for at least two weeks and reintroduce them one at a time, noting any problems that may occur. If a particular food is causing problems, then that food should be avoided. Just be sure that you are eating properly, substituting one food for another if need be.

For those children who are being bottle-fed and who are experiencing colic, the problem could be that the formula is made of cow's milk, one of the most common foods that babies react to. It may be that the child is lactose-intolerant. Babies born to families with histories of eczema, asthma, and hay fever are more likely to experience a reaction to milk.

Herbal Help for Colic

Herbal help for colic comes from herbs such as chamomile, caraway seeds, catnip, cinnamon, dill seeds, fennel seeds, anise, lemon balm, marshmallow, and slippery elm. Anne McIntyre recommends giving any of the above herbs as a tea in 1 oz portions before each feeding. Use 1/4 to 1/2 tsp of the herb and infuse in 4 oz of boiling water. After feeding, if the baby still seems uncomfortable, give some of the tea again. The herbs mentioned are anti-flatulents, soothing herbs that can also stop spasms. If the baby seems particularly tense, try using chamomile,

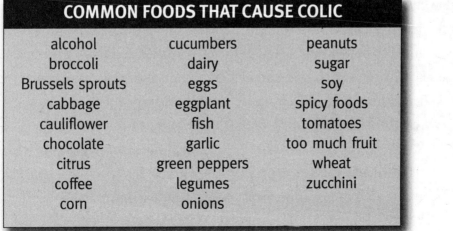

COMMON FOODS THAT CAUSE COLIC

alcohol	cucumbers	peanuts
broccoli	dairy	sugar
Brussels sprouts	eggs	soy
cabbage	eggplant	spicy foods
cauliflower	fish	tomatoes
chocolate	garlic	too much fruit
citrus	green peppers	wheat
coffee	legumes	zucchini
corn	onions	

catnip, or lemon balm, which also help the baby relax. When eighty-eight babies with colic were given either a placebo or 2 ml per kilogram of a liquid made from powdered extracts of the herbs chamomile, fennel, and lemon balm for seven days, the babies on the placebo cried for an average of 170 minutes per day, while the babies given the herbs cried for only 77 minutes per day. More than 85 per cent of the babies on the herbs had a 50 per cent or greater decrease in crying, compared to only 49 per cent of the placebo group[2].

Bove recommends that breast-feeding mothers drink herbal teas made out of catnip, cinnamon, dill, fennel, lemon balm, or crampbark. The medicinal properties of the herbs will pass into the breast milk and through to the child. These same teas can be given in weaker forms directly to the baby by the dropperful every fifteen minutes. Fennel, caraway, anise, and dill can also be infused, 1 tbsp to 8 oz of water, allowed to steep for ten minutes and mixed with 3 oz of vegetable glycerine. Bove suggests using 1/4 to 1/2 tsp every half hour if colic is present, or give it fifteen minutes before each feeding. Many of these herbs come already prepared, ready to use, in tincture form for children's and babies' colic and can be found in health-food stores.

Catnip can also be used as a warm compress on the child's stomach. Catnip works particularly well as a compress since it is an antispasmodic (relieves cramping) and a carminative (relieves gas). It can also make the baby less tense and help him to sleep. Other useful herbs for making a warm fomentation include lavender and lobelia. Make a warm infusion, soak a cloth in it, and apply over the tummy area of the child with a wrapped hot-water bottle. These herbs will encourage relaxation and relieve spasms and gas. Or rub a few drops of these herbs in essential-oil form, diluted, onto the baby's tummy. Chamomile, fennel, and anise seed will also work well as essential oils applied to the child's tummy area.

Baths are a particularly good place to make use of these herbs. All of the herbs mentioned can also be used in the baby's bath water, in stronger forms, to help soothe cramping, gas, and tension. If tension is a particular problem, try relaxing herbs in the bath, such as hops, lemon balm, chamomile, catnip, skullcap, vervain, passionflower, and wild oats. Or add a few drops of the essential oils from these herbs to the baby's bath water. Herbal baths and essential oils often are of great benefit before a feeding since they relax the child and help to allay any cramping quickly and easily, making feedings easier.

After a feeding, if the baby is sleepy, try laying him on his side with a hot-water bottle in a towel close to his tummy. You may even want to apply a few drops of one of the diluted essential oils mentioned above to the child's tummy to help him sleep better and to relieve any cramping that the feeding may have caused.

With a little care, attention to diet and atmosphere, and with the help of a few herbs, soon you and your child will be sleeping through the night, waking up well-rested, happier, and eager to start your day with each other.

Chapter Endnotes

1. Hill, D.J., et al. 'Effect of a low-allergen maternal diet on colic among breastfed infants: A randomized, controlled trial.' *Pediatrics*, 2005; 116:e709'e715.

2. Savino, F., et al. 'A randomized double-blind placebo-controlled trial of a standardized extract of *Matricariae recutita, Foeniculum vulgare* and *Melissa officinalis (ColiMil)* in the treatment of breastfed colicky infants.' *Phytotherapy Research*, 2005; 19:335'40.

CHILDHOOD CONSTIPATION

Even breast-fed babies can become constipated. They become irritable and crampy, and they may lose their appetites and even vomit, while their little abdomens become distended. Organic causes have been ruled out and still the baby cannot seem to pass a stool. When the baby does pass a stool, it seems to hurt him, making him scared to try again.

Causes of constipation

Causes of constipation in infants are many: poor diet on the part of the mother or of the child if he is beyond nursing, lack of friendly flora in the gut, stress, lack of exercise, and lack of fluids.

When is a child actually constipated? When the child has trouble passing a stool, and any stool passed is hard. Not all babies pass a stool every day. When a child does pass a stool, if it looks and smells normal, if she did not have trouble passing it, and if not too much time has gone by since her last stool, then the child is likely not constipated.

The most common culprit producing constipation in children is diet. Food allergies, either in a breast-feeding mother or in the child if he is eating, can cause constipation. Common allergens are wheat, dairy, tomato, and citrus fruits that carry mould. Try to determine which foods are causing the problem and then eliminate them from the diet, for at least two weeks. Then re-introduce them, one at a time, every few days, and note symptoms if they appear. Any foods that are found to be causing the problem should be eliminated entirely. Eliminating milk and other dairy products will cure childhood constipation about 70 per cent of the time. Also, a diet low in fibre and high in sugar can cause constipation. So try to make sure that the diet that your baby gets, whether through breast milk or food, is free of sugar and high in fibre. Eat more vegetables, fruits, whole grains, and legumes—just be careful

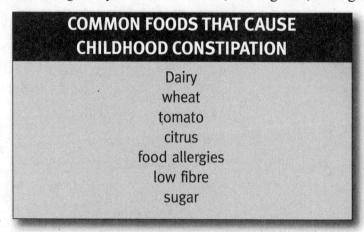

COMMON FOODS THAT CAUSE CHILDHOOD CONSTIPATION

Dairy
wheat
tomato
citrus
food allergies
low fibre
sugar

of allergens. If the child is old enough, try adding natural fibre to the diet, such as ground flaxseeds and psyllium, to help increase the moistness of the stools, making them easier to pass while increasing peristaltic movement in the intestines.

Relieving Constipation

Try to eat foods rich in vitamin C and magnesium if you are breast-feeding, or even supplement them, since lack of these two nutrients has been found to cause constipation. Lack of folic acid has also been linked to constipation. If your child is eating on his own, be sure to supply lots of vegetables, since these three nutrients are found in abundance in vegetables.

Also, be sure to give your child plenty of fluids such as pure water and diluted herbal teas and juices, since a lack of fluids can cause constipation. Give the extra fluids between feedings to ensure that the baby still eats at meal times and is not full. Good herbal teas to try are licorice, which helps to clean the baby out, dandelion root, which stimulates bile, increasing peristaltic movements in the intestines; flaxseed tea, which adds moisture to the stools, making them easier to pass, senna, use only if needed, mixed with cloves or fennel to prevent gripping and only for short periods of time; relaxant teas, such as lemon balm, catnip, chamomile, to prevent spasming in the intestines and mucilaginous herbs, such as marshmallow or slippery elm tea to soothe sore intestines.

If your child has very sore intestines, try mixing 1 tsp of slippery elm powder with 1 tbsp of warm water with a pinch of cinnamon. Mix this into a kind of gruel and feed to the child. The slippery elm gruel acts as a soother to irritated surfaces and will also provide more nutrients than porridge. Depending on the age of your child, the usual dose for teas is 1 to 2 tsps, 3 times a day, but she can have more if needed. These teas can be drunk by the mother as well if she is breast-feeding, and their properties will be passed through the breast milk. The mother should drink one cup 3 to 4 times a day. If stools are green and no parasites have been found, try having the baby sip raspberry leaf tea, which is good for clearing out unwanted matter in the intestines. Diluted pure prune, and fig, juice are also good for short periods of time to increase peristaltic movement in the intestines, just to get things moving.

A good formula to help is 1/4 oz each of bruised cloves and powdered cinnamon, 1/2 oz of senna leaves, and 4 ozs of prunes. Bruise the prunes and simmer in 1 1/2 pints of water for twenty minutes. Strain and give 1/2 to 1 tsp as needed. Do not, however, rely on this formula for long periods of time. It should only be used to establish regular movements until other changes can be made. Do not give senna to children with blocked bowels.

Many babies have a flora imbalance in their guts that can cause constipation, so it is a good idea whenever constipation strikes to replenish friendly flora using acidophilus and bifidus supplements specially designed for children. They come in flavoured liquids that are easy to administer. Over-use of antibiotics, either in the breast-feeding mother or the child, can cause this flora imbalance, leading to constipation.

Often a baby has passed a particularly hard or large stool that caused pain, making the child afraid to pass stool again. If this problem has occurred, the relaxant herbs can help, as can herbs such as flaxseed tea, which moisten stool, making it softer and easier to pass. Try to keep the environment as stress-free as possible, since stress is a major factor in causing constipation.

Exercise your baby's legs, bending them and bringing the knees up to the stomach; this too can encourage the stool to move along. Any kind of bending at the abdomen can help to force the stool through the intestines and out the rectum. You can help the stool along by massaging the infant's abdomen daily, using diluted, warmed fennel oil. Put a few drops of fennel oil in warmed castor oil and massage the baby's abdomen in a clockwise direction daily to encourage the natural direction of elimination. You can also use diluted ginger, peppermint, or lobelia oil. Use the massage time as a playtime and a time of cuddling that will help to make your child feel secure and happy.

Finally, be sure to get a stool sample analyzed to be sure that there is no blood in the stools and also no parasites. For instance, pinworms can cause constipation and hard, itching stools in infants. Roundworm can also cause constipation and cramping in the intestines, and over one million North Americans have roundworm.

DIAPER RASH

Many babies will get diaper rash: it is extremely common, yet it does not have to be. To treat it, we must look at what causes it.

What Are the Causes of Diaper Rash?

When urine and stool are left in the diaper for too long, the bacteria in the stool break down the urine to release ammonia, which irritates the skin. A red rash appears around the genitals, and it can get worse if untreated, leading to sores. Bacteria breed in an alkaline environment, which can be a result if the child is bottle-fed, as opposed to breast-fed. If the rash is only on the skin around the top of the thighs, it is often due to not drying the baby well enough. Diapers made from fabrics that have been washed in detergent may cause an allergic reaction, so use a natural washing cleanser.

This kind of rash will cover the area that the diaper is on. Thrush, caused by candida, can also be a cause. Check the mouth for signs of thrush. The rash will usually spread from the anus over the buttocks and onto the thighs. Small blisters can indicate other problems, such as a herpes infection. Diarrhea can make rashes worse, so check the child for food allergies or check your own diet if still breast-feeding if diarrhea is a problem. Plastic pants and/or elastic pants can also cause a rash since the child may be sensitive to plastic; also, plastic holds in more moisture. Diaper rash also occurs in babies who have sensitive skin and can indicate the beginning of eczema or seborrhea.

Treatment

Try taking baby's diaper off sometimes to let her skin get some air and sunlight. Keep your baby's skin dry. You should always towel-dry the skin,

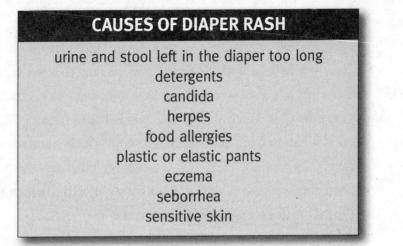

CAUSES OF DIAPER RASH

urine and stool left in the diaper too long
detergents
candida
herpes
food allergies
plastic or elastic pants
eczema
seborrhea
sensitive skin

and allow it to totally dry before putting on a diaper. You can even dry the bottom with a blowdryer to make sure it is totally dry before putting a diaper on. Change the diaper frequently to prevent moisture from sitting too long.

At each change, wash the baby's skin with witch hazel and dry it thoroughly. Apply one of the creams given below, using calendula or chamomile cream, or a diluted tincture of myrrh or indigo, or oregano oil, if you think there is an infection. You can also use the essential oils mentioned below to stop the rash. Make sure all fabric diapers are sterilized and rinsed free of any detergent. Avoid plastic pants; use unbleached disposable diapers if necessary. Use fabric liners, which let urine pass through to the diaper and leave baby's skin dry and comfortable. If oral thrush is present, treat for thrush (see section on Thrush). If the rash is particularly bad, try using tea made from calming herbs, such as chamomile or catnip or valerian, to soothe the baby.

Use only natural ingredients on your baby's skin. Make your own baby powder out of arrowroot, white clay, slippery elm, and either calendula or comfrey powder. These herbs help both to soothe and to prevent diaper rash. Arrowroot helps to absorb moisture, as does clay, which also detoxifies; slippery elm is a demulcent, so it soothes irritated skin; calendula and comfrey both help to soothe the skin and clear up rashes, and calendula is also antifungal. Add lavender or chamomile essential oils to this mixture to help sterilize and soothe infections.

Mary Bove, N.D., says that calendula, chickweed, and plantain all make great herbal salves for diaper rash. Again, calendula is antifungal and heals rashes; chickweed heals rashes, and plantain helps to draw matter out and to heal. Herbalist Rosemary Gladstar says to use a salve of St. John's wort, comfrey leaf and root, and calendula. St. John's wort helps to soothe irritated surfaces and to heal.

Anne McIntyre, author of *The Herbal for Mother and Child*, recommends washing the baby's bottom with a herbal infusion of lavender, chamomile, rosewater, or calendula. She recommends a cream of either chamomile, chickweed, comfrey, or calendula to soothe, heal, and protect the skin. These herbs will also protect the skin against the corrosive effects of urine or stool. She adds that you can also use oils such as St. John's wort, lavender, or chamomile in a base of almond oil or grape or sesame oil. She recommends avoiding regular talcum powder because it cakes on the skin, holding in the damp, and it can collect bacteria, leading to a worse rash and even a secondary infection. Aloe vera applied topically is also good. It heals bacterial infections and fungus, and it soothes rashes and irritated skin as it heals.

Rosemary Gladstar also recommends giving your baby children's acidophilus. This treatment will help if the rash is caused by yeast, or if the baby's system is weak. Bove says to use oregano oil in calendula cream to clear up rashes caused by yeast. As mentioned, rashes can be a sign that the baby has yeast and needs to have it treated. If this is the case, give your child acidophilus and/or take it yourself if you're still breast-feeding. Avoid sugar, yeast, mould, and dairy in your diet and your child's diet (see Candida section on diet). Try taking, or giving your child, raspberry tea, tincture of myrrh or indigo, or any age-appropriate suggestions from the Candida section. It is often best to give herbs to the mother and have them pass through the breast milk.

An old-time remedy, according to Anne McIntyre, is to apply egg white thickly and repeatedly to the affected area before putting on a diaper. The egg white encourages a protective coating of albumen to form, allowing the baby's bottom to heal.

Amanda McQuade Crawford, M.N.I.M.H., author of *Herbal Remedies for Women*, recommends adding 1/4 cup of apple cider vinegar to the rinse cycle of diapers.

Most importantly, don't wait for a rash to get worse. Treat immediately at the first sign to prevent a secondary or worse infection from settling in.

EAR INFECTION

Most kids we grew up with had recurring ear infections. And the same can be said for kids today. On average, children have one ear infection in each of their first three years, and 93 per cent of all children will have at least one by the time they are seven. And ear infections are excruciatingly painful. Untreated, they can lead to complications.

What Are Some of the Causes of Ear Infections?

Allergies and viruses are the most common causes of ear infections. Ear infections are rarely caused by bacteria. Nonetheless, ear infections are still the most common reason for prescribing antibiotics to kids: 50 per cent of all antibiotics given to kids are for ear infections. They are still prescribed despite the fact that there is absolutely no evidence of any benefit to using antibiotics for ear infections, according to a review of seven placebo-controlled studies[1].

Allergies and Other Causes

Recurrent ear infections are strongly associated with bottle-feeding. Breast-feeding, on the other hand, protects against ear infections[2]. Ear infections are also associated with pacifiers[3] and second-hand smoke[4].

The major cause of ear infections, though, is allergies. Most sufferers of ear infections have allergies, and most get better when the allergies are eliminated[5]. Dairy is the worst allergy for ear infections, followed by wheat, eggs, peanuts, soy, and corn[6]. Many children improve dramatically, even completely, when allergens are removed from their diet.

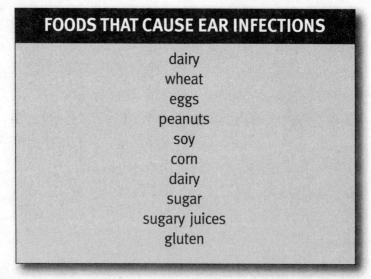

FOODS THAT CAUSE EAR INFECTIONS

dairy
wheat
eggs
peanuts
soy
corn
dairy
sugar
sugary juices
gluten

What Else Can You Do to Help an Ear Infection?

To avoid ear infections and to clear them up if you or your child has one, support the immune system by avoiding sugar, including sugary juices. Also avoid dairy and, for some, gluten. These foods make mucous, which yeast and viruses thrive in. Avoid untested chlorinated pools, as many contain bacteria that can cause ear infections.

Herbal Eardrops

Herbal eardrops are incredible for ear infections. Traditionally, garlic, mullein, calendula, and St. John's wort have been used in olive oil, with the drops being put in both ears. And now, science has proven the effectiveness of these herbal eardrops.

In one study, eardrops made of garlic, mullein, calendula, and St. John's wort in olive oil were compared to an anaesthetic eardrop in 103 children with ear infections. When five drops were placed in their ears three times a day, both groups had significant relief from ear pain. The treatments were equally effective, and all the children were successfully treated[7].

Recently, a similar herbal eardrop containing garlic, mullein, calendula, St. John's wort, lavender, and vitamin E in olive oil was compared to an anaesthetic eardrop, an anaesthetic eardrop used with with antibiotics, and the herbal eardrop

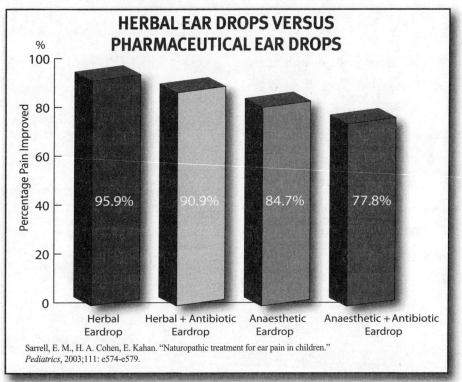

HERBAL EAR DROPS VERSUS PHARMACEUTICAL EAR DROPS

%
Percentage Pain Improved

- Herbal Eardrop: 95.9%
- Herbal + Antibiotic Eardrop: 90.9%
- Anaesthetic Eardrop: 84.7%
- Anaesthetic + Antibiotic Eardrop: 77.8%

Sarrell, E. M., H. A. Cohen, E. Kahan. "Naturopathic treatment for ear pain in children." *Pediatrics*, 2003;111: e574-e579.

used with antibiotics. Again, the children were given five drops three times a day. Not only was the herbal eardrop more effective than the anaesthetic eardrop, but while the average level of ear pain dropped by 95.9 per cent in the herbal eardrop group, it dropped by a lesser 90.9 per cent in the group that got the antibiotic in addition to the herbal eardrops, showing that the addition of antibiotics is not helpful[8].

Mary Bove, N.D., says that goldenseal and lobelia can also be effective in eardrops. Tea tree oil, diluted, and grapefruit-seed extract, diluted, have also been used.

Other Help

Bove also recommends using immune-supporting herbs such as echinacea, astragalus, garlic, chamomile, and wild indigo.

Herbalist Rosemary Gladstar suggests tinctures of goldenseal, echinacea, usnea, garlic, and ginger. She also suggests supplementing acidophilus.

Many causes of recurrent ear infections are actually yeast related, especially if the child has been on antibiotics. So it is a good idea to give acidophilus and yeast-killers such as indigo, goldenseal, raspberry leaf, usnea, and garlic to get rid of the yeast and the ear infection.

Michael Murray N.D., and Joseph Pizzorno, N.D., recommend supplementing a multivitamin/mineral, beta-carotene, vitamin C, bioflavonoids, zinc, and echinacea for ear infections.

Acupuncture is also a great idea for ear infections. As is a poultice made of herbs such as mullein, garlic, and calendula.

And don't forget relaxing herbs to help the child sleep and to help get rid of her pain. Use herbs such as chamomile, valerian, poppy, hops, skullcap, catnip, and lemon verbena.

Chapter Endnotes

1. Froom, J., et al. "Antimicrobials for acute otitis media? A review from the International Primary Care Network." *BMJ*, 1997; 315:98'102.

2. Saarinen, U.M. 'Prolonged breast feeding as prophylaxis for recurrent otitis media.' *Acta Ped Scand*, 1982; 71:567'571.

3. Niemela, M., M. Uhari, A. Hannuksela. "Pacifiers and dental structure as risk factors for otitis media." *Int J Pediatr Otorhinolaryngol*, 1994; 29:121-27; Niemela M., M. Uhari, M. Mottonen. "A pacifier increases the risk of recurrent acute otitis media in children in daycare centers." *Pediatrics*, 1995; 96:884-88; Jackson, J. M., A.P. Mourino. "Pacifier use and otitis media in infants twelve months of age or younger." *Pediatr Dent*, 1999; 21:256-261; Warren, J. J., et al. "Pacifier use and the occurrence of otitis media in the first year of life." *Pediatr Dent*, 2001; 23:103-107.

4. Ethel, R. A., et al. "Passive smoking and middle ear effusion among children in day care." *Pediatr*, 1992; 90:228-232; Ilicali, O. C., et al. "Evaluation of the effect of passive smoking on otitis media in children by an objective method: urinary continence analysis." *Laryngoscope*, 2001; 111:163-167.

5. Nsouli, T. M., et al. "Role of food allergy in serous otitis media." *Ann Allerg*, 1994; 73:215-9; McGovern J. P., T. H. Haywood, A. A. Fernandez. "Allergy and secretory otitis media." *JAMA*, 1967; 200:134-8; Roukonen J., A. Pagnaus, H. Lehti. "Elimination diets in the treatment of secretory otitis media." *Internat J Pediatr Otorhinolaryngol*, 1982; 4:39-46.

6. Nsouli, T. M., *et al*. Role of food allergy in serous otitis media. *Ann Allerg*, 1994; 73:215-219.

7. Sarrell, E. M., A. Mandelberg, H. A. Cohen. "Efficacy of naturopathic extracts in the management of ear pain associated with acute otitis media." *Arch Pediatr Adolesc Med*, 2001; 155:796-799.

8. Sarrell, E. M., H. A. Cohen, E. Kahan. "Naturopathic treatment for ear pain in children." *Pediatrics*, 2003;111: e574-e579.

HEAD LICE

Head lice are always a problem in school-age children. They are quickly becoming an epidemic because the lice are developing immunity to conventional treatment.

Head lice move from one child to another by close contact. Lice can live for twenty-four hours away from the body. They are hard to see, as they are a pale greyish-brown colour. They are most easily found at the back of the neck. The white eggs that the female lays, called nits, hatch in eight days and live for about five weeks. The lice bite the scalp several times a day to feed, causing itching and inflammation that can lead to infection if the child scratches a lot or if the infestation is high. Signs of infection include swollen lymph nodes in the throat and redness and swelling.

Treatment

One old-time treatment that is very effective is to soak the child's hair and scalp in olive oil that has been mixed with essential oils and leave this on the hair and scalp overnight. Essential oils that are especially toxic to lice include eucalyptus, rosemary, marjoram, and pennyroyal[1]. Wash out thoroughly in the morning. Protect bedclothes with towels. While the hair is saturated with olive oil, carefully comb out all the white nits. Using vinegar on the comb helps to get them out.

Recipe for removing head lice

25 drops of lavender oil

10 drops of geranium oil

25 drops of rosemary oil

1 dessert teaspoon of eucalyptus oil

2 teaspoons of tea tree oil

*Anne McIntyre, *The Herbal for Mother and Child*

Mix with olive oil, almond, or sunflower oil. Apply each night for five nights, then repeat for two nights after a week. Clean all hairbrushes and hair apparel, too.

Others suggest using pure tea tree oil mixed with the olive oil. Or use herbal shampoos and conditioners mixed with tea tree oil to treat and prevent lice.

One study found that citronella lotion worked better than a placebo lotion[2].

For infections, use supplements such as echinacea, astragalus, garlic, licorice, elderberry, vitamin C, and zinc at age-appropriate doses.

Chapter Endnotes

1. Yang, Y. C., *et al.* "Insecticidal activity of plant essential oils against *Pediculus humanus capitis* (Anoplura: Pediculidae)." *J Med Entomol*, 2004; 41:699-704.

2. Mumcuoglu, K. Y., S. Magdassi, J. Miller, *et al.* "Repellency of citronella for head lice: double-blind randomized trial of efficacy and safety." *Isr Med Assoc J*, 2004; 6:756-759.

TEETHING

Teething affects everybody. You don't remember, but you went through it, too.

Two great teething remedies are the herbs catnip and chamomile. Both herbs will be beautifully soothing to your baby. But they go beyond soothing. Herbalist Rosemary Gladstar says that catnip will also relieve pain and help take care of any fever that comes along with it. Mary Bove, N.D., adds that since it is also an immune-supporting herb, catnip will help prevent any secondary infections that may accompany teething. Other good immune boosting herbs to use during teething, according to Bove, are lemon balm and echinacea. Like catnip and chamomile, lemon balm is a great soothing herb. The beautiful gentleness of all three of these herbs makes them ideal remedies for children.

If your child doesn't like taking chamomile or catnip as teas or tinctures, then surprise him or her with a frozen herbal sucker. The frozen sucker is not only a fun way to deliver the healing properties of the herbs, the cold will also help numb the gums and relieve the pain. You can either make a strong herbal tea and then freeze it into an ice cube or popsicle, or you can mix it with an equal part of fruit juice first.

Canadian herbalist Terry Willard recommends a general calming formula for children that can be used during teething. He suggests combining catnip, chamomile, and lemon balm with peppermint, hyssop, and elder.

Homeopathic remedies for teething can also be helpful. Let your baby chew on a licorice or marshmallow root: both taste sweet, as modern-day snack foods still affirm.

Or try diluted oil of clove, topically, to dull the pain.

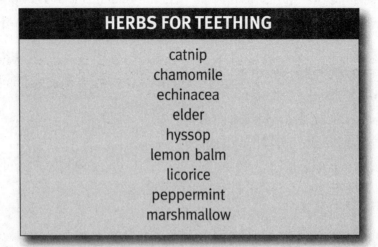

HERBS FOR TEETHING

catnip
chamomile
echinacea
elder
hyssop
lemon balm
licorice
peppermint
marshmallow

THRUSH

Thrush is a condition that occurs mostly in babies, but children and adults can get it, too. The throat, mouth, and/or tongue can become coated with white matter. Little white sores may form.

How Does Your Baby Get Thrush?

Thrush is believed to result from an overgrowth of yeast-causing candida. It is usually caused by antibiotics or nutritional deficiencies, such as lack of iron and zinc. Poor eating habits or a weak immune system can also contribute to thrush. If a mother is breast-feeding and her child has thrush, it could be that her diet is poor. According to Joy Gardner, author of *Healing Yourself During Pregnancy*, if a mother who has candida gives birth, the child could get it, too, in the digestive system, where it is known as thrush.

Candida can cause a whole host of symptoms (see Candida section). But, at the very least, the child will have reduced ability to absorb nutrients,

and digestion will be poor. He may also feel tired, sore, and ill.

How Do You Get Rid of Your Baby's Thrush?

Treatment is aimed at getting rid of the yeast. It is a good idea to give probiotics, such as acidophilus, since the white coating is seen as a sign that candida is present. Adults should take 20 billion live cultures a day, and children should take a dosage appropriate to their weight. Also, all sugar, dairy, and white refined carbohydrates should be avoided, as should mould and yeast foods, until the problem clears up. (See Candida section and follow the dietary suggestions given there). Yoghurt with live culture may be given, but for those sensitive to dairy, it is still best to avoid it.

The yeast must be killed and the system flushed out, and the immune system should be supported.

Excellent choices for thrush include tincture of

HERBS FOR THRUSH

astragalus	goldenseal root	probiotics
calendula	marjoram	rosemary
echinacea	marigold	sage
garlic	myrrh	tea or oil
licorice	oregano	thyme
grapefruit seed extract	pau d'arco	wild indigo

myrrh, and/or wild indigo. You can use them straight or diluted with water and sprayed directly into the mouth and throat several times a day. Use one part herb to five parts water. These herbs kill the yeast, support the immune system, and purge the surfaces of bad matter.

Sage tea or tincture is also a good choice to use. Other possible good choices include goldenseal-root tincture or tea, oregano tea or tincture or oil, and echinacea to support the immune system. These herbs help to kill and/or dry up the yeast and support the immune system.

Try other good anti-candida herbs, or good herbs for throat problems, such as garlic, thyme, oleic acid from olive oil, marjoram, marigold, rosemary, licorice, and immune-supporting herbs such as astragalus.

Herbalist Anne McIntyre, author of *The Herbal for Mother and Child*, recommends using a mouthwash made from an infusion of calendula, sage, or thyme. Allow it to cool and add one drop of essential oil of either thyme, marjoram, or oregano to each cup. Use two or three times a day. Or use 1/4 to 1/2 tsp of tincture of goldenseal, calendula, myrrh, or sage diluted in a little water. She adds that lemon juice diluted with equal parts of water is also useful.

Amanda McQuade Crawford, M.N.I.M.H., author of *Herbal Remedies for Women*, suggests using mashed garlic and live yoghurt applied directly to the problem area. She also suggests trying live yoghurt on its own and avoiding sugar for both mother and child. Or, she says, try rinsing the mother's nipples with diluted calendula tincture or tea before and after every feeding.

Other good candida fighters include grapefruit seed extract and pau d'arco.

If digestive symptoms are a problem, try giving the child slippery elm or marshmallow tea to help ease the digestive distress.

Old-time herbalists used a strong infusion of raspberry leaf tea to clear up this problem. Pour 1/2 pint of boiling water over 1 oz of the raspberry leaves. Cover and let stand for twenty minutes. Strain and give every two hours, 1 to 3 tbsp for a child, and 8 oz, four times a day for an adult.

The bowels were also cleansed in old-time herbalism using a combination of 1/4 oz bruised cloves, 1/4 oz powdered cinnamon, 1/2 oz senna leaves, and 4 ozs prunes. Simmer everything in 1 1/2 pints of water for forty minutes. Strain and give 1/2 to 1 tsp as often as needed. You can also take buckthorn, cascara sagrada, aloe, triphala, or senna to get the bowels moving. Fibre, such as psyllium or flax seed, is also a good idea to help clear out the system.

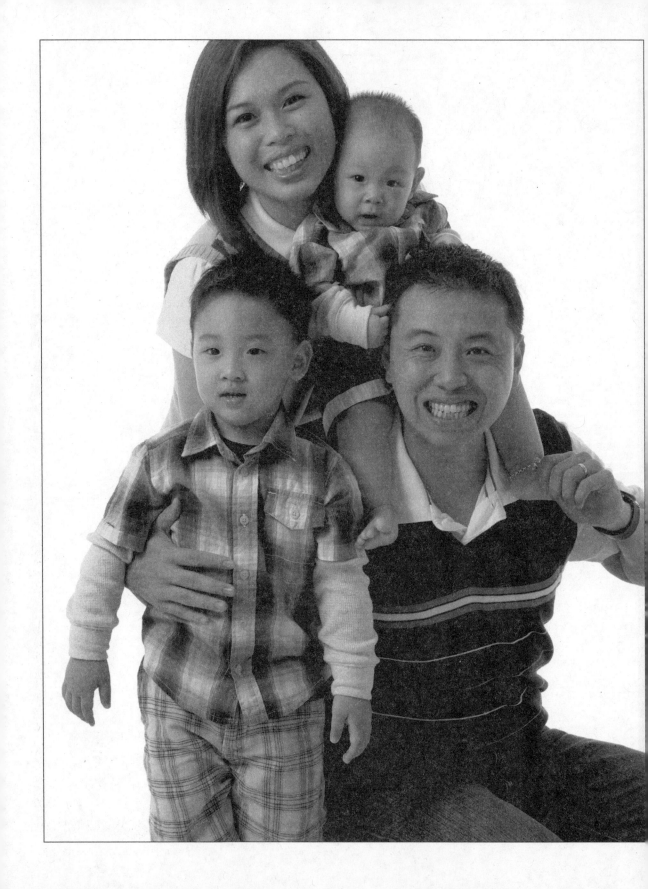

HEALTH FOR THE FAMILY

Something for everyone. This large section of the book contains information that the whole family can use to help them enjoy good health. This section is here because we are all people, and, so, we face many of the same health concerns.

In this section of the book, you will find easy, how-to advice for the whole family. Whether you are young or old, male or female, looking for help from everything from the common cold to addictions, you will find information here that can help the whole family. It is your family's natural health reference section, for the most common health concerns.

And best of all, it is all in one place: not a separate book for every problem. You will find information on nutrition, vitamins, minerals, supplements, herbs and other natural health information. And you will learn how to treat issues that affect everyone. You will also find research, personal and clinical experience, folklore, expert and cultural information, included in the upcoming chapters, all designed to help you understand the health problem that you are trying to solve.

This section will look at colds and flus, sinusitis and runny nose, allergies, pain and injuries, bronchitis, asthma, migraine, skin health, eczema, candida, nail fungus, urinary tract infections (including kidney stones), cigarettes and alcohol addiction and insomnia, depression, anxiety, stress, ulcers, celiac disease, multiple sclerosis, anemia, HIV/AIDS, Crohn's and colitis, and carpal tunnel syndrome.

ADDICTIONS

Cigarettes

Cigarette-smoking is the number-one cause of death in North America. On average, smokers live seven to eight years less than non-smokers. And smoking gets them in a number of ways. It hugely increases their risk of heart disease, several kinds of cancer—including about 90 per cent of all cases of lung cancer—bronchitis, and emphysema. Less well-known are the facts that cigarettes contribute to bone loss, double your chance of losing your teeth, add wrinkles to your skin, and increase the chance of your hair falling out. Smoking also contributes to depression. Nicotine is highly addictive. Quite simply, it is one of the most harmful and addictive substances there is. Quitting is hard, but nature can help.

Though it may not be the first thing you would think of, diet can help reduce the cravings. Elson Haas, M.D., says research shows that alkalinizing your body by increasing the fruits, vegetables, and whole grains in your diet and decreasing the amount of fat can help.

Hass also recommends giving up other addictive substances such as alcohol, caffeine, and sugar, since they can all increase the desire to smoke.

A number of herbs have been used traditionally to help people stop smoking. One really interesting stop-smoking herb is lobelia. The lobeline in lobelia has a chemical structure much like that of nicotine and with similar physiological effects, but it's not addictive. So lobelia satisfies the craving for nicotine while you wean yourself off it. There is some research to support the traditional use of this herb.

Oat seed, or *Avena sativa*, is another herb that helps. It is also an effective herb for withdrawal from opium and other drugs. Though not all studies have been positive, a double-blind study found that heavily addicted smokers smoked way fewer cigarettes when given a fresh oat-seed extract than when given a placebo[1].

Oats, like many herbs that help you quit, is a nervine, a relaxant herb that tones, calms and nourishes the nervous system. Another such herb is skullcap. Other nervines can help reduce the depression, anxiety, and irritability that can come along with withrawal. Nervines that can be used to help break all kinds of addiction include vervain, chamomile, linden, lemon balm, and California poppy. Eric Yarnell, N.D., *et al*, include oats, skullcap, passionflower, and catnip in this list. They also say that kava kava may help with the anxiety and that St. John's wort may help with the depression. New research suggests that St. John's wort may do way more than that. Though small and uncontrolled, a new study offers the exciting possibility that St. John's wort can actually help you quit smoking. When twenty-four people who smoked an average of twenty cigarettes a day for the past twenty-two years were given 900 mg of St. John's wort a day, 54 per cent had successfully quit at the three-week mark, and 37.5 per cent of them were still successfully cigarette-free after twelve weeks[2]. The researchers pointed out that this success rate is better than that achieved with the drug bupropion (Wellbutrin). Bupropion had a 30 per cent success rate after twelve weeks in one study and has significant side effects.

Also try 5-HTP (5-Hydroxytryptophan) and S-AMe (S-adenosyl-methionine) to improve anxiety and depression. Again, try them for breaking all kinds of addiction.

If you get the urge to put a cigarette in your mouth, put a piece of licorice root in instead. It will help keep a cigarette out of your hands while reducing your stress level and supporting your adrenals, both of which will help you quit. Licorice also has many benefits for lungs, cough, and congestion—a bonus for smokers.

Haas also says to drink the following herbal tea several times throughout the day when you feel cravings: 3 parts each of lemon grass and dandelion root, 2 parts each of raspberry leaf, red clover, alfalfa, peppermint, and mullein leaf; and 1 part each of valerian and catnip. He adds that high doses of the ascorbate form of vitamin C can help reduce cravings. And the extra antioxidant punch certainly won't hurt anyway since smoking depletes antioxidants. A B-complex vitamin may

also help, as it helps the body deal with stress. A calcium/magnesium complex may help for the same reason.

Counselling and acupuncture can also help a great deal.

Alcohol

What about giving up alcohol? Here again, diet can help. And, once again, you want to focus on vegetarian foods to alkalinize your body. Drink lots of water and herbal teas, too. It is very important when quitting alcohol to stabilize your blood-sugar. So eliminate sugar and limit refined carbs while increasing complex carbs. There is research to back this idea. A 1991 study found that restricting sugar, increasing complex carbs, and eliminating caffeine reduced cravings for alcohol[3]. A second study found that only 38 per cent of those on a hospital diet were still sober after six months. But when they were put on a diet that included fruit and wheat germ, and eliminated coffee, junk food, dairy, and peanut butter, 81 per cent of them remained sober[4].

The other lifestyle change that helps people stay sober is an increase in exercise[5].

One really exciting nutrient for alcoholism is L-glutamine. One double-blind study found that 1 gram of glutamine in divided doses with meals decreases the desire to drink[6].

B-vitamin deficiencies are common in alcoholics and a B-complex vitamin may help reduce cravings. It is known that B1 deficiencies result in greater consumption of alcohol, and preliminary research suggests that niacin (B3) may help alcoholics stop drinking[7].

Given the importance of balancing blood-sugar, it is not surprising that chromium can help with cravings, as well.

The most exciting new supplement to help you stop drinking is the herb kudzu. Though the research is new, the use isn't. In traditional Chinese medicine, kudzu is used to diminish intoxification from alcohol. And now a new study has verified this use. Heavy drinkers were given either 1,000 mg of kudzu or a placebo three times a day for a week, then they were allowed to drink up to six bottles of their favourite beer. The people in the kudzu group drank significantly less beer than the people in the placebo group, and they also experienced a slight reduction in the urge to drink[8].

Another herb that can help is skullcap. Herbalist Michael Tierra says that skullcap is one of the best herbs for alcohol withdrawal. Try any of the nervines; they can be helpful.

Also try 5-HTP, SAMe, calcium and magnesium—all nutrients that can help control anxiety and depression.

Acupuncture and counselling can also be helpful.

Other Addictions

Natural remedies may offer some help in withdrawal from other drug addictions. Tierra says that skullcap is not only a great herb for alcohol withdrawal, but for drug withdrawal, as well. Another nervine that, as we have seen helps with quitting smoking is passionflower. And it looks as though it can help with withdrawal from opiate drugs such as morphine and codeine. Though the drug clondine is used for the physical symptoms of withdrawal from opiates, it does nothing for the psychological symptoms such as anxiety. When clondine was combined with passionflower, though, it reduced the psychological symptoms significantly more than when it was combined with a placebo[9].

Eric Yarnell reports that practitioners have found that the herb chastetree berry can decrease cravings for heroin, as can B-complex vitamins. Oats and passionflower once again appear as calming herbs that help.

The appearance of chastetree berry, a herb better known for balancing women's hormones, is especially interesting because in 2002, Ernest Hawkins reported in *HerbalGram* that chastetree berry bonds to dopamine-2 receptors. These receptors control a system that might be involved in addictive behaviour, raising the possibility that chastetree berry could help people with addictive personalities[10]. And now there are testimonies turning up saying that the herb helps with heroin addiction. Perhaps chastetree berry will turn out to be an important addiction herb.

Chapter Endnotes

1. Anand, C.L. "Effect of Avena sativa on cigarette smoking." *Nature*, 1971; 233:496.

2. Lawvere, S., M. Mahoney, K.M. Cummings, *et al.* "A phase II study of St. John's wort for smoking cessation." *Complement Ther Med*, 2006; 14:175'84.

3. Biery, J. R., J. H. Williford, E. A. McMullen. "Alcohol craving in rehabilitation: assessment of nutrition therapy." *J Am Diet Assoc*, 1991; 91:463-66.

4. Guenther, R. M. "Role of nutritional therapy in alcoholism treatment." *Int J Biosoc Res*, 1983; 4:5-18.

5. Sinyor, D., *et al.* "The role of a physical fitness program in the treatment of alcoholism." *J Stud Alcohol*, 1982; 43:380'66.

6. Rogers, L. L., R. B. Pelton. "Glutamine in the treatment of alcoholism." *Q J Stud Alcohol*, 1957; 18:581-87.

7. Smith, R. F. "A five-year field trial of massive nicotinic acid therapy of alcoholics in Michigan." *J Orthomolec Psychiatry*, 1974; 3:327-31.

8. Lukas, S. E., D. Penetar, J. Berko, et al. "An extract of the Chinese herbal root kudzu reduces alcohol drinking by heavy drinkers in a naturalistic setting." *Alcohol Clin Exp Res*, 2005; 29:756-62.

9. Akhondzadeh, S., *et al.* "Passionflower in the treatment of opiates withdrawal: a double-blind randomized controlled trial." *Journal of Clinical Pharmacy and Therapeutics*, 2001; 26:369'73.

10. Hawkins, E. B. "Conference Report: Third International Congress on Phytomedicine." *HerbalGram*, 2002; 55:61.

The great outdoors: the smells, the sneezing; the warmth of the sun, the itching skin; the beauty of the flowers, the red, runny eyes. We all love the nicer weather and being outside, the relief from the drab, dreary, dark days of winter; but for many of us, the nicer weather brings with it allergies, forcing us to stay inside, looking longingly at the sun-filled world outside. Fortunately, there is help for allergy suffers; for some there is even complete relief.

We do not say this lightly. Ted used to suffer from outdoor allergies so badly that he simply could not go out in the woods. Chemical antihistamines provided no relief for him. It wasn't until he completely detoxified his body and became a vegetarian that his allergies disappeared. Yes, that's right: completely disappeared.

A vegetarian diet puts fewer toxins into the body, and less arachidonic acid, a fatty acid found only in animal products that causes inflammation and allergies. Vegetarian diets are very anti-inflammatory.

Ancient Wisdom: Detoxifying

There is a good reason why the ancients used to detoxify in the spring: They knew that not only did the spring provide the perfect ingredients to do a cleanse, dandelions for example, but also that by cleansing in the spring they would suffer from fewer health problems, including allergies, in the months to come. And in traditional Chinese medicine, spring is the time of the liver—one of the

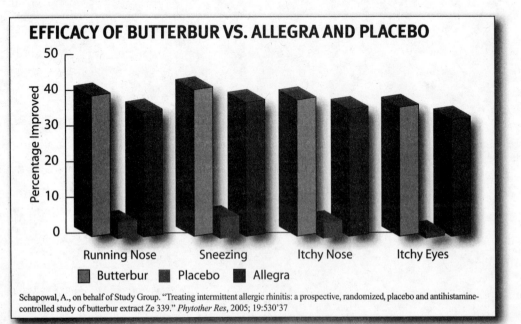

EFFICACY OF BUTTERBUR VS. ALLEGRA AND PLACEBO

Butterbur ▪ Placebo ▪ Allegra

Schapowal, A., on behalf of Study Group. "Treating intermittent allergic rhinitis: a prospective, randomized, placebo and antihistamine-controlled study of butterbur extract Ze 339." *Phytother Res*, 2005; 19:530'37

most important organs of detoxification.

Ancient people such as the Celts and Teutonics, people from Africa, Melanesia, New Guinea, and Polynesia, made use of sweat baths to cleanse. In the Americas, the Aztecs used sweat baths to help almost every sickness, for they knew, as modern herbalists know today, that sweating the body, cleansing the body, frees it of toxins, which is the first step to healing, among other things, allergies. The First Nations people of North America used sweat baths, adding all kinds of herbs to aid in the cleansing and purifying process.

But sweat baths are not the only way to cleanse. There are many herbs that can aid in cleansing, such as milk thistle,. dandelion, artichoke, and boldo for the liver; echinacea, mullein, cleavers, and red root for the lymph system; cascara sagrada, buckthorn, and senna for the digestive tract; coltsfoot, elecampane, licorice, and goldenseal for the lungs; uva ursi, buchu, and parsley for the urinary tract; burdock for the skin; and many cleansers and alternatives, such as sarsaparilla, yellow dock, Oregon grape root, and nettle, which slowly purify the bloodstream, thereby affecting the whole body. This list is only partial and is meant as a suggestion. Get a good cleansing kit or go to a herbalist and get a program designed for you, paying special attention to the liver, since this is the most important organ to cleanse in helping with allergies.

Herbal Relief for Allergies

Herbal expectorants such as lobelia, licorice, skunk cabbage, wild-cherry bark, mullein, horehound, and anise are very helpful for allergies. Expectorant herbs encourage the expulsion of excess mucous from the throat and lungs. An old-time herbal recipe for treating allergies is to combine mau huang with expectorants.

Another herb that has been shown to provide relief, even in people who are sensitive to pollens, dust, food, and animal dander is dong quai. Used traditionally in Chinese medicine, dong quai seems to work by inhibiting the production of allergic antibodies.

Proven to be an effective anti-inflammatory and anti-allergy agent in numerous studies[1], licorice also has one other advantage, it tastes good and is, therefore, easy to take. It seems to work partially by increasing the half-life of cortisol, leading to increased anti-inflammatory action of this hormone. It also contains substances that are structurally similar to the corticosteroids released by the adrenal glands.

Onions and garlic have been shown in studies to reduce inflammatory reactions, and they contain quercetin and mustard oils. Quercetin is a powerful anti-inflammatory, and mustard oils offer protection when dealing with allergies.

You can also get quercetin in supplement form. It is possibly the best choice for treating allergies. Quercetin works by inhibiting the release of histamine and other inflammatory agents within the body and, unlike conventional chemical antihistamines (which do not prevent the release of histamine within the body, but block its binding to receptor sites), quercetin will not cause unpleasant side effects. The problem with allergies is the histamine your body releases—that's why doctors prescribe antihistamines. Antihistamines block the binding of histamine. Quercetin actually has the amazing ability to inhibit histamine from being released at all[2]. Quercetin also helps fight hay fever by inhibiting other inflammatory compounds such as prostaglandins and leukotrienes and by acting as a powerful antioxidant. Quercetin has been shown to inhibit the release of mast cells and the manufacture of allergy-related compounds, including leukotrienes. Quercetin also helps vitamin C in the body.

It is a good idea to take 400 to 500 mg of quercetin twenty minutes before each meal, combined with the powerful anti-inflammatory bromelain to help increase absorbtion. Start taking quercetin as soon as the allergy season starts and continue taking it until the season is over. Food sources of quercetin include blue-green algae, garlic, onions, broccoli, grapefruit, and summer squash.

Another herb that has a long history of use is lobelia. Lobelia is an expectorant and a bronchial relaxer that also promotes the release of adrenal hormones, making it useful for treating allergies.

Herbalist Michael Tierra calls lobelia an expectorant and antispasmodic and recommends it during an asthma attack.

Other useful herbs include chilli peppers, skunk cabbage, and Chinese skullcap. Chilli peppers are used for their ability to reduce sensitivity to chemical irritants; skunk cabbage is an expectorant and respiratory sedative that makes it useful in the treatment of allergies; Chinese skullcap has powerful anti-inflammatory action.

Or perhaps you would like to try a remedy that has been used in India for years to clear away allergies. Brew a tea made of black peppercorns, cloves, ginger, mustard seeds, and cardamom, and drink daily.

In North America, old-time herbalists used nettle tea to reduce allergy problems, and modern herbalists still do. Nettle is a good source of quercetin, as well as being a good detoxifier. Linda get very good results clinically, for even the worst allergy sufferers by using freeze-dried nettle and quercetin together.

Dr. Andrew Weil has said that he knows of nothing as dramatic as the allergy relief offered by freeze-dried nettle leaf. A double-blind, placebo-controlled study found significant relief in 70 per cent of allergy and hay fever sufferers when they were given freeze-dried nettle leaf[3].

Nettle is traditionally drunk daily as a tea. Freeze-dried nettle capsules are particularly effective.

Butterbur is another very effective herb for allergies. Butterbur has been clinically shown to reduce allergy symptoms. One hay-fever study compared butterbur to the antihistamine cetirizine and found that it worked just as well. In fact, the advantage went to the herb because, even though cetirizine is supposed to be a non-sedating antihistamine, some people still experienced drowsiness on the drug, while no one did on the herb[4].

In another study, 330 people with hay fever were given either the herb butterbur, the antihistamine Allegra, or a placebo in a double-blind, placebo-controlled study. The herb and the drug both worked significantly better than the placebo. The butterbur and the Allegra were equally effective, but the nod goes to the herb because it was safer than the drug[5].

Ginkgo biloba is also effective.

Don't Forget Your Vitamins

A key nutrient for relief of allergies is vitamin C. Vitamin C reduces histamine levels[6], helping to reduce allergy symptoms. Vitamin C prevents the secretion of histamine by white blood cells and increases the detoxification of histamine.

Other key nutrients include carotenes, which help protect the respiratory linings, and vitamin E, which has recently been shown to reduce the sneezing, runny nose, stuffiness, and itchiness of allergies[7].

Among the most important supplements you can take for allergies are essential fatty acids, especially flaxseed oil, which is rich in omega-3 fatty acids. Flaxseed oil can help to reduce the arachidonic acid in the body, reducing inflammation that can cause allergies. Take 1 to 2 tbsps a day.

With a little time and persistence, you'll soon be outside enjoying all of that nice weather as it was meant to be enjoyed.

Chapter Endnotes
1. Okimasu, E., *et al.* "Inhibition of phospholipase A2 and platelet aggregation by glycyrrhizin, and anti-inflammatory drug." *Acta Med Okayama*, 1983; 37:385'91.

2. Middleton, E., G. Drzewieki. "Flavonoid inhibition of human basophil histamine release stimulated by various agents." *Biochem Pharmacol*, 1984; 33:3333'38; Busse, W. W., D. E. Kopp, E. Middleton. "Flavonoid modulation of human neutrophil function." *J Allergy Clin Immunol*, 1984; 73:801'09.

3. Mittman, P. "Randomized double-blind study of freeze-dried Urtica dicia in the treatment of allergic rhinitis." *Planta Med*, 1990; 56:44'47.

4. Schapowal, A. "Randomised controlled trial of butterbur and cetirizine for treating seasonal allergic rhinitis." *BMJ*, 2002; 324:1'4.

5. Schapowal, A., on behalf of Study Group. "Treating intermittent allergic rhinitis: a prospective, randomized, placebo and antihistamine-controlled study of butterbur extract Ze 339." *Phytother Res*, 2005; 19:530'37.

6. Johnston, C. S., L. J. Martin, X. Cai. "Antihistamine effect of supplemental ascorbic acid and neutrophil chemotaxis." *J Am Coll Nutr*, 1992; 11:172'76.

7. Pollack, S., E. Shahar, G. Hassoun. "Effect of vitamin E supplementation on the regular treatment of seasonal allergic rhinitis." *Annals of Allergy, Asthma, & Immunology*, 2004; 92:654'58.

ANEMIA

Anemia means that the blood is deficient in red blood cells or in hemoglobin, the iron-containing part of red blood cells. When this deficiency happens, not enough oxygen is carried to the body's tissue and the person experiences tiredness, weakness, paleness and weakened resistance to infection. Other possible symptoms of anemia include irritability, poor concentration and cognitive ability, shortness of breath, heart palpitations, intolerance to cold, loss of appetite and a general lack of well being.

Causes of Anemia

Anemia can be caused by excessive blood loss from ulcers, heavy menstrual bleeding or aspirin. If this is why you are anemic, you can use astringent herbs like shepherd's purse, oak bark, yarrow, witch hazel or squaw vine to control the bleeding and should treat the underlying condition. Iron deficiency can not only be a result of excessive menstrual bleeding but, ironically, a cause of it. For both these reasons, iron is often included in premenopausal women's multivitamin/mineral formulae.

Anemia can also result from a deficiency of B12, folic acid or, most commonly, iron. Iron deficiency is one of the most common deficiencies in the world.

In addition to excessive blood loss, iron deficiency can be the result of parasites, infection or not getting enough iron in your diet. If you are getting enough iron in your food, and you are still anemic, you may not be absorbing enough of what you get.

Eating for Iron

If you're not getting enough in your diet, start eating more iron rich foods. Green leafy vegetables are perfect for people with anemia. They are rich in iron, folic acid, vitamin C, betacarotene and

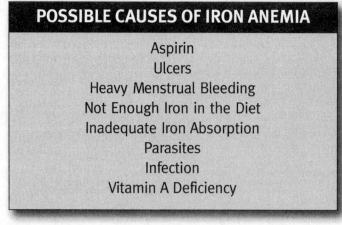

POSSIBLE CAUSES OF IRON ANEMIA

Aspirin
Ulcers
Heavy Menstrual Bleeding
Not Enough Iron in the Diet
Inadequate Iron Absorption
Parasites
Infection
Vitamin A Deficiency

chlorophyll. Chlorophyll stimulates hemoglobin and red blood cell production. The fat-soluble chlorophyll found in green plants is also very similar to the hemoglobin in red blood cells and is good for anemia. The blue-green algae spirulina is a rich source of fat-soluble chlorophyll, as well as iron, folic acid, B12 and betacarotene, and is great for treating anemia. Spirulina has been successfully used to treat anemia in Japan. For anemia, you may want to double the normal spirulina dose of 10g and take 20g a day. Chlorella is also good, since it is one of the richest source of chlorophyll.

Other good foods for uping the iron content of your diet include legumes, whole grains, beets, alfalfa, cherries, prunes, apricots, wheat germ, brewer's yeast, seeds and nuts.

Absorbing the Iron You Eat

If you're not absorbing enough of the iron you do get, you could be low in hydrochloric acid. If this is the case, take hydrochloric acid with your meals. Poor absorption can also be caused by chronic diarrhoea, antacid use, parasites, high intake of calcium, tea, coffee, egg yolk or wheat bran.

Vitamin A is also important for iron absorption[1]. Sometimes iron deficiency anemia is not because of not enough iron or loss of iron, but because there is a deficiency of vitamin A, which leads to defective iron transport. Perhaps that is why one study found that vitamin A taken with iron is more helpful than iron taken alone[2]. Bitters, like yarrow, yellow dock root, dandelion root and gentian will also stimulate the digestion of iron.

Another vitamin that should be taken with your iron supplement is vitamin C. Vitamin C has been shown to increase the absorption of iron[3]. 500-1,000mg of vitamin C with each meal could be enough to increase your body's iron stores.

Supplementing Iron

And, of course, if you are iron deficient, you can always supplement your diet with iron. Take 30mg twice a day between meals, or three times a day with meals if it bothers your stomach, for six months to a year until your serum ferritin tests are normal. Even then a maintainance dose of 18mg a day may be necessary.

The form of iron that is, unfortunately, most commonly dispensed, ferrous sulfate, can cause constipation, nausea and bloating. Instead, go for the superior forms of iron: ferrous succinate, fumerate or glycine amino acid chelates. These forms not only do not cause these problems, but are better absorbed anyway.

Easily Absorbed Herbal Sources of Iron

There are also tons of easily absorbed iron rich herbs. You can try nettle, burdock root, red clover, horsetail, rose hips, alfalfa, parsley and watercress. Dandelion leaf is loaded in iron as well as vitmains C and A. Yellow dock root is a specific for anemia. Other herbs that receive mention include motherwort, red clover and dong quai. Seaweeds like kelp are also good. Unrefined black strap molasses is also good, as is chlorella.

B12 and Folic Acid Deficiency Anemia

If your anemia is not caused by a deficiency in iron, but in B12, then try taking 2,000mcg a day of B12 for one month, and then 1,000mcg a day after that.

If your anemia is the result of a folic acid deficiency, then supplement 1,000mcg three times a day. Folic acid deficiencies can result from alcoholism, pregnancy, cancer drugs, birth control pill, chronic diarrhoea, celiac or Crohn's disease.

Foods that are rich in folic acid include dark green leafy vegetables, beans, asparagus, whole grains, broccoli and nuts.

When Not to Take Iron

Just like you, bacteria need iron. One of the ways your body fights infection is by reducing iron. So don't supplement iron during an infection unless iron supplementation is essential to you. In fact, in general, people who are not iron deficient should not supplement iron unless they are menstruating.

Chapter Endnotes

1. Semba R. D., *et al*. Impact of vitamin A supplementation on hematological indicators of iron metabolism and protein status in children. *Nutr Res* 1992;12:469–78; Suharno D, *et al*. Supplementation with vitamin A and iron for nutritional anemia in pregnant women in West Java, Indonesia. *Lancet* 1993;342:1325–8.

2. Mejia L. A., Chew F., Hematological effect of supplementing anemic children with vitamin A alone and in combination with iron. *Am J Clin Nutr* 1988;48:595–600.

3. Ajayi O. A., Nnaji U. R., Effect of ascorbic acid supplementation on haematological response and ascorbic acid status of young female adults. *Ann Nutr Metab*

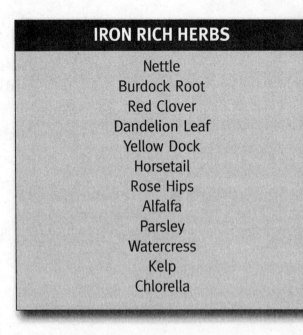

IRON RICH HERBS

Nettle
Burdock Root
Red Clover
Dandelion Leaf
Yellow Dock
Horsetail
Rose Hips
Alfalfa
Parsley
Watercress
Kelp
Chlorella

ANXIETY

Anxiety is a generalized uneasy feeling or fear that something is going, or is going to go, wrong in the absence of an identifiable cause. When anxiety is severe, panic attacks can result. Anxiety and panic attacks are surprisingly common.

The most important physical imbalance in people who suffer from anxiety and panic attacks is elevated levels of lactate. So the first step in the natural treatment of anxiety is bringing those levels down. And the first step in doing that is eliminating alcohol, sugar and caffeine.

Lowering Lactate

Caffeine both causes[1] and aggravates[2] anxiety. It interferes with a brain chemical called adenosine that is one of your body's natural relaxants. Just eliminating caffeine can go a long way in relieving anxiety[3].

Alcohol also causes anxiety. Men given alcohol in a study suffered significant increases in anxiety compared to men given a placebo[4].

There are not only things to avoid, but things to add if you want to bring down levels of lactate. The B vitamins are important antianxiety vitamins. B1 deficiency can increase anxiety by allowing lactate levels to rise, and B3 and B6 are also important because they may lower lactate levels.

Putting the B's to the test, when 23 people were given high dose general supplements and mega doses of any B vitamins they were deficient in, 19 out of 23 improved and 11 of those 19 were totally panic attack free[5].

In another study, inositol, another member of the B vitamin family, was able to control panic attacks in people with anxiety[6].

Also crucial for bring down lactate levels are calcium and magnesium. Calcium deficiencies can make anxiety worse and deficiencies of magnesium increase both lactate levels and anxiety.

Herbs that Soothe and Calm

By far the best treatment for anxiety, natural or pharmaceutical, is the herb kava kava. It has been proven in double-blind research to be as good as

---

HERBS PROVEN TO BE AS GOOD OR BETTER THAN BENZODIAZEPINES

Kava kava
Passionflower
Valerian

benzodiazepines while being safer[7].

But, although it is still available in the States, kava is no longer legal in Canada. Based on twenty-eight case studies in Europe of people who have used kava suffering liver toxicity, Health Canada pulled the herb. But at least four separate analyses of the case reports have now concluded that there is no evidence that the liver damage was caused by the kava and that kava is a safe alternative for the treatment of anxiety. Many of the cases can be explained by preexistent liver disease and simultaneous use of alcohol or drugs that are known to be liver toxins. Several toxicological studies on kava show no evidence that kava has any liver toxicity.

So while kava still tops the list in the States, with the unfortunate and ridiculous unavailability of kava in Canada, now topping the Canadian list of antianxiety herbs is passionflower. Passionflower has gone head to head with the leading drugs and won. It works every bit as well as benzodiazepines, but the benzodiazepines impair daily functioning significantly more than the herb[8].

The great sleep herb valerian is also as good as the drugs for anxiety. When researchers compared valerian to benzodiazepines for insomnia, they found an unexpected side result: the herb not only equalled the drug for insomnia, it also equalled it on anxiety scores, and with fewer side effects[9]. Combining valerian and passionflower is also effective[10].

One double-blind study also found that the great depression herb St. John's wort reduces anxiety[11]. And it may not be a complete surprise to find that the great calming herb chamomile has antianxiety properties. And now a double-blind, placebo-controlled study of chamomile and generalized anxiety disorder has shown that when people with generalized anxiety disorder are given either chamomile extract or a placebo, the ones given the chamomile have significantly greater improvement on the Hamilton Anxiety scale. The chamomile was very safe, producing even fewer

LACTIC ACID	
Factors That Increase Lactic Acid	Factors That Decrease Lactic Acid
Caffeine	Vitamin B1
Alcohol	Vitamin B3
Sugar	Vitamin B6
	Calcium
	Magnesium

side effects than the placebo[12].

But there are also some more surprising herbs on the list. The Indian herb gotu kola has antianxiety powers. When people were given either gotu kola or a placebo and then subjected to a startle response test used to study anxiety disorders, the startle response was significantly lower in those given the herb, indicating antianxiety activity for gotu kola[13].

And reishi, the great immune mushroom, has the amazing ability to calm the nerves while revitalizing them. Herbalist Christopher Hobbs recommends reishi as a calming herb for people with nervousness, anxiety and sleeplessness who have weak adrenals.

The remarkable herb Rhodiola has been shown to significantly improve anxiety in people with generalized anxiety disorder[14]. Earlier research has also shown that it decreases mental fatigue and anxiety while increasing work capacity and general well-being.

Other great calming herbs include skullcap and

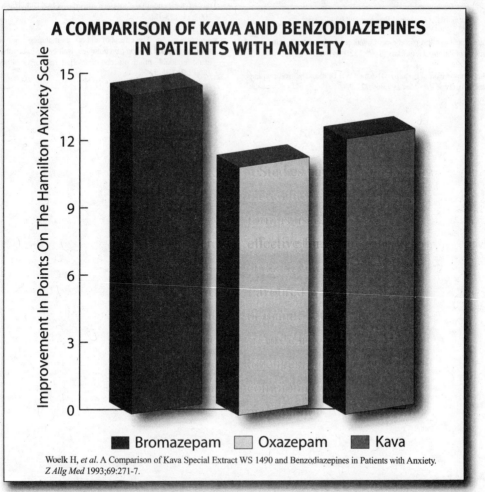

A COMPARISON OF KAVA AND BENZODIAZEPINES IN PATIENTS WITH ANXIETY

Improvement In Points On The Hamilton Anxiety Scale

■ Bromazepam ☐ Oxazepam ■ Kava

Woelk H, *et al*. A Comparison of Kava Special Extract WS 1490 and Benzodiazepines in Patients with Anxiety. *Z Allg Med* 1993;69:271-7.

lemon balm.

And don't forget your multivitamin/mineral: double-blind research shows the multi's ability to significantly reduce anxiety[15].

Chapter Endnotes

1. Uhde TW, *et al*. Caffeine and behavior: Relation to psychopathology and underlying mechanisms. Caffeiene: Relationship to human anxiety, plasma MHPG and cortisol. *Psychopharm Bull* 1984;20:426-30.

2. Charney D. S., *et al*. Increased anxiogenic effects of caffeine in panic disorders. Arch Gen Psychiat 1985;42:233-43; Bruce M., *et al*. Anxiogenic effects of caffeine in patients with anxiety disorders. *Arch Gen Psychiatry* 1992;49:867-9.

3. Bruce M., Lader M., Caffeine abstention in the management of anxiety disorders. *Psychol Med* 1989;19:211-14.

4. Montiero M. G., *et al*. Subjective feelings of anxiety in young men anfter ethanol and diazepam infusions. *J Clin Psychiatry* 1990;51:12.

5. Abbey L. C., Agoraphobia. *J Orthomol Psychiat* 1982;11:243-59.

6. Benjamin J., *et al*. Double-blind, placebo-controlled, crossover trial of inositol treatment for panic disorder. *Am J Psychiatry* 1995;152:1084-6.

7. Woelk H, *et al*. A comparison of kava special extract WS 1490 and benzodiazepines in patients with anxiety. *Z Allg Med* 1993;69:271-7.

8. Akhondzadeh S., *et al*. Passionflower in the treatment of generalized anxiety: a pilot double-blind randomized controlled trial with oxazepam. *J Clin Pharm Ther* 2001;26:363-7.

9. Dorn M. Efficacy and tolerability of Baldrian versus oxazepam in non-organic and nonpsychiatric insomniacs: a randomized, double-blind, clinical, comparative study. *Forsch Komolementarmed Klass Naturheilkd* 2000;7:79-84.

10. Brown D. Valerian root: Non-addictive alternative for insomnia and anxiety. *Quart Rev Nat Med* 1994;Fall:221-4.

11. Witte B., *et al*. Treatment of depressive symptoms with a high concentration Hypericum preparation. A multicenter placebo-controlled double-blind study. *Fortschr Med* 1995;113:404-8.

12. Amsterdam J. D., *et al*. Randomized, double-blind, placebo-controlled trial of Matricaria recutita (Chamomile) extract therapy for generalized anxiety disorder. *J Clin Phsycopharmacol* 2009;29: 378-382.

13. Bradwein J., *et al*. A double-blind, placebo-controlled study of the effects of gotu kola (Centella asiatica) on acoustic startle response in healthy subjects. *Journal of Clinical Psychopharmacology* 2000;20:680-684.

14. Bystritsky A., Kerwin L., Feusner J. D., A pilot study of Rhodiola rosea (Rhodax®) for generalized anxiety disorder (GAD). *J Altern Complement Med* 2008;14: 175-180.

15. Carroll D., *et al*. The effects of an oral multivitamin combination with calcium, magnesium, and zinc on psychological well-being in healthy young male volunteers: a double-blind placebo-controlled trial. *Psychopharmacology* (Berl) 2000;150:220-5.

ASTHMA

Asthma is on the attack. And we're losing. The number of people suffering from asthma is rapidly increasing. So is the number of people dying of it. The news media and the TV news have been all over a report that in some parts of North America, the number of kids suffering from asthma is four times higher than twenty years ago. In Canada, an unbelievable 20 per cent of boys and 15 per cent of girls between eight and eleven have asthma. That's incredible. So what's to be done?

Strange New Causes of Asthma

First, look to the causes of the rise in asthma. Increased pollution and increasingly poor diet shoulder much of the blame, but so do some unexpected causes. When researchers surveyed the parents of 456 children, they found that antibiotics were a significant risk factor for asthma. When the antibiotics were used in the first year, the risk was even greater[1]. And this study was not the first to find this result: One year earlier, researchers found that antibiotic use in the first two years of life was associated with an increased risk of asthma[2].

Vaccinations might also be a problem. A 1994 study reported in the *Journal of the American Medical Association* found that while only 1.97 per cent of kids who had not had the pertussis vaccine had asthma, the number leapt to 10.69 per cent among those who had. Three per cent of the kids who had had other vaccines had asthma, while only 1 per cent of those who had had no vaccines did[3].

Obesity is also on the rise, and that is another reason for the rising rates of asthma, because being overweight is significantly associated with asthma[4]. One study found that asthma is an incredible 73 per cent more common in kids with the highest body mass index than in kids of nor-

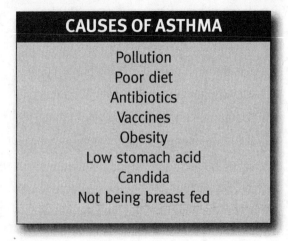

CAUSES OF ASTHMA

Pollution
Poor diet
Antibiotics
Vaccines
Obesity
Low stomach acid
Candida
Not being breast fed

mal weight[5]. The good news is that when overweight asthmatics lose weight, their breathing improves significantly and they use significantly less medication[6].

And there are still other causes of asthma. Many asthmatics have low stomach acid. One very early study found that as many as 80 per cent of children with asthma have low stomach acid[7]. If low stomach acid is a problem, supplementing with betaine HCl can help.

Another cause of asthma that is not usually thought of is candida. Treating the candida—including taking acidophilus—can significantly improve the asthma.

Breast-feeding is another important consideration. When breast-feeding is a part of the child's diet for the first nine to twelve months, asthma is dramatically reduced[8].

What You Eat Affects How You Breathe

Diet affects asthma in many ways. For starters, don't add salt to your food. Increasing salt worsens asthma[9], and decreasing salt seems to improve it[10].

Try to watch artificial colours and preservatives, as they, too, can be a problem[11].

A vegan diet can also help. When asthmatics made lifestyle changes that especially included adopting a vegan diet that eliminated all animal products, 92 per cent of them improved significantly after one year[12]. The vegan diet probably helps for many reasons, as Michael Murray N.D. and Joseph Pizzorno, N.D., have pointed out: It eliminates food allergies, increases antioxidants, and reduces inflammation by eliminating the highly inflammatory arachidonic acid found in animal fats.

Vitamin C

When children with asthma eat a diet high in vitamin C-rich fruit, they wheeze less[13]. And asthmatics had less severe and less frequent attacks when they were given one gram of vitamin C a day for fourteen weeks in a double-blind study[14]. Overall, seven out of eleven studies have shown a significant improvement in asthma when one to two grams of vitamin C a day are taken[15]. James Duke, Ph.D. says that a review of about forty good studies shows that one gram of vitamin C a day helps prevent asthma attacks. A recent study found that one gram of vitamin C a day allows asthmatics to reduce the amount of inhaled corticosteroids they use without losing any control of their symptoms[16]. This discovery about vitamin C is very important because reducing the dose of corticosteroids reduces their side effects, including bone loss, immune suppression, and cataracts.

Other Antioxidants

Other antioxidants, such as selenium, carotenes, and vitamin E can also be helpful. Several studies have shown that people with low levels of selenium are at high risk of asthma. One double-blind study found that six out of eleven asthmatics improved when they were given 100 mcg a day of selenium, while only one out of ten improved when they were given a placebo[17]. And in a pilot study, 200 mcg of selenium reduced the need for corticosteroids[18].

Lycopene, a member of the carotene family, might also help. Asthma attacks are often triggered by exercise. But when people with exercise-induced asthma were given either 30 mg of lycopene a day or a placebo for a week, the lycopene group had significantly fewer asthma symptoms[19].

Pycnogenol is another powerful antioxidant. Children with mild to moderate asthma were given 1 mg pycnogenol per pound of body weight. After supplementing for three months, they had significantly fewer and less severe attacks while needing to take less medication. Children who were given a placebo instead got no better at all[20].

B6
Vitamin B6 may also help. One study found that 200 mg of B6 a day for two months significantly reduced the severity of asthma in children while reducing the amount of medication they needed[21]. A second study produced a dramatic improvement in the frequency and severity of attacks with 50 mg of B6 taken twice a day[22]. A third study, however, found no benefit[23].

Another B vitamin, B12, may also be important, according to Jonathan Wright, M.D., especially for those who react to sulfites.

Magnesium
Magnesium is also important. Levels of magnesium are often low in asthmatics[24]. Population studies show that when the intake of magnesium goes down, the number of asthma cases goes up[25].

Many double-blind studies have shown that intravenous magnesium can quickly stop an acute asthma attack. Until recently, no studies had been done on magnesium supplements. But now at least three have been done. In a small study, 300 mg of magnesium taken for thirty days lessened bronchial reactivity in adults with asthma[26].

A double-blind study found significant improvement in symptoms but not in objective measures when 400 mg of magnesium was taken for three weeks[27].

The third, and most recent study differed from the first two because it looked at children. When youngsters with asthma added either 300 mg of magnesium or a placebo to their regular medication, the ones given magnesium had significantly fewer asthma attacks. They also had to turn to their inhalers as rescue medication less often[28].

Herbal Help for Asthmatics
There are many herbs that help asthma. Three of the most promising are boswellia, khella, and but-

terbur.

Boswellia is not very well known. But perhaps asthmatics should get to know it better. When asthmatics were given either 300 mg of boswellia or a placebo three times a day for six weeks, the number of attacks was significantly lower in the boswellia group. Objective measures of breathing capacity improved significantly on the herb. Overall, 70 per cent of the boswellia group improved, compared to only 27 per cent of the placebo group[29].

One of the least known and most amazing herbs for asthma is the Egyptian herb, khella. Herb authority Rudolf Fritz Weiss, M.D., says that khella's powerful antispasmodic action in the small bronchials makes it the perfect treatment for asthma. Khella probably is of little help during an attack, but Daniel Mowrey, PH.D, says it does prevent attacks. As a preventative to take between attacks, Weiss calls khella the treatment of choice.

The newest discovery for asthma is the herb butterbur. Butterbur proved its ability to decrease both the number and the severity of asthma attacks in a recent study[30]. Ninety-five per cent of the asthmatics in this study found that the butterbur was effective in treating their asthma. As many as two-thirds had clinically significant improvements in breathing. Among those taking medication during the study, 43 to 48 per cent of them were able to reduce the amount of meds they needed when taking the herb.

Of the many things that *Ginkgo biloba* can help, one of the less well known is asthma. Ginkgo is great at inhibiting platelet-activating factor, which is responsible for triggering inflammation, asthma, and the bronchoconstriction of asthma. Michael Murray, N.D., reports that Ginkgo has been shown in many double-blind studies to have anti-asthma effects. Donald Brown, N.D., endorses Ginkgo as a good long-term treatment for asthma.

Other Supplements that Help

With its anti-inflammatory, anti-allergy, expectorant, and cortisol-like activity, it is no surprise that licorice can help. The powerful antispasmodic and expectorant lobelia can also help. Nettle is an excellent antihistamine, and anise and fennel are excellent expectorants. Turmeric and ginger can also help, and an uncommon herb called coleus forskohlii can relieve bronchial muscles and inhibit histamine. Also, quercetin is one of the best anti-inflammatories in nature. Eat lots of garlic and onions. Onions have been shown to be an excellent anti-asthma food[31].

Other good herbs for asthma include thyme, mullein, elecampane, celandine, wild cherry bark, coltsfoot, and comfrey.

Yoga and acupuncture can also be helpful.

Chapter Endnotes

1. Wickens, K., N. Pearce, J. Crane, R. Beasley. "Antibiotic use in early childhood and the development of asthma." *Clin Exp Allergy*, 1999; 29:766'71.

2. Farooqu, I. S., J. M. Hopkin. "Early childhood infection and atopic disorders." *Thorax*, 1998; 53:927'32.

3. Odent, M. R., E. E. Culpin, T. Kimmel. "Pertussis vaccination and asthma. Is there a link?" *JAMA*, 1994; 272:592'93.

4. Camarqo, C. A., Jr., S. T. Weiss, S. Zhang, et al. "Prospective study of body mass index, weight change, and risk of adult-onset asthma in women." *Arc Intern Med*, 1999; 159:2582'88.

5. Von Mutius, E., J. Schwartz, L.M. Neas, et al. "Relation of body mass index to asthma and atopy in children: the National Health and Nutrition Examination Study III." *Thorax*, 2001; 56:835-38.

6. Stenius-Aarniala, B., T. Poussa, J. Kyarnstrom, et al. "Immediate and long term effects of weight reduction in obese people with asthma: randomized controlled study." *BMJ*, 2000; 320:827'32.

7. Bray, G. W. "The hypochlorhydria of asthma in childhood." *Quart J Med*, 1931; 24:181'97.

8. Wright, A. L., C. J. Holberg, et al. "Breast feeding and lower respiratory tract illness in the first year of life." *Br Med J*, 1989; 299:946'49.

9. Burney, P. G. J. "A diet rich in sodium may potentiate asthma: epidemiological evidence for a new hypothesis." *Chest*, 1987; 91:143'48; Javaid, A., M. J. Cushley, M. F. Bone. "Effect of dietary salt on bronchial reactivity to histamine in Asthma." *BMJ*, 1988; 297:454; Fogarty, A., J. Britton. "The role of diet in the aetiology of asthma." *Clin Exp Allergy*, 2000; 30:615'27.

10. Burney, P. G. J., J. E. Neild, C. H. Twort, *et al.* "Effect of changing dietary sodium on the airway response to histamine." *Thorax*, 1989; 44:36'41; Carrey, O. J., C. Locke, J. B. Cookson. "Effect of alterations of dietary sodium on the severity of asthma in men." *Thorax*, 1993; 48:714'18; Medici, T. C., T. Z. Schmid, M. Jacki, W. Vetter. "Are asthmatics salt-sensitive? A preliminary controlled study." *Chest*, 1993; 104:1138'43; Gotshall, R. W., T. D. Mickleborough, L. Cordain. "Dietary salt restriction improves pulmonary function in exercise-induced asthma." *Med Sci Sports Exerc*, 2000; 32:1815'19.

11. Freedman, B. J. "A diet free from additives in the management of allergic disease." *Clin Allergy*, 1977; 7:417'21.

12. Lindahl, O., L. Lindwall, A. Spangberg, *et al.* "Vegan diet regimen with reduced medication in the treatment of bronchial asthma." *J Asthma*, 1985; 22:45'55.

13. Forastiere, F., R. Pistelli, P. Sestini, *et al.* "Consumption of fresh fruit rich in vitamin C and wheezing symptoms in children." SIDRIA Collaborative Group. *Thorax*, 2000; 55:283'88.

14. Anah, C. O., L. N. Jarike, J. A. Baig. "High dose ascorbic acid in Nigerian asthmatics." *Trop Geogr Med*, 1980; 32:132'37.

15. Bielory, L., R. Gandhi. "Asthma and vitamin C." *Annals Allergy*, 1994; 73:89'96.

16. Fogarty, A., *et al.* "Corticosteroid sparing effects of vitamin C and magnesium in asthma: a randomized trial." *Respiratory Medicine*, 2006; 100:174-79.

17. Hasselmark, L., *et al.* "Selenium supplementation in intrinsic asthma." *Allergy*, 1993; 48:30'36.

18. Gazdik, F., J. Kadrabova, K. Gazdikova. "Decreased consumption of corticosteroids after selenium supplementation in corticoid-dependent asthmatics." *Bratisel Lek Listy*, 2002; 103:22'25.

19. Neuman, I., H. Nahum, A. Ben-Amotz. "Reduction of exercise-induced asthma oxidative stress by lycopene, a natural antioxidant." *Allergy*, 2000; 55:1184'89.

20. Lau, B., S. Riesen, K. Truong, *et al.* "Pycnogenol as an adjunct in the management of childhood asthma." *J Asthma*, 2004; 41(8):825'32.

21. Collip, P. J., S. Goldzier, III, N. Weiss, *et al.* "Pyridoxine treatment of childhood bronchial asthma." *Ann Allergy*, 1975; 35:93'7.

22. Reynolds, R. D., C. L. Natta. "Depressed plasma pyridoxal-5-phosphate concentrations in adult asthmatics." *Am J Clin Nutr*, 1985; 41:684'88.

23. Sur, S., M. Camara, A. Buchmeier, *et al.* "Double-blind trial of pyridoxine (vitamin B6) in the treatment of steroid dependent asthma." *Ann Allergy*, 1993; 70:141'52.

24. Haury, V. G. "Blood serum magnesium in bronchial asthma and its treatment by the administration of magnesium sulfate." *J Lab Clin Med*, 1940; 26:340'44.

25. Soutar, A., A. Seaton, K. Brown. "Bronchial reactivity and dietary antioxidants." *Thorax*, 1997; 52:166'70.

26. Rylander, R., C. Dahlberg, E. Rubenowitz. "Magnesium supplement decreases airway responsiveness among hyperreactive subjects." *Magnesium-Bulletin*, 1997; 19:4'6.

27. Jill, J., A. Micklewright, S. Lewis, J. Britton. "Investigation of the effect of short-term change in dietary magnesium intake in asthma." *Eur Respir J*, 1997; 10:2225'29.

28. Contijo-Amaral, C., et al. "Oral magnesium supplementation in asthmatic children: a duoble-blind randomized placebo-controlled trial." *Eur Gr J Clin Nutr* 2007; 61: 54-60

29. Gupta, I., V. Gupta, A. Parhar, et al. "Effects of Boswellia serrata gum resin in patients with bronchial asthma: results of a double-blind, placebo-controlled, 6-week clinical study." *Eur J Med Res*, 1998; 3:511'14.

30. Danesch, U. "Petasites hybridus (butterbur root) extract in the treatment of asthma—an open trial." *Alternative Medicine Review*, 2004; 9(1):54'62.

31. Dorsch, W. "Anti-asthmatic effects of onions. Alk(en)ylsufino thioic acid alk(en)yl-esters inhibit histamine release, leukotriene and thromboxane biosynthesis in vitro and counteract PAF and allergen-induced bronchial obstruction in vivo." *Biochem Pharmacol*, 1988;,37(23):4479'86.

BRONCHITIS

Bronchitis is a painful, annoying, clinging condition that just won't go away. So what can you do to make it go away?

Don't Take Antibiotics for Bronchitis

Don't smoke, don't eat any sugar, and stay away from dairy. That's what you can *not* do to get rid of it. And, in most cases, don't take antibiotics; usually they are useless. More than 90 per cent of cases of acute bronchitis are viral and so antibiotics are not recommended. At least ten placebo-controlled studies have demonstrated that antibiotics offer no help for acute bronchitis.

Natural Immune Boosters

As for what you *can* do, some of the best-known immune boosters are great for bronchitis. Start with the excellent immunity herb echinacea to fight the infection. Since echinacea does its work not as an antibiotic but by supporting your immune system's own efforts, it continues to work in viral conditions when antibiotics cannot.

Add some garlic and goldenseal. Goldenseal fights infection, thins the mucous, and heals the mucous membrane. Wild indigo, elderberry, astragalus, lomatium, myrrh, and oregano oil are also very good immune herbs to try. Wild indigo is one of the best natural antibiotics that there is.

Bromelain for Bronchitis

Bromelain may seem like a surprising entry in a section on bronchitis. It's much better known as a digestive aid. But bromelain has many uses, and it is great for chronic bronchitis. Bromelain helps with the cough while it thins the material that is coughed up. It also improves lung function[1].

Herbal Expectorants

Herbs that thin the phlegm and help you to get it out of your throat and lungs are called expectorants. Some of the best expectorants are licorice, lobelia, wild cherry bark, horehound, coltsfoot, thyme, anise, pleurisy root, and mullein. These herbs can all be combined.

Licorice will not only act as an expectorant, but will also help your immune system and soothe your throat and lungs while it helps eliminate phlegm. Thyme is anti-microbial and antispasmodic in addition to being an expectorant, and mullein is also a demulcent herb that soothes the irritated tissue. Other demulcents that help bronchitis include plantain, slippery elm, and marshmallow.

Another expectorant herb that has long been used in Europe but is hardly known in North America is ivy leaf. Ivy leaf is a good expectorant that also eases coughs. One double-blind study showed ivy leaf to be as effective as the drug ambroxol for chronic bronchitis[2]. Try taking 5 ml of the liquid extract three times a day.

Eucalyptus oil is also a good expectorant. You can inhale the vapours by rubbing it on your chest. You can also take advantage of eucalyptus's expectorant properties by drinking a tea made from the leaf.

Or try a mustard pack, a very useful remedy to clear congestion.

Comfrey is also good for lung troubles. Black cohosh is also used for its antispasmodic and expectorant properties. Elecampane is also considered a specific for chronic coughs and mucous. It is an expectorant and is very good for chronic bronchitis and even the asthma it can often trigger in those susceptible.

The Most Exotic Herb for Bronchitis

One of the most promising but least known herbs for bronchitis is a South African herb called *Pelargonium sidoides*. This herb has been extensively studied for acute bronchitis and is commonly used in Germany. The Zulus have long used it to treat coughs, upper respiratory infections, and tuberculosis. Recently, a double-blind study gave either *Pelargonium sidoides* or a placebo to 124 people suffering from acute bronchitis. Bronchitis scores improved significantly more in the herb group than in the placebo group: 90.6 per cent of people given the herb had a rapid recovery, compared to 41.7 per cent in the placebo group. In the herb group, 84.4 per cent had a major improvement or a complete recovery, compared to only 30 per cent in the placebo group. The herb was as safe as the placebo[3]. A previous double-blind, placebo-controlled study of 468 people with acute bronchitis also found *Pelargonium sidoides* to be significantly better than a placebo[4].

Don't Forget the Vitamin C

Not only herbs but also vitamins and other nutrients can help you fight off bronchitis. It is not surprising that the great cold fighter vitamin C helps bronchitis. People with bronchitis get better faster when they take vitamin C. In a double-blind study of elderly people suffering from bronchitis, vitamin C helped significantly more than the placebo did[5].

Other Helpful Nutrients

N-acetylcysteine (NAC) works as an expectorant that also eases coughs. A review of thirty-nine studies concluded that 400 to 600 mg of NAC a day is a safe and effective treatment for chronic bronchitis[6]. Zinc lozenges, flavonoids and beta-carotene can also help.

Diet and Bronchitis

Diet can help, too. Eating more fruits and vegetables reduces your risk of getting bronchitis[7]. Getting plenty of essential fatty acids in your diet may also help, since your diet will be more anti-inflammatory.

And finally, avoiding dairy helps because it will decrease mucous production, but also because allergies to milk are associated with bronchitis in kids[8].

Chapter Endnotes

1. Rimoldi, R., F. Ginesu, R. Giura. "The use of bromelainin pneumological therapy." *Drugs Exp Clin Res*, 1978; 4:55'66.

2. Meyer-Wegner, J. "Ivy versus ambroxol in chronic bronchitis." *Zeits Allegemeinmed*, 1993; 69:61-6.

3. Chuchalin, A., B. Berman, W. Lehmacher. "Treatment of acute bronchitis in adults with Pelargonium sidoides preparation (EPs 7630): a randomized, double-blind, placebo controlled trial." *Explore!*, 2005; 1:437'45.

4. Matthys, H., *et al.* "Efficacy and safety of an extract of Pelargonium sidoides (EPs 7630) in adults with acute bronchitis. A randomized, double-blind, placebo-controlled trial." *Phytomed*, 2003; 10 Suppl 4:7'17.

5. Hunt, C., *et al.* "The clinical effects of vitamin C supplementation in elderly hospitalised patients with acute respiratory infections." *Int J Vitam Nutr Res*, 1994; 64:212-19.

6. Stey, C., *et al.* "The effect of oral N-acetylcysteine in chronic bronchitis: a quantitative systematic review." *Eur Respir J*, 2000; 16:253-62.

7. La Vecchia, C., A. Decarli, R. Pagano. "Vegetable consumption and risk of chronic disease." *Epidemiology*, 1998; 9:208-10.

8. Hill, D. J.. "Clinical manifestations of cows' milk allergy in childhood. II. The diagnostic value of skin tests and RAST." *Clin Allergy*, 1988; 18:481-90; Cohen, G.A., et al. "Severe anemia and chronic bronchitis associated with a markedly elevated specific IgG to cow's milk protein." *Ann Allergy*, 1985; 55:38-40; Hide, D.W., B.M. Guyer. "Clinical manifestations of allergy related to breast and cows' milk feeding." *Arch Dis Child*, 1981; 56:172-75.

CANDIDA

It is estimated that as much as two-thirds of the population have at least some overgrowth of candida. This overgrowth of yeast can cause a whole host of health problems, such as low energy, digestive problems, skin issues, memory loss, mood imbalances, immune problems, fungal, bacterial, and viral infections, yeast infections, sinus infections and urinary tract infections, jock itch, toenail infections, allergies, and chemical sensitivities, just to name a few.

What Is Candida?

Candida is an overgrowth of yeast in the body that is not being held in check by friendly flora that live in the intestines. Everyone has some candida yeast; it is only when it grows out of proportion that the problem begins.

Fortunately, there is help for this common problem. There are several natural remedies that have been shown to be safer than drugs.

Causes of Candida

Antibiotics promote candida[1]. They wipe out both the bad bacteria they are targeting and also the good bacteria. Antibiotics also increase the virulence of candida infections and accelerate the conversion of *candida albicans* from its yeast form to its more invasive fungal form. According to Michael Murray N.D., and Joseph Pizzorno, N.D., use of antibiotics is the most important factor in

CANDIDA DIET		
Things to Include:		
vegetables	amaranth	pears
legumes	teff	plums
seeds	buckwheat	peaches
nuts	millet	berries
quinoa	brown rice	complex carbohydrates
	apples	
Things to Eliminate:		
sugar	peanuts	dairy
refined carbohydrates	cashews	oranges
fruit juice	melons	grapes
honey	alcohol	tropical fruits
maple syrup	vinegar	gluten,
yeast	dried fruit	food allergens

the development of candida, since antibiotics suppress the normal intestinal bacteria, allowing the yeast overgrowth and suppressing the immune system. A person with a low immune system is more likely to develop candida and bacterial infections; these are often treated with more antibiotics, leading to more candida. For many, it can be a vicious cycle.

And there are other drugs, such as corticosteroids, cortisone, and prednisone, oral contraceptives, such as the pill, and ulcer medicines that also cause candida. People who have been on ulcer medications such as Zantac® and Tagamet® actually develop candida overgrowth in the stomach[2], making it very clear that hydrochloric acid (HCL) is very important in preventing candida, since these medicines suppress HCL. To correct low stomach acid, try supplementing your diet with HCL or take Swedish bitters, which also promote HCL in the stomach, helping to prevent candida.

A diet high in sugar or refined carbs can also lead to candida; sugar is the primary nutrient of candida. Eliminating sugar is the first step to eliminating candida[3].

Help the Liver to Help You

The liver of a person with candida may not function properly. This can cause sensitivity to chemicals and, often, can lead to P.M.S. and skin problems, since the liver isn't doing its job of filtering blood properly. A damaged liver allows candida overgrowth and, worse, when the overgrowth is being treated, when on a candida program, dying candida produce toxins that require a strong liver to filter them. It is, therefore, very important to support the liver as part of a candida program. Supporting the liver helps with digestive function, which helps to kill off candida. Correcting any lack of HCL, protease, and bile insufficiencies is crucial. Use liver-supporting herbs to help, such as milk thistle, gentian, Swedish bitters, artichokes, and dandelion root. Jerusalem artichokes are also high in FOS (fructo- oligosaccharides), another key ingredient in fighting off candida.

What Diet Should You Follow to Get Rid of Candida?

Follow a diet that avoids simple carbohydrates, refined sugars, fruit juices, honey, maple syrup, yeast, or foods with mould (such as peanuts, cashews, and melons), alcohol, vinegar, dried fruit, and milk and milk products—since they contain lactose, or milk sugar—and antibiotics. Eliminate or reduce intake of high-carbohydrate foods such as potatoes, yams, squash, and corn. You can freely eat all other vegetables, legumes, seeds and raw nuts, and whole non-glutenous grains—gluten can aggravate the colon and weaken the immune system, and for many people it is an allergen. Eat grains such as quinoa, amaranth, teff, buckwheat, millet, and brown rice. You can even eat some fruits, such as apples, pears, plums, peaches, and berries, but limit it to two or three servings a day. Avoid oranges, grapes, melon, and tropical fruits. And, of course, avoid all known or suspected food allergens, since they can weaken the immune system, allowing candida to overgrow. Canadian herbalist Terry Willard, PH.D., adds that during the first six weeks of a candida diet, all soy products should also be avoided and then may be eaten freely. He also says to avoid flour foods for the first month or two. But eat complex carbs. A diet rich in complex carbohydrates helps to treat candida because it favourably alters the balance of intestinal flora.

WHAT SHOULD YOU TAKE TO GET RID OF CANDIDA?

Probiotics

One of the best things you can do to fight candida is take a supplement containing friendly flora such as *Lactobacillus acidophilus*. Acidophilus is crucial since it will help to replace the friendly flora in the gut, favourably altering Ph levels, enabling the yeast to be killed off, and improving digestion and absorption of nutrients, as well as helping to correct a weakened immune system and any nutritional deficiencies that can cause candida. Take 20 billion live cells a day. Look for acidophilus with *Bifidobacterium bidfidum*, another crucial probiotic.

FOS

Also look for acidophilus with FOS (fructo-oligosaccharides), as FOS will feed the friendly flora, enabling more of it to reach the gut. Studies show that FOS increases the good bifidobacteria and lactobacilli, while it reduces the bad. It also improves liver function and improves the elimination of toxic compounds, which is crucial in treating candida. It is usually recommended that you use 1/2 tsp of straight FOS a day (2,000 to 3,000 mg) in powder form, since is it more absorbable. It also tastes like cotton candy, and, therefore, may enable candida sufferers to deal with their sweet tooth withdrawal.

Grapfruit Seed Extract

Another very good choice in fighting candida is grapefruit seed extract. It can be used safely for three to six months at a time. It is useful for getting rid of the candida yeast that has spread throughout the body. Medical doctors Michael Rosenbaum and Murray Susser, authors of *Solving the Puzzle of Chronic Fatigue Syndrome*, say grapefruit seed extract has a powerful action on candida. The usual dosage is 5 to 15 drops three times a day in water. Doctors Leo Gall and Charles Ressenger say grapefruit seed extract is as powerful as the drug nystatin. It does not, however, have any unwanted side effects. If you suffer from internal cold, it is a good idea to mix grapefruit seed extract with a little ginger powder.

Goldenseal

Another good choice for fighting off candida is goldenseal. It is a fantastic digestive tonic that is high in berberine, which is effective against candida and many bacterial infections, including urinary tract infections. So if you are susceptible to urinary tract infections and candida, this one herb can do both jobs and help you avoid antibiotics, which can weaken the system and lead to candida. Goldenseal improves immune function, helping to destroy viruses, yeast, and bacteria. It also normalizes intestinal flora and helps with digestive problems. Goldenseal can also help to alleviate the diarrhoea that can come with candida, since it is a powerful antidiarrheal and digestive tonic. Barberry and Oregon grape root have similar properties. Murray recommends 1 to 2 g of the dried root or 1 to 1.5 tsps of the tincture three times a day.

Garlic

Garlic, an extremely powerful antibacterial and anti-fungal agent, has been shown to be more effective than nystatin, the most common anti-candida drug, in treating candida[4]. It can even be applied diluted to tampons and used as a vaginal insert to get rid of vaginitis.

Pau d'arco

Or try pau d'arco, a South American herb that has been shown to have potent anti-candida effects[5]. Michael A. Weiner, PH.D., and Janet A. Weiner, in their book, *Herbs that Heal*, also say that anecdotal evidence suggests pau d'arco is effective in fighting candida. They suggest making a decoction of the bark by steeping 1/2 oz of pau d'arco in 2 cups of boiling water for 15 minutes. Cool and drink 1 tbsp at a time, using 2 to 4 cups per day.

Other Candida Killers

Michael and Janet Weiner also talk about a little-known herb called mathake, or tropical almond. It is commonly used in the South Pacific and is supposed to be one of the most effective anti-fungal agents there is. William Crook also suggests it in his book, *The Yeast Connection and the Woman*, and Rosenbaum and Susser mention it in *Solving the Puzzle of Chronic Fatigue Syndrome*. In 1984, Weiner introduced mathake to several physicians who later reported that it had strong activity against candida. Weiner says it may work by enhancing the immune system or by directly killing off the yeast. This herb can be used for up to three months at a time and can be prepared as a pleasant-tasting tea. The parts used are the leaves and the bark.

Or you may want to try fatty acids derived from olives or castor beans, which contain oleic acid, since they have also been found to be useful, according to the authors of *Alternative Medicine*. Herbalist Anne McIntyre suggests using some in your salad each day.

Caprylic acid and bentonite clay are also commonly used. The caprylic acid kills off the candida[6] and the clay helps to escort toxic matter from the intestines by binding to the waste and removing it.

Other herbs that are excellent candida fighters are oregano, marjoram, sage, thyme, and peppermint, either as the herb itself or in an oil form. A recent study proved oregano oil to be more than a hundred times more effective than caprylic acid for killing off candida[7] and the volatile oils of thyme, peppermint, tea tree, and rosemary have all been shown to kill candida *in vitro*[8].

Or try chamomile[9], uva ursi[10], aloe vera, ginger, cinnamon, rosemary, and licorice, which are all good for killing off candida as are black walnut, myrrh, raspberry, usnea, and spilanthes. Murray and Pizzorno, in their book, *Encyclopedia of Natural Medicine*, also mention ginger, cinnamon, balm, and rosemary as among the most effective fungus fighters. Anne McIntyre also suggests using thyme, fennel, hyssop, and marigold as antifungal agents. She prefers infusing the herbs and using them as teas, three times a day.

Fibre

Also, be sure to consume plenty of fibre to ensure clean bowels. Undigested material that is left to sit in the colon can ferment, leading to an overgrowth of yeast and the absorption of toxic matter into the system. Low fibre diets[11] that are high in saturated fat and protein are a cause of candida. You may wish to add 1tbsp of flaxseeds, pectin, or psyllium each day to your diet to keep the bowels clean. Fibre also positively affects the balance of good and bad bacteria.

Support The Immune System

To strengthen your immune system and to prevent the reoccurrence of vulvovaginal candida, try adding echinacea purpurea to your candida regime[12]. McIntyre also says that you may want to try using other immune-enhancing herbs like astragalus, dong quai, and wild indigo to keep your immune system strong, thereby preventing candida.

It is also crucial to support the thymus gland to improve your immune function. Take echinacea, B6, zinc, vitamin C, beta-carotene, vitamin E, and selenium to aid the thymus gland. Be sure to supplement your diet with vitamins and minerals to help correct any nutritional deficiencies that may have weakened your immune system, allowing candida to take over your body, or that may have been caused by the candida.

Stopping Candida from Returning: Resealing the Gut

It is also crucial to rebuild the gut and intestinal walls to prevent candida from coming back. Many candida sufferers fail to do this step in their candida program and find themselves succumbing once gain. The best method that Linda has found clinically for rebuilding the gut is to supply extra B-vitamins and vitamin C, minerals, and essential fatty acids. Also try MSM. MSM reseals the gut and prevents food allergies by stopping toxic matter from entering the bloodstream. Other good gut-sealing nutrients include DGL (licorice), slippery elm, marshmallow, chamomile, and L-glutamine.

As for the traditional drugs that are used against candida, Dr. Virender Sodhi says the most popularly used drug, nystatin, does not get rid of candida, even after being used for one year, but only causes it to mutate into another species of yeast, and that nystatin lingers in the intestine and can kill helpful organisms[13]. Murray says that nystatin is not capable of getting rid of candida that is firmly entrenched in the lining of the gastrointestinal tract.

Chapter Endnotes

1. Caruso, L. J. "Vaginal moniliasis after tetracycline therapy." *Am J Obstet Gynecol*, 1964; 90:374; Reid, G., A.W. Bruce, R. L. Cook. "Effect on urogenital flora of antibiotic therapy of urinary tract infection." *Scand J Infect Dis*, 1990; 22:43'47; Nord, C. E., C. Edlund. "Impact of antimicrobial agents on human intestinal microflora." *J Chemother*, 1990; 2:218'37.

2. Buero, M., *et al.* "Candida overgrowth in gastric juice of peptic ulcer subjects on short- and long-term treatment with H2-receptor antagonists." *Digestion*, 1983; 28:158'63.

3. Horowitz, B. J., S. Edelstein, L. Lippman. "Sugar chromatography studies in recurrent Candida vulvovaginitis." *J Reprod Med*, 1984; 29:441-43.

4. Arora, D. S., J. Kaur. "Anti-microbial activity of spices." *Int J Antimicrob Agents*, 1999; 12:257-62.

5. Gershon, H., L. Shanks. "Fungitoxicity of 1,4-naphthoquinones to Candida albicans and trichophyton mentagrophytes." *Can J Microbiol*, 1975; 21:1317'21; De Lima, O.G., et al. Rev Inst Antibiot (Recife), 1971; 11:21'26; Oswald, E.H. *Br J Phytother*, 1993/1994; 3:112'17.

6. Keeney, E. L. "Sodium caprylate: a new and effective treatment of moniliasis of the skin and mucous membrane." *Bull Johns Hopkins Hosp*, 1946; 78:333'39; Neuhauser, I., E.L. Gustus. "Successful treatment of intestinal moniliasis with fatty acid resin complex." *Arch Intern Med*, 1954; 93:53'60.

7. Stiles, J. C. "The inhibition of Candida albicans by oregano." *J Applied Nutr*, 1995; 47:96-102.

8. Hammer, K. A., C.F. Carson, T.V. Riley. "In-vitro activity of essential oils, in particular Melaleuca alternafolia (tea tree) oil and tea tree oil products, against Candida albicans." *J Antimicrobial Chemother*, 1998; 42:591-95.

9. Aggag, M. E., R. T. Yousef. *Planta Med*, 1972; 22:140'44.

10. Holopainen, *et al. Acta Pharm Fenn*, 1988; 97:197'202.

11. Burkitt, D. P. "Relationship between diseases and their etiological significance." *Am J Clin Nutr*, 1977; 30:262'67.

12. Coeugniet, E., R. Kuhnast. "Recurrent candidiases: Adjuvant immunotherapy with different formulations of Echinacin." *Therapiewoche*, 1986; 36:3352'58.

13. The Burton Goldberg Group. *Alternative Medicine: The Definitive Guide.* Fife WA: Future Medicine, 1993.

CARPAL TUNNEL SYNDROME

With more and more of us spending practically the entire day on the computer keyboard, carpal tunnel syndrome is becoming more and more of a problem. Carpal tunnel syndrome is a painful condition caused by a compression of the nerve in the wrist as a result of repetitive work with the hands. The nerve compression causes pain when gripping, weakness, numbing, burning and tingling in the palm and fingers. The pain may extend all the way up the arm to the shoulder.

Vitamin B6

The most important treatment of carpal tunnel syndrome is supplementation with vitamin B6. Deficiencies of B6 are very common in carpal tunnel syndrome[1]. And several double-blind studies have proven that B6 can effectively treat carpal tunnel syndrome[2], though a few studies have not been positive. Taking the larger dose of 300mg may be the difference in some of these studies. B6 may even effectively reduce pain when there is no B6 deficiency[3].

Research has also shown that vitamin B2 can help carpal tunnel syndrome and that the effect is even greater when B2 and B6 are combined[4]. Adding B2 may help because it is necessary for the conversion of B6 (pyridoxine) into its active form (pyridoxal 5'-phosphate). Though we are not aware of any studies looking at the effect of adding magnesium, magnesium also plays a role in that conversion. If you are adding B2, try a dose of 10mg a day.

You should start taking B6 at a dose of 50mg a day and increase to 100mg-300mg as needed. The therapy may take up to three months. Even George Phalen M.D., who first described carpal tunnel syndrome and invented its surgical treatment, has said that, in the future, B6 may be the treatment of choice for carpal tunnel syndrome[5].

Taking Vitamin B6

Start taking B6 at a dose of 50mg a day. If you need to increase the dose, don't buy a pill with more in it. The liver cannot deal with doses of B6 greater than 50mg at a time. So take your 100mg-300mg dose divided into 50mg doses.

As we have already seen, B2 and magnesium help to convert B6 into its active, pyridoxal 5'-phosphate form. For most people, the regular B6 form is fine. However, the active form may be even better, especially if you have liver disease, and you should try using it if the regular form has not produced any results after six weeks of supplementation.

Some things can interfere with your body's ability to use B6. Some of the more important ones are alcohol, excessive protein, birth control pills, dopamine, penicillamine, and the food colouring FD&C yellow #5.

Is There a Hormonal Component?

Though it doesn't seem to come up in discussions of carpal tunnel syndrome, we wonder if there may be some hormonal component to the syndrome, since it is more common amongst women, and since risk factors include being menopausal, being pregnant and being on the birth control pill[6].

Other Natural Treatments

Hydrotherapy may help carpal tunnel syndrome. Immersing the hand in hot water for three minutes followed by cold water for thirty seconds three to five times can increase the circulation to the hand. The increased circulation can help with the inflammation and edema that are present in carpal tunnel syndrome and, by doing so, reduce the pain.

Immobilizing the wrist with a splint day and night may also help.

Research also suggests that flexing the wrist and fist with arms extended before work and during breaks might help[7].

And, as is so often the case, acupuncture can be of great help. In one study, thirty-five of thirty-six people with carpal tunnel syndrome were helped by acupuncture, even though fourteen of them were not helped by surgery[8].

Anti-inflammatories can also be helpful. Good natural anti-inflammatories include bromelain, turmeric (curcumin), quercetin and flaxseed oil.

Chapter Endnotes

1. Ellis J. M., *et al*. Response of vitamin B6 deficiency and the carpal tunnel syndrome to pyridoxine. *Proc Natl Acad Sci USA* 1982;79:7494-8; Fuhr JE, Farrow A, Nelson Jr HS. Vitamin B6 levels in patients with carpal tunnel syndrome. *Arch Surg* 1989;124:1329-30.

2. Ellis J. M., Vitamin B6 deficiency in patients with a clinical syndrome including the carpal tunnel defect. Biochemical and clinical response to therapy with pyridodxine. *Res Comm Chem Path Pharm* 1976;13:743-57; Ellis J. M., *et al*. Survey and new data on treatment with pyridoxine of patients having a clinical syndrome including the carpal tunnel and other defects. *Res Comm Chem Path Pharm* 1977;17:165-77; Ellis J. M., *et al*. Clinical results of a cross-over treatment with pyridoxine and placebo of the carpal tunnel syndrome. *Am J Clin Nutr* 1979;32:2040-46; Ellis JM, *et al*. Response of vitamin B6 deficiency and the carpal tunnel syndrome to pyridoxine. *Proc Natl Acad Sci USA* 1982;79:7494-8; Ellis J. M., Treatment of carpal tunnel syndrome with vitamin B6. *South Med J* 1987;80:882-4; Folkers K., Ellis J., Successful therapy with vitamin B6 and vitamin B2 of the carpal tunnel syndrome and need for determination of the RDA's for vitamin B6 and B2 disease states. *Annals NY Acad Sci* 1990;585:295-301; Ellis JM, Folkers K. Clinical aspects of treatment of carpal tunnel syndrome with B6. *Annals NY Acad Sci* 1990;585:302-20.

3. Bernstein A. L., Dinesen J. S., Brief communication: effect of pharmacologic doses of vitamin B6 on carpal tunnel syndrome, electronencephalographic results, and pain. *J Am Coll Nutr* 1993;12:73-6

4. Folkers K. A., *et al*. Enzymology of the response of carpal tunnel syndrome to riboflavin and to combined riboflavin and pyridoxine. *Proc Nat Acad Sci* 1984;81:7076-8.

5. Phalen G. S., The birth of a syndrome, or carpal tunnel syndrome revisited. *J Hand Surg* 1981;6:109-10.

6. de Krom MCTFM, *et al*. Risk factors for carpal tunnel syndrome. *Am J Epidemiol* 1990;132:1102-10; Sandez S. C., Carpal tunnel syndrome. *Am Fam Phys* 1981;24:190-204.

7. Seradge H., Splints aren't enough; hand exercises improve carpal tunnel treatment. *Modern Med* 1996;64:14-15.

8. Chen G. S., The effect of acupuncture treatment on carpal tunnel syndrome. *Am J Acupunct* 1990;18:5-9.

CELIAC DISEASE

Unfortunately, this article is important to a lot more people than used to be thought. Recent research reveals the startling fact that nearly one in a hundred people suffer from celiac disease[1].

Celiac disease is a dietary disease. It is an autoimmune response to gluten, the protein found in certain grains, that destroys the intestinal villi needed for absorbing your food. So to get rid of the symptoms, you have to get rid of the gluten. That means total avoidance of all forms of wheat—including kamut and spelt—as well as barley and rye. Couscous and bulgar are both made from wheat.

As for the other grains, there is much confusion out there. But the confusion is easy to clear up. Rice and buckwheat are okay. Corn and millet do not cause celiac disease, but may aggravate symptoms in sensitive people. Some sources feel that even rice and buckwheat can do this: so watch for symptoms.

The real confusion is over oats. Most sources continue to list this grain with wheat, rye and barley. But recently, better designed studies have shown that most celiacs actually do tolerate oats[2]. 1996 research found that most celiacs are fine with moderate amounts of oats[3], and another study showed that 95 per cent of celiacs tolerated 50g of oats a day for up to a year[4].

So why the confusion? Because oats often does seem to cause problems for celiacs. But the problem is not the oats. The problem is that it is incredibly common for commercial oats products found in the mass market to be contaminated with

THE ROLE OF GLUTEN INTOLERANCE IN OTHER CONDITIONS

Lack of Muscle Coordination
Tingling and Numbness
Migraine-like Headache
Female Infertility
Male Infertility
Type I Diabetes
Thyroiditis
Arthritis
Autism
ADHD
Depression
Hair Loss
Congenital Heart Disease
Cystic Fibrosis
Dyspepsia
Epilepsy
Irritable Bowel Syndrome
Fibromyalgia
Osteoporosis
Schizophrenia
Short Stature
Delayed Puberty
Lupus
Early Dementia

[From Helms S. Celiac disease and gluten-associated diseases. *Alt Med Rev* 2005;10;3:172-92]

aggravating gluten[5]. When people who thought they were on a gluten free diet were put on a truly gluten free diet, 77 per cent of them improved[6]!

So read labels carefully, and look for the many specialty gluten free celiac foods available in health food stores. We know the celiac diet is a challenging one to strictly follow, with grain and gluten hidden in so many things. But it's the only way to treat the disease. And, if you truly do eliminate gluten from your diet, research shows that symptoms will usually start going away really fast: even within one week. Michael Murray, N.D., says 30 per cent will start responding in as little as three days. Another 50 per cent will respond within a month, and another 10 per cent within one more month. 10 per cent will, unfortunately, take much longer. If you don't get better, and you really do have celiac disease, and you really aren't eating unknown gluten, than get tested for zinc deficiency. Murray says that celiacs do not respond to a gluten free diet if there is a zinc deficiency. And zinc deficiencies are common among celiacs.

After two to three months on the strictest of diets, millet and corn can be carefully reintroduced one at a time, according to Stephen Helms, N.D. Murray says that milk and all milk products should also be eliminated until the intestines return to normal. Actually, giving milk early in a child's life is a major causative factor in celiac disease[7]. Breast milk, on the other hand, protects against celiac disease[8]. So breast feeding and holding off on the introduction of milk and grains is a good strategy for reducing the risk of celiac.

Because celiac disease leads to malabsorption, celiacs often develop deficiencies of nutrients. The most common deficiencies are vitamins E, D, K, B12 and folic acid, iron, selenium, zinc, calcium, magnesium, carnitine and essential fatty acids. So a high potency multivitamin/mineral is a very good idea. Additional supplementation of particular deficiencies may also be necessary. Because women with celiac are at much higher risk of having babies with neural tube defects[9], the gluten free diet must be supplemented with folic acid during the child bearing years.

Because of these deficiencies, celiacs are at increased risk of osteoporosis[10]. Amazingly, a gluten free diet can increase bone mineral density to about normal in only a year[11], and staying on the celiac diet will keep it normal[12].

There are a few other nutrients that can help celiacs. Glutamine helps to rebuild the damaged intestines. Helms recommends 2-4g daily in divided doses. Probiotics help to reestablish healthy microflora.

Papain, the protein digesting enzyme from papaya, seems to be able to digest gluten and render it harmless to celiacs[13]. So it may be a good insurance policy to take 500-1,000mg with meals in case of hidden gluten. That dose may allow some celiacs to tolerate gluten[14].

Chapter Endnotes

1. National Institute of Health consensus development conference statement on celiac disease. *Gastroenterol* 2005;128:S1-9.

2. Janatuinen E. K., *et al*. No harm from five year ingestion of oats in coeliac disease. Gut 2002;50:332-5; Högberg L., *et al*. Oats to children with newly diagnosed coeliac disease: a randomised double blind study. *Gut* 2004;53:649-54; Kemppainen T. A., *et al*. Unkilned and large amounts of oats in the coeliac disease diet: a randomized, controlled study. *Scand J Gastroenterol* 2008;43:1094–101.

3. Srinivassan U, *et al*. Absence of oats toxicity in adult coeliac disease. *BMJ* 1996;313:1300–1.

4. Jantauinen E. K., *et al*. A comparison of diets with and without oats in adults with celiac disease. *N Engl J Med* 1995;333:1033–7.

5. Thompson T., Gluten contamination of commercial oat products in the United States. *N Engl J Med* 2004;351:2021-2.

6. Faulkner-Hogg K. B., Selby W. S., Loblay R. H., Dietary analysis in symptomatic patients with coeliac disease on a gluten-free diet: the role of trace amounts of gluten and non-gluten food intolerances. *Scand J Gastroenterol* 1999;34:784–9.

7. Fallstrom SP, Winberg J, Anderson HJ. Cow's milk malabsorption as a precursor of gluten intolerance. Acta Paediatrica Scand 1965;54:101-15; Auricchio S. Gluten-sensitive enteropathy and infant nutrition. J Ped Gastroenterol Nutr 1983;2:S304-9; Cole SG, Kagnofff MF. Celiac disease. *Ann Rev Nutr* 1985;5:241-66.

8. Auricchio S., *et al*. Does breast feeding protect against the development of clinical symptoms of celiac disease in children? *J Pediatr Gastroenterol Nutr* 1983;2:428–33; Ivarsson A. Breast-feeding protects against celiac disease. *Am J Clin Nutr* 2002;75:914-21.

9. Dickey W., *et al*. Screening for coeliac disease as a possible maternal risk factor for neural tube defect. *Clin Genet* 1996;49:107-8.

10. West J., *et al*. Fracture risk in people with celiac disease: a population-based chort study. Gastroenterology 2003;125:429-36; Stenson WF, *et al*. Increased prevalence of celiac disease and need for routine screening among patients with osteoporosis. *Arch Intern Med* 2005;165:393-9.

11. Mora S., *et al*. Reversal of low bone density with a gluten-free diet in children and adolescents with celiac disease. *Am J Clin Nutr* 1998;67:477–81; Kavak US, *et al*. Bone mineral density in children with untreated and treated celiac disease. *J Pediatr Gastroenterol Nutr* 2003;37:434-6; McFarlane XA, Bhalla AK, Robertson DAF. Effect of a gluten free diet on osteopenia in adults with newly diagnosed coeliac disease. *Gut* 1996;39:180–4.

12. Mora S., *et al*. Bone density and bone metabolism are normal after long-term gluten-free diet in young celiac patients. *Am J Gastroenterol* 1999;94:398–403.

13. Messer M., Anderson C. M., Hubbard L. Studies on the mechanism of destruction of the toxic action of wheat gluten in coeliac disese by crude papain. *Gut* 1964;5:295-303.

14. Messer M., Baume P. E., Oral papain in gluten intolerance. *Lancet* 1976;2:1022.

CROHN'S AND COLITIS

Unfortunately, inflammatory bowel disease is on the rise. Yet in countries where people eat a more primitive diet of whole grains, fruits and vegetables and less refined processed food, inflammatory bowel disease is almost unheard of.

Crohn's and colitis, the two kinds of inflammatory bowel diseases, share many common features. People who suffer from either have diarrhoea with abdominal pain. There can be fever, weight loss, blood loss, gas, and nutritional deficiencies. Ulceration can also develop, leading to fistulas and lesions.

Who gets inflammatory bowel disease? Caucasians are more likely to get inflammatory bowel disease than noncaucasians, and if you're Jewish your chances are even greater. Also, females are more susceptible than males.

Common Causes of Inflammatory Bowel Disease

What causes inflammatory bowel disease? There are several possible causes of inflammatory bowel disease. Antibiotics have been linked to Crohn's disease. Other known causes of inflammatory bowel disease are genetic predisposition, infectious agents, abnormalities of the immune system and dietary factors. Smoking is also linked to Crohn's disease and to disease relapse[1].

Many viruses are thought to be potentially responsible for inflammatory bowel disease, like Epstein Barr, chlamydia, rotavirus and many more. Since the 1950's, inflammatory bowel disease has greatly increased, and in the 1950's antibiotics were made widely available. As more antibiotics were prescribed, more people developed inflammatory bowel disease. Statistics have

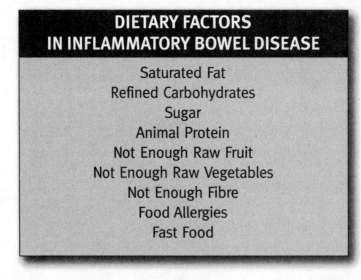

DIETARY FACTORS IN INFLAMMATORY BOWEL DISEASE

Saturated Fat
Refined Carbohydrates
Sugar
Animal Protein
Not Enough Raw Fruit
Not Enough Raw Vegetables
Not Enough Fibre
Food Allergies
Fast Food

shown that when antibiotics are used early in large quantities, the incidence of inflammatory bowel disease is quite high. Immune system abnormalities are also found in inflammatory bowel disease patients but are likely secondary.

One of the most important factors in inflammatory bowel disease is diet. When I see clients with inflammatory bowel disease, the very first thing that I do is get food allergy testing done and clean up their diets. The incidence of inflammatory bowel disease is continuing to increase in countries where people eat a diet high in saturated fats, refined carbohydrates and refined sugar, while it is almost unheard of in countries where people eat more fibre and less refined food[2]. Typically, people who go on to develop Crohn's disease eat more sugar[3] and less raw fruit, vegetables and fibre than most people. Though not all the earlier studies got the same result, recent studies are finding that consuming lots of sugar is also associated with colitis[4]. Diets high in animal protein and fat are linked to inflammatory bowel disease[5].

Food allergy is also important. Studies that have used an elemental diet, intravenous nutrition or an exclusion diet have shown great success in treating inflammatory bowel disease[6]. And this success is likely because these diets give the system a rest from food allergies.

People with Crohn's disease have trouble metabolizing histamine[7]. There is a lot of histamine in yeast and some cheeses. Baker's yeast can be a trigger for Crohn's disease[8]. There is also preliminary evidence that eating fast food twice a week or more more than triples the risk of developing Crohn's and colitis[9], again showing the importance of a healthy diet.

Stress also plays a key role in inflammatory bowel disease.

Treatment of Inflammatory Bowel Disease

So how do you treat inflammatory bowel disease? The natural treatment is aimed at correcting nutritional factors, healing the gut, reducing stress and improving the immune system. Conventional medicine often uses harsh and toxic drugs to control inflammatory bowel disease, while the natural approach seeks to heal the gut through safe and non toxic means.

What are some of the nutrients used to heal inflammatory bowel disease? Even before you look to supplements to help with inflammatory bowel disease, first and foremost get proper food allergy testing done and avoid known allergens. Eat a diet that is high in fibre[10] and essential fatty acids, and avoid carrageenan, which is linked to inflammatory bowel disease. Supplementing fibre, like psyllium, may also help[11].

Correct Nutritional Deficiencies

Then there are many supplements that can help. Take a high dosage multivitamin/mineral supplement that helps to replenish lost nutrients. Most people with inflammatory bowel disease suffer from many nutritional deficiencies due to the poor absorption that the disease itself causes, to poor nutrition caused by lack of appetite and often to the drugs and surgery that are used for inflammatory bowel disease that interfere with nutrient absorption. Extra iron, calcium, magnesium, zinc, vitamins C, D, E, K, betacarotene and B vitamins are frequently needed. Blood loss through bloody diarrhoea often increases the need for iron. Calcium and magnesium, at the very least, are needed to build strong bones, since those with inflammatory bowel disease are more at risk for bone disease because of the steroids and other drugs used to treat the disease and because of poor absorption. It is amazing how many people with Crohn's and colitis come into the clinic on prednisone without ever having been sent for bone density tests even though the drug causes decreases in most of the major bone building nutrients, including calcium, zinc, vitamins C, D, B6 and folic acid. That is why one out five people who take corticosteroids like prednisone long term will break a bone due to osteoporosis. In fact, one out five people in the U.S. who have osteoporosis have it because they take corticosteroids. Vitamins C and E and betacarotene are needed to help heal the gut, to keep the immune system strong and to increase antioxidants.

Why do people with inflammatory bowel disease need to take B vitamins? As many as 64 percent of patients with inflammatory bowel disease are low in folic acid, a B vitamin. Often the drug sulfasalazine, frequently used in inflammatory bowel disease, causes a folate deficiency. Lack of folic acid causes malabsorbtion and diarrhoea. B12 is also often low in people with inflammatory bowel disease, since it is absorbed where the damage often is present: the last part of the small intestine[12]. B5 and B6 are needed to help the body deal with the stress of the illness. So it is a good idea to take a B-complex to make sure every one of the B vitamins are supplied.

Patients with inflammatory bowel disease are often also low in zinc[13]. As many as 45 per cent of patients with inflammatory bowel disease are low in zinc. Since zinc is crucial for healing the gut, keeping the immune system strong and preventing many of the other problems that inflammatory bowel disease leads to, it is crucial to take zinc.

To help digest your food and absorb nutrients, it is a good idea to use a full spectrum digestive enzyme. It is also good to use protein digesting enzymes like papaya and bromelain. Herbal bitters, like milk thistle, wild yam and dandelion root, that tone the entire digestive tract can also be helpful.

Balancing Friendly Flora

To correct underlying friendly flora problems in the gut, use probiotics like acidophilus and bifidus, and take supplements that wipe out bacteria, viruses and parasites but don't destroy the friendly flora the way antibiotics do. Try grapefruit seed extract, goldenseal, oregano oil, echinacea, sterols, and wild indigo. These herbs also help to support the immune system, which is crucial to those with inflammatory bowel disease.

Healing and Soothing

Use soothing demulcent herbs, like slippery elm, marshmallow, licorice, flaxseeds and small dosages of aloe and comfrey, to reduce inflammation and ulceration and promote healing. Wild yam is also wonderful for reducing inflammation. Astringent herbs, like goldenseal root, cransebill root, oakbark, agrimony and bayberry, are wonderful for safely and naturally stopping bleeding and diarrhoea.

Reducing Inflammation

Crohn's and colitis are inflammatory diseases, so it is crucial to address the inflammation. It is a good idea to take essential fatty acids, like flaxseed oil, to reduce inflammation and promote healing. Flaxseed oil can also reduce pain and intestinal cramping.

Curcumin, the active component of the anti-inflammatory herb turmeric, was shown in one small study to help Crohn's disease[14], and the anti-inflammatory herb boswellia was shown in a small study to help 82 per cent of people with colitis compared to 75 per cent taking sulfasalazine[15]. A second small study has also found that boswellia works at least as well as sulfasalazine[16]. In a double-blind study, people whose colitis was in remission had a 20.5 per cent rate of relapse when given a placebo, but a relapse rate of only 4.7 per cent whe given curcumin[17].

You should also reduce animal products, as these increase the inflammatory process in the body.

More Herbal Help

Try using carmative herbs, like anise, fennel, dill, licorice, caraway and peppermint, that get rid of cramping, gas and gripping. It may also be necessary to add nervines and antispasmodics like lemonbalm, chamomile—which also heals ulceration—valerian, passionflower, hops and 5-HTP to help balance mood. Anxiety and stress play a big role in inflammatory bowel disease, and it is crucial to get these emotions under control. Try acupuncture, relaxation techniques and other stress reducing methods as well.

One study gave a herbal combination of dandelion, St. John's wort, lemon balm, calendula and fennel to twenty-four people with colitis. Twenty-three of them had their pain completely resolved by the fifteenth day[18].

A plecebo-controlled study found that wheat grass led to clinical improvement in 78 per cent of colitis sufferers compared to only 30 per cent of those on a placebo[19].

In a double-blind study, 47 per cent of people with colitis who took aloe vera juice experienced improvement or complete remission compared to only 14 per cent of those who took a placebo[20].

I often combine herbs to cover all of the various parts of the illness that need to be taken into account for each person individually.

Chapter Endnotes

1. Cottone M., Rosselli M., Orlando A, et al. Smoking habits and recurrence in Crohn's disease. Gastroenterol 1994;106:643–8.

2. Grimes D. S., Refined carbohydrate, smooth-muscle spasm and diseases of the colon. Lancet 1976;1:395-7; Thornton JR, Emmett P. M., Heaton K. W., Diet and Crohn's disease: Characteristics of the pre-illness diet. Br Med J 1979;279:762-4; Mayberry JF, Rhodes J, Newcombe RG. Increased sugar consumption in Crohn's disease. Digestion 1980;20:323-6; Jarnerot J, Jarnmark I., Nilsson K., Consumption of refined sugar by patients with Crohn's disease, ulcerative colitis, or irritable bowel syndrome. Scand J Gastroenterol 1983;18:999-1002; Mayberry J. F., Rhodes J. Epidemiological aspects of Crohn's disease: a review of the literature. Gut 1984;886–99; Levi AJ. Diet in the management of Crohn's disease. Gut 1985;26:985-8.

3. Mayberry J. F., Rhodes J. Epidemiological aspects of Crohn's disease: a review of the literature. Gut 1984;886–99.

4. Reif S., et al. Pre-illness dietary factors in inflammatory bowel disease. Gut 1997;40:754–60; Tragnone A., et al. Dietary habits as risk factors for inflammatory bowel disease. Eur J Gastroenterol Hepatol 1995;7:47–51.

5. Kono S. Dietary and other risk factors of ulcerative colitis. A case-control study in Japan. J Clin Gastroenterol 1994;19:166–71; Shoda R., et al. Epidemiologic analysis of Crohn's disease in Japan: increased dietary intake of n-6 polyunsaturated fatty acids and animal protein relates to the increased incidence of Crohn's disease in Japan. Am J Clin Nutr 1996;63:741–5; Reif S., Klein I, Lubin F., et al. Pre-illness dietary factors in inflammatory bowel disease. Gut 1997;40:754–60.

6. Rowe A., Uyeyama K. Regional enteritis—its allergic aspects. Gastroenterol 1953;23:554-71;Workman EM, et al. Diet in the management of Crohn's disease. Human Nutr 1984;38A:469-73; Jones VA, et al. Crohn's disease: maintenance of remission by diet. Lancet 1985;2:177-80.

7. Wantke F., Gotz M., Jarisch R. Dietary treatment of Crohn's disease. Lancet 1994;343:113.

8. Alic M., Baker's yeast in Crohn's disease—can it kill you? Am J Gastroenterol 1999;94:1711.

9. Persson P. G., Ahlbom A, Hellers G. Diet and inflammatory bowel disease: a case-control study. Epidemiology 1992;3:47–52.

10. Heaton K. W., Thornton JR, Emmett PM. Treatment of Crohn's disease with an unrefined-carbohydrate, fibre-rich diet. BMJ 1979;2:764–6.

11. Fernandez-Banares F., et al. Randomized clinical trial of Plantago ovata seeds (dietary fibre) as compared with mesalamine in maintaining remission in ulcerative colitis. Am J Gastroenterol 1999;94:427–33.

12. Rosenberg I. H., Bengoa J. M., Sitrin MD. Nutritional aspects of inflammatory bowel disease. Ann Rev Nutr 1985;5:463-84; Filipsson S, Julten L, Lindstedt G. Malabsorption of fat and vitamin B12 before and after intestinal resection for Crohn's disease. Scand J Gastroenterol 1978;13:529-36.

13. Fleming C. R., et al. Zinc nutrition in Crohn's disease. Dig Dis Sci 1981;26:865-70.

14. Holt P. R., Katz S, Kirshoff R. Curcumin therapy in inflammatory bowel disease: a pilot study. Dig Dis Sci 2005;50:2191–3.

15. Gupta I., et al. Effects of Boswellia serrata gum resin in patients with ulcerative colitis. Eur J Med Res 1997;2:37–43.

16. Gupta I., et al. Effects of gum resin of Boswellia serrata in patients with chronic colitis. Planta Med 2001;67:391-5.

17. Hanai H., et al. Curcumin maintenance therapy for ulcerative colitis: randomized, multicenter, double-blind, placebo-controlled trial. Clin Gastroenterol Hepatol 2006;4:1502–6.

18. Chakurski I., et al. Treatment of chronic colitis with an herbal combination ot Taraxacum officianale, Hypericum perforatum, Melissa officinalis, Calendula officinalis, and Foeniculum vulgare. Vutr Boles 1981;20:51-4.

19. Ben-Arye E., et al. Wheat grass juice in the treatment of active distal ulcerative colitis: a randomized double-blind placebo-controlled trial. Scand J Gastroenterol 2002;37:444–9.

20. Langmead L., et al. Randomized, double-blind, placebo-controlled trial of oral aloe vera gel for active ulcerative colitis. Aliment Pharmacol Ther 2004;19:739–47.

COLDS AND FLUS

Having a healthy immune system can make all the difference to your health and the number of illnesses you succumb to. Viruses are around all the time, and yet only some of us catch them. Why? Because if your immune system is strong, it will fight them off before you get them, whereas those whose systems are not as strong will get sick more frequently.

Conventional medicine tries to kill everything to prevent our getting sick and does little to help the overall immune system, whereas natural medicine tries to strengthen the overall system so that we can fight illnesses off, no matter what kind they are. It's like a pond that is infested with mosquitoes. You can spray the pond and kill the insects, but the pond is still stagnant and the mosquitoes will come back. But if you drain the pond and clean the water, then it won't matter if the mosquitoes come back because the pond is no longer a good place for them to live and breed. Just like your immune system: strengthen it and it won't matter what you come into contact with—you'll have a better chance of fighting it off.

Some Simple and Effective Ways to Avoid Getting Sick

What you eat or don't eat can make all the difference to a weakened immune system. To prevent illness, drink plenty of fluids—dehydrated mucous surfaces are a better breeding ground for viruses—but avoid sugar and sugary fruit juices. Sugar depresses immune functions[1]. This depression happens because glucose and vitamin C compete for transport sites into the white blood cells (one of your body's main defences against illness). Increased levels of sugar decrease vitamin C levels and may result in a reduction in white blood cell function. Even fruit juices, such as orange juice, can depress immune function; studies show that sugar of all kinds impairs the ability of white blood cells to kill bacteria, and that it weakens the immune system and competes with vitamin C.

As well as avoiding sugar it is equally important to avoid dairy and other mucous-forming foods such as gluten, for those susceptible to illnesses such as colds and sinusitis. The mucousy surface these foods create allows bacteria and viruses to thrive, since they tend to like that atmosphere.

It is important to watch what you eat to prevent illness, but it is also important to pay attention to other bodily needs such as rest. Go to bed early and stay there if you are not feeling well. During deep sleep, strong immune-enhancing compounds are released and many immune functions are greatly increased.

HERBS THAT HELP STRENGTHEN THE IMMUNE SYSTEM

Goldenseal

This herb is native to North America and was used extensively by First Nations people. It was primarily used to soothe the mucous linings of the respiratory, digestive, and urinary tract. It was used in cases of allergy and infection. One of the components found in goldenseal, berberine, has been well studied and found to be a powerful antibiotic as well as an immune enhancer. It exerts wide anti-microbial activity, effective against bacteria, protozoa, and fungi, including such species as *staphylococcus, streptococcus, chlamydia, salmonella, entamoeba histolytica, giardia, candida, trichomonas,* and many more. According to Michael Murray, N.D., goldenseal actually exerts a stronger action than the antibiotics that are commonly used in the treatment of some of the diseases that these pathogens cause. Also, unlike chemical antibiotics, berberine inhibits the growth of the candida yeast. Chemical antibiotics can actually stimulate the growth of yeast.

Goldenseal also not only kills bacteria, but it prevents bacteria from sticking to host cells, preventing them from gaining a hold. Goldenseal promotes blood supply to the spleen, releasing immune compounds. It also enhances macrophage activity. Macrophages are white blood cells that engulf bacteria, viruses, and fungi. And goldenseal can lower a fever. Thus, goldenseal also helps to improve overall immunity.

ANDROGRAPHIS VERSUS PLACEBO FOR TREATING UPPER RESPIRATORY TRACT INFECTIONS

Symptom	Andrographis Significantly Better than Placebo Day 2	Andrographis Significantly Better than Placebo Day 4
Headache		√
Tiredness	√	√
Earache		√
Sleepiness	√	√
Sore Throat	√	√
Nasal Secretion	√	√
Phlegm		√
Cough		√

Source: Caceres DD, et al., Use of visual analogue scale measurements (VAS) to assess the effectiveness of standardized Andrographis paniculata extract SHA-10 in reducing the symptoms of common cold. A randomized, double-blind, placebo study. Phtyomed 1999;6:217-23

Licorice

Licorice is one of the most extensively used and studied herbs, and has been used for thousands of years in both the east and west. It is a demulcent (which means it soothes irritated surfaces) and an expectorant. Licorice also increases production of interferon, the body's natural antiviral compound. It blocks viruses, activates macrophage and natural killer cell activity, helping to get your immune system working. And it has antibiotic activity against *staphylococcus, streptococcus,* and *candida,* among others. It also acts as a natural cortisone in the body to help fight off allergies. And licorice helps the body cope with stress, which is crucial when fighting off illness.

Astragalus

Astragalus has a long history of use in the east and has been used a lot lately in the west. It strengthens the defences of the body. It is used to treat colds, flus, fevers, and infections. Astragalus works in a number of ways to strengthen the immune system. It induces interferon production, which prevents viruses from gaining a hold on the respiratory system, and it binds to cells' surfaces and stimulates the synthesis of proteins that prevent viral infection. It also increases white blood cells when they are low. Studies show that astragalus reduces the incidence and shortens the duration of colds. In one study, bronchitis sufferers were shown to have a reduction in symptoms when using astragalus[2]. It is also used to fight off all kinds of illnesses from colds to cancer. According to Daniel Mowrey, Ph.D., astragalus is used to treat all immune system breakdowns, colds, fevers, and infections.

Another study of 1,137 people found that astragalus combined with interferon was more effective in combatting the cold virus than interferon alone. Studies in China have proven that astragalus reduces the incidence of, and shortens the duration of, the common cold.

Echinacea

Perhaps the best-known immune herb of all is echinacea. Echinacea was originally used by First Nations healers for many things, including snake bites. Aboriginal people of the plains used this plant more than any other for illness and injury. The root was used externally for wounds, burns and abscesses, and insect bites, and internally for infections, toothache, and joint pain. In 1870, H. C. F Meyer, a German lay healer, introduced it to Americans as a cure for almost everything. He wasn't far wrong. Research has found echinacea—both the *angustiofolia* and *purpurea* species—to aid the immune system. In fact, there have been over three hundred studies on echinacea's immune-enhancing properties. Since some active parts of the plant are water soluble and some are better extracted in alcohol; a product that combines both the fresh juice and an alcohol extract is best, using both species of plant and the above-ground portion of the plant as well as the root.

Science has found all kinds of reasons this great immune modulator works. It stimulates the production of immune cells and then increases their ability to devour invading pathogens. It also has an interferon-like effect. Interferon is your body's own immune-enhancing virus fighter. It then turns on a secondary immune system in your body, called the alternate complement pathway, that is triggered when antibodies start destroying invaders. And, if that's not enough, echinacea has the amazing ability to disable the virus's mechanism for spreading throughout your body.

Interestingly, the common belief that echinacea is an immune-system stimulant that can only be used short-term is confused. It is true that the tincture of echinacea is an immune enhancer, best used at the beginning of an infection, but the whole herb or the powdered root as a capsule or tablet is an immune system modulator that balances immunity in either direction—increasing it when too low and sedating it when too high. So capsules or tablets of the whole herb or the root can be taken daily, in doses of 250 to 500 mg as a preventative for people exposed to viruses.

Eleuthero

Another great immune herb that is best known for its ability to give energy is eleuthero (formerly known as Siberian ginseng). This herb hails from the east, where it is commonly used to support the adrenal glands in times of stress and for increased energy; yet, according to Daniel Mowrey, Ph.D., it also has been proven to reduce fevers. It is known to support the immune system by stimulating phagocytosis (phagocytes are the garbage collectors of the body that devour invading microorgansims, bacteria, and viruses) and modifying interferon responses (the body's own immune-boosting antiviral and anticancer substance).

Eleuthero has been used to tone the immune system and prevent colds and flus. It has been used by athletes not only for its ability to increase energy, but also for preventing illnesses. In 1987, a study was done using eleuthero on thirty-six healthy volunteers. The results of the study proved that eleuthero augments the human immune system by increasing the absolute number of immune cells, especially T lymphocytes[3].

Another large study found a 40 per cent drop in flus, colds, and other infections when eleuthero was taken every day in November and December. Yet another also found a huge reduction in respiratory disease and flu with daily eleuthero.

Elderberry

This herb was originally popular with the Roma people, and it is one of the few herbs that tastes good. If you're thinking of getting the flu shot, you may want to look at elderberry extract first. This herb has been found to be effective against ten strains of viruses, compared to the common flu shot, which is only effective against two to three strains of viruses. Elderberry works by preventing viruses from penetrating into cells, preventing them from replicating. Elderberries are also potent sources of anthocyanins, strong antioxidants that also enhance immune function.

How good are these berries? Research found that while a placebo group took six days to get over the flu, 90 per cent of the elderberry group was better in three[4]. In a more recent study, people with the flu were given either a placebo or 15 ml of standardized elderberry extract syrup four times a day. On a scale of 1 to 10, most of the people on elderberry had improved to near 10 by the third or fourth day. But the people on the placebo did not achieve that level until after seven or eight days. By day four, the people on elderberry had all reached a score higher than 9 for aches, pains, sleep quality, and congestion. Those on placebo were still at or below 1 on the scale[5].

In another recent study, people were given lozenges containing 175 mg of elderberry extract or a placebo lozenge four times a day. After two days, no one in the elderberry group had a fever, while most on the placebo had not improved. 78 per cent of the elderberry group were rid of their headaches, while headaches in the placebo group got worse. 50 per cent of the herb group had no increased nasal congestion, while most of the placebo group were worse. The elderberry lozenges were also significantly better at improving coughs. The researchers concluded that elderberry rapidly relieves flu symptoms and that the results were similar or superior to antiviral drugs for flu[6].

Elderflowers can also be used. The flowers induce sweating and mild fever, which kicks in the immune system and fights infection. This property of herbs is known as diaphoretic. Traditional herbalists suggest combining elderflower with two other diaphoretics: peppermint and/or yarrow. Boneset is another good diaphoretic.

Garlic

This herb keeps many things away. Perhaps that is how it got its reputation for keeping vampires away. Garlic enhances the immune system. It is also an antibiotic and expectorant and encourages sweating. It has a wide range of activity against bacteria and viruses, including *streptococcus*, *staphylococcus*, and *klebsiella*. In one study, when 146 people took garlic from November to January, they had only twenty-four colds, compared to the placebo group, which had sixty-five. And when they did get a cold, it went away a lot faster: in one and a half days compared to five[7]. Garlic can be used for everything from colds and urinary-tract infections to cancer. Garlic in olive oil can be placed in the ears to help fight off ear infections.

Wild Indigo

A little-discussed herb that deserves more attention is wild indigo. This antimicrobial, anti-inflammatory immune booster is one of the best herbs for fighting infection. Several studies have shown a combination of wild indigo, echinacea, and thuja to be very effective[8]. It is great for thinning mucous, too.

Androgaphis

This herb comes from India. It is a wonderful herb for both preventing and treating colds. One double-blind study found that after four days, cold symptoms were much better when people were given andrographis than when they were given a placebo[9]. In another study, it was found to be better than a placebo in those with colds and sinusitis[10]. In a very impressive double-blind study, 208 people with upper respiratory tract infections were given either andrographis or a placebo. By the second day, the herb group had a significant reduction in cold symptoms, such as runny nose and sore throat, compared with the placebo group. By day four, they also had significant improvement in cough, headache, earache, and fatigue[11]. But that's not all! It also helps to prevent illness. When 107 healthy children were given andrographis or a placebo for three months during the winter months, the kids on the herb had a significantly (2.1 times) lower risk of catching a cold[12].

Androgaphis combined with eleuthero (formerly known as Siberian ginseng) has been shown in a study to outperform a placebo in the treatment of sinusitis and acute upper respiratory infections such as laryngitis, bronchitis, and the common cold[13].

Cat's Claw

This herb comes from South America and has traditionally been used to fight off infection and boost immunity. Cat's claw has anti-inflammatory, anticancer, and immune-stimulating properties. German researchers discovered that alkaloids found only in cat's claw had a huge effect on the immune system. The alkaloids enhanced the white blood cells' ability to engulf and destroy bacteria, tumour cells, and dead matter—a process known as phagocytosis.

Also try pau d'arco another excellent South American herb for fighting colds and stimulating the immune system.

Shiitake, Maitake, and Reishi Mushrooms

These mushrooms are a must on any list to help improve overall immunity. They help to fight everything from the common cold to cancer and HIV. These mushrooms have antibacterial activity, antiviral activity, anti-candida activity, are antioxidants, and they enhance the immune system.

Nutrients for the Immune System

There are also many nutrients to help strengthen the immune system.

To strengthen immunity, you have to support the thymus gland—the body's chief gland of the immune system. To strengthen the thymus gland, it is a good idea to take a multivitamin to improve immunity and reduce infections[14]. Other key nutrients needed to support the immune system include antioxidants to prevent free-radical damage that can shrink the thymus gland (thymic involution). Take nutrients such as vitamins E, C, selenium, and zinc. B6 is also crucial to support the thymus gland.

A study found that people given a multivitamin/mineral with probiotics had 14 per cent fewer colds than people given a placebo. Their colds also didn't last as long, and they had significantly fewer and milder fevers and headaches[15].

Vitamin C and Zinc

Vitamin C supplementation has been shown to reduce the severity of and shorten the length of the common cold in numerous studies. Vitamin C is antiviral and antibacterial and possesses an ability to enhance host resistance. It is able to enhance the immune system, including enhancing white-blood-cell production, antibody responses, and interferon levels.

When a review looked at twenty-one studies that used one to eight grams of vitamin C, it discovered that in every single one of them the vitamin C reduced the length and severity of the cold by over 23 per cent[16]. But you have to take at least a gram, and subsequent research shows that two grams work better than one[17].

What's new in vitamin C research is the discovery that it not only helps get rid of a cold, but that taking it every day helps prevent colds, too. And that's even better! A new study gave either 50mg or 500mg of vitamin C to 244 people for five years. The 50mg dose acted as a placebo. The 500 mg group was an amazing 70 per cent less likely to catch one or more colds per year[18].

Zinc is a nutrient that is crucial for optimal immune function. It encourages healing and builds immunity. Zinc effects direct antiviral activity against several of the viruses that cause the common cold.

Studies have shown that zinc lozenges possess incredible ability to kill colds. When an effective form is used, zinc lozenges work every time. The effective forms are zinc gluconate, zinc acetate, and zinc gluconate-glycine. Other forms or those flavoured with citric acid, tartaric acid, sorbitol, or manitol don't work as well.

An early double-blind study proved zinc lozenges' ability to shorten the duration of the common cold to four days, compared to eleven days without[19]. Recent studies have found the same. Zinc gluconate lozenges taken every two waking hours killed colds in 4.4 days versus 7.6

on placebo[20]. Zinc acetate lozenges containing only 12.8 mg of zinc given every two to three waking hours killed the cold in four and a half days; people on placebo continued to suffer for eight. The zinc also significantly decreased the severity of the colds[21].

This high dose of zinc is more than is usually taken, and you should not take it for more than a week. But, as you can see, you won't need to!

B Vitamins and Beta-carotene

Folic acid and B12 also help the immune system. A deficiency of these vitamins can lead to thymic involution and to a reduction of white blood cell production and function. B1, B2 and B5 are also crucial for immunity.

Or try beta-carotene, which protects mucous surfaces and encourages healing. Carotenes are important antioxidants that help protect the thymus gland. They also increase the number and activity of immune cells.

Traditional Healing for Colds

Traditional herbalists treated colds using diaphoretic (sweating) herbs to increase the heat of the body, stimulating the immune system. They would use, alone or in combination, herbs such as elderberry, yarrow, peppermint, and linden, and brew a tea that would increase sweating, helping to burn the cold out. One method we have found to be particularly helpful is to soak four crushed whole cayenne pepper pods in the juice of one freshly squeezed orange or grapefruit. Let sit for half an hour and then take by the tablespoon every half an hour until symptoms are gone.

If sinuses are particularly clogged, try using a steam inhaler. In a bowl of boiling water, put 15 drops each of eucalyptus and lavender essential oil. Lean over the bowl and drape your head with a towel; breathe the steam into the sinuses, being careful not to burn yourself. Also see the Sinusitis section of the book for other good ideas.

And avoid stress. Stress depresses immune function. Rent a comedy DVD at least once a week. Laughter improves immune function.

Chapter Endnotes

1. Sanchez, A., et al. "Role of sugar in human neutrophilic phagocytosis." *Am J Clin Nutr*, 1973; 26:1180'84; Ringsdorf, W., E. Cheraskin, R. Ramsay. "Sucrose, neutrophil phagocytosis, and resistance to diseases." *Dent Surv*, 1976; 52:46'48; Bernstein, J. et al. "Depression of lymphocyte transformation following oral glucose ingestion." *Am J Clin Nutr*, 1977; 30:613.

2. Yunde, H., et al. "Effect of *radix astagali seu hedysari* on the interferon system." *Chinese Medical Journal*, 1981; 94:35'40.

3. Bohn, B., C. T. Nebe, C. Birr. "Flow-cytometric studies with Eleutherococcus senticosus extract as an immunomodulatory agent." *Arzneimittel-forschung*, 1987; 37:1193'96.

4. Zakay-Rones, Z., et al. "Inhibition of several strains of influenza virus in vitro and reduction of symptoms by an elderberry extract (*Sambucus nigra L.*) during an outbreak of influenza B Panama." *J Altern Compliment Med*, 1995; 1:361'69.

5. Zakay-Rones, Z., et al. "Randomized study of the efficacy and safety of oral elderberry extract in the treatment of influenza A and B virus infections." *J International Med Res*, 2004; 32:132-40.

6. King H. F. "Pilot clinical study on a proprietary elderberry extract: efficacy in addressing influenza symptoms." *Online Journal of Pharmacology and Pharmacokinetics* 2009;5: 32-43.

7. Josling, P. "Preventing the common cold with a garlic supplement: a double-blind, placebo-controlled survey." *Adv Ther*, 2001; 18:189'93.

8. Forth, H., N, Beuscher. "Influence of Esberitox on the frequency of the common cold." *Zeutschrift fur Allgemeinmedizin*, 1981; 57:2272'75; Vorberg, G. "For colds, stimulate the nonspecific immune system." *Arztl Prax*, 1984; 35:97'98; Reitz, H. D. "Immunomodulation with phytotherapeutic agents: a scientific study on the example of Esberitox." *Notebene Medici*, 1990; 20:362'66 Henneicke-von Zepelin, H.H., *et al.* "Efficacy and safety of a fixed combination phytomedicine in the treatment of the common cold (acute viral respiratory infection): Results of a randomized, double-blind, placebo-controlled, multicenter study." *Current Med Res Opinion*, 1999; 15:214-27

9. Hancke, J., et al. "A double-blind study with a new monodrug Kan Jang: Decrease of symptoms and improvement in recovery from common cold." *Phytother Res*, 1995; 9:559'62.

10. Melchior, J., S. Palm, G. Wikman. "Controlled clinical study of standardized Andrographis paniculata extract in common cold-a pilot trial." *Phytomed*, 1996; 3:315'18.

11. Caceres, D. D., *et al.* "Use of visual analogue scale measurements (VAS) to assess the effectiveness of standardized *Andrographis paniculata* extract SHA-10 in reducing the symptoms of common cold. A randomized, double-blind, placebo study." *Phtyomed*, 1999; 6:217'23.

12. Caceres, D. D., et al. "Prevention of common colds with *Andrographis paniculata* dried extract. A Pilot double-blind trial." *Phytomedicine*, 1997; 4:101'04.

13. Panossian, A., et al. "Effect of Andrographolide and Kan Jang—fixed combination of extract SHA-10 and extract SHE-3—on proliferation of human lymphocytes, production of cytokines and immune activation markers in the whole blood cells culture." *Phytomedicine*, 2002; 9:598'605.

14. Chandra, R. K. "Effect of vitamin and trace-element supplementation immune responses and infection in elderly subjects." *Lancet*, 1992; 340:1124'27.

15. Winkler, P., *et al.* "Effect of a dietary supplement containing probiotic bacteria plus vitamins and minerals on common cold infections and cellular immune parameters." *International Journal of Clinical Pharmacology and Therapeutics*, 2005; 43:327'34.

16. Henuka, H. "Does vitamin C alleviate the symptoms of the common cold?—A review of current evidence." *Scand J Infect Dis*, 1994; 26:1'6.

17. Hemilä, H. "Vitamin C supplementation and common cold symptoms: factors affecting the magnitude of the benefit." *Med Hypotheses*, 1999; 52:171-78.

18. Sasazuki, S., *et al.* "Effect of vitamin C on common cold: randomized controlled trial." *European Journal of Clinical Nutrition*, 2006; 60:9-17.

19. Eby, G. A., D. R. Davis, W. W. Halcomb. "Reduction in duration of common colds by zinc gluconate lozenges in a double-blind study." *Antimicrob Agents Chemother*, 1984; 25:20'24.

20. Sherif, B., *et al.* "Zinc gluconate lozenges for treating the common cold: A randomized, double-blind, placebo-controlled study." *Ann Intern Med*, 1996; 125:81'88.

21. Prasad, A. S., *et al.* "Duration of symptoms and plasma cytokine levels in patients with the common cold treated with zinc acetate." *Ann Intern Med* 2000;133:245-52.

DEPRESSION

Depressingly, depression is becoming a virtual epidemic. The U.S. National Institute of Mental Health says 6.7 per cent of adults suffer from major depression in any given year. Health Canada says that between 7.9 per cent and 8.6 per cent of adults will experience major depression in their lifetime. And although conventional medicine has come up with many pharmaceutical drugs to treat depression, none are without troubling side effects. The real crime is that several natural remedies work at least as well, without the side effects, but are almost never recommended.

The three most powerful natural antidepressants are St. John's wort, 5-HTP and SAMe.

St. John's Wort

"When treating patients with mild to moderate depression, Hypericum (St. John's wort) should be considered as one of the first treatment options based on both efficacy and safety, particularly in cases where treatment is a choice between fluoxetine (Prozac) and Hypericum"[1]. This was the authors' conclusion after showing that the low dose of only 500mg of St. John's wort—instead of the normal dose of 900mg—worked slightly better than Prozac, with significantly more people responding to it, while being way safer.

And this is not the only study to prove the superiority of St. John's wort over the leading class of pharmaceutical antidepressants, the selective serotonin reuptake inhibitors (SSRI's). In fact, St. John's wort has consistently defeated Prozac and its SSRI relatives. St. John's wort has equaled Prozac in a second comparison, while being safer[2], and bettered it—again despite being deliberately handicapped by a very low 500mg dose—in a third. And, once again in this study, St. John's wort was not only more powerful, but safer: 72 per cent of the side effects occurred in the Prozac group, and the few side effects that did occur in the St. John's wort group were way less serious[3].

Against the SSRI Zoloft, St. John's wort has fared just as well, equaling the drug in one study[4] and beating it in two[5].

St. John's wort has continued to triumph over any SSRI antidepressant pharmaceutical medicine wants to throw at it. It easily defeated Paxil. While 70 per cent improved on the herb, only 60 per cent improved on the drug, the ones on the herb improved more and 50 per cent of them had their depression completely resolved compared to only 35 per cent on the drug. As always, St. John's wort was also safer[6]. St. John's wort also beat the SSRI Celexa in a recent study by more safely working just as well: while the improvement on the Hamilton Depression scale was identical for both treatments, there were three times as many side effects in the Celexa group[7].

The latest news on St. John's wort is two recent meta-analyses. The first was conducted by the highly respected Cochrane Database of Systemic Reviews. This meta-analysis of double-blind studies on major depression looked at eighteen studies that compared St. John's wort to a placebo and seventeen that compared it to a drug. The herb came out significantly better than a placebo and equal to, but safer than, the drugs[8]. The second put together thirteen double-blind studies that compared St. John's wort to SSRI antidepressants in major depression. St. John's wort won this toughest of challenges too because it equaled the drugs with less people having to drop out of the studies[9].

The really impressive thing about St. John's wort is that it works at least as well as the best antidepressant drugs while being way safer. Notice that both meta-analyses found that the herb was safer than the drugs.

St. John's wort, standardized for hypericin, and sometimes for hyperforin, is usually taken at a dose of 900mg a day. For more severe depression, double the dose.

5-HTP

For some reason, 5-hydroxytryptophan, or 5-HTP for short, has never gotten the attention it deserves. It works well, and it works fast: faster than drugs. And, like St. John's wort, it has beaten the drugs repeatedly in studies.

In one difficult test, researchers sought out to see if 5-HTP could help people who had not been helped by any of the antidepressant drugs: any of them! Incredibly, 43 per cent of them had their depression cured completely and another 8 per cent improved significantly[10]. The study's author observed that he had never seen an antidepressant that worked so fast, that so completely restored the person to whom they had previously been and that was so entirely without side effects. He concluded that 5-HTP "merits a place in the front ranks of the antidepressants".

Several studies have proven that 5-HTP works as well or better than drugs with fewer and less severe side effects. When 5-HTP got its chance to go up against an SSRI, the leading class of antidepressant drug, it also came out on top. More people responded to it, they responded faster, and they responded more. By the end of the study, 60.7 per cent had responded to the 5-HTP versus 56.1 per cent to the drug. 5-HTP was also safer: there were more side effects in the drug group, and those side effects were more severe. More people in the drug group were also forced to drop out[11].

The starter dose of 5-HTP for depression is 50mg three times a day. If after two weeks you are not satisfied with the results, increase the dose to 100mg three times a day.

SAMe

Another antidepressant with overwhelming scientific support that is often ignored is S-adenosyl methionine, or SAMe. A large body of research proves that SAMe is one of the top antidepressants available today.

Your brain needs SAMe to make serotonin and other antidepressant neurotransmitters. Overall, in all kinds of studies, SAMe has crushed placebo treatments, working 78 per cent of the time compared to just 4 per cent for the placebo. In overall matches against tricyclic antidepressant drugs, SAMe has also proven significantly more effective[12].

In a review of forty-seven studies on mild to moderate depression, SAMe brought about an improvement on the Hamilton Depression Scale that was significantly better than placebo and every bit as good as drugs[13]. No significant side effect has ever been reported!

The dose of SAMe should gradually be increased from 200mg twice a day, to 400mg twice a day on day three, then 400mg three times a day on day ten, and finally 400mg four times a day on day twenty.

More Help: B Vitamins and EFA's

Many people who suffer from depression are deficient in folic acid[14], and, if you are deficient in B12, you are at higher risk for depression[15]. Correcting these deficiencies can improve depression.

Depressed people are also often low in B6, which is not surprising, since B6 is necessary for the body to make serotonin, melatonin and dopamine. Research shows that the lower the level of B6 in depressed people, the worse the depression[16].

Inositol, another member of the B vitamin family, can also offer significant help[17].

And the essential fatty acids seem to be essential for depression too. While not getting enough omega-3 fatty acids in your diet has been linked to depression[18], diets high in omega-3 fatty acids are associated with lower rates of depression. Omega-3 fatty acids have been shown in double-blind studies to significantly help depression[19]. A small, recent study found more than 50 per cent improvement in 70 per cent of depressed children when they were given omega-3 supplements. 40 per cent of the kids got completely better, while none of them had much improvement on the placebo[20].

Still More Help

More help may come from the mineral zinc. A small double-blind study has found that adding 25mg of zinc to antidepressant medication brings about significant improvement in depression compared to adding a placebo[21].

The Latest in Antidepressant Herbs: Rhodiola and Saffron

Rhodiola rosea is an exciting, but little known herb that has already been shown to increase both mental and physical energy while calming you at the same time. And now, in a brand new study, people with mild to moderate depression were given either 340mg or 680mg of Rhodiola extract or a placebo for six weeks. The depression scores went down from 24.5 to 16 on one scale and from 12.2 to 7.1 on another in the low dose Rhodiola group. They went down from 23.8 to 16.7 and from 10.4 to 4.8 in the high dose group. They didn't go down at all in the placebo group. The Rhodiola was as safe as it was effective[22].

And here's an unusual one. That expensive yellow herb that you use to colour your Spanish rice may just be the next big antidepressant. Saffron has long been used for depression in traditional Persian medicine. And now at least three small double-blind studies have supported that use. A 30mg extract of saffron petals given for six weeks proved to be significantly better than a placebo at treating mild to moderate depression[23].

But how does saffron stack up against a drug? When people with major depression were given either 10mg of saffron extract or 100mg of imipramine for six weeks, the improvement was significant and equal in the two groups. But the saffron produced fewer side effects[24].

But can it compete with the big SSRI's like Prozac? When people with major depression were given 15mg of saffron petal extract or 10mg of Prozac twice a day for eight weeks, the herb produced a significant effect that was equal to the drug's[25].

Diet and Lifestyle

In fighting depression, it is also important to eat well and to eliminate smoking and alcohol. Nicotine and alcohol both increase cortisol output. Increased cortisol decreases the amount of tryptophan delivered to your brain. Tryptophan is the precursor to serotonin, the brain's natural antidepressant. Less tryptophan in the brain means less serotonin in the brain, and less serotonin in the brain means more depression. Cortisol also contributes to depression by decreasing the sensitivity of serotonin receptors in the brain.

Caffeine is also a factor in depression.

You should also eliminate food allergies[26] and exercise regularly[27]. Amazingly, studies show that exercise is as effective as drugs and psychotherapy[28].

Acupuncture also helps.

Chapter Endnotes

1. Schrader E., Equivalence of St John's wort extract (Ze117) and fluoxetine: a randomized, controlled study in mild-moderate depression. *International Clin Psychopharmacol* 2000;15:61-8.

2. Harrer G., *et al*. Comparison of equivalence between the St. John's wort extract LoHyp-57 and fluoxetine. *Arzneimittelforschung* 1999;49:289–96.

3. Fava M., *et al*. A Double-blind, randomized trial of St John's wort, fluoxetine, and placebo in major depressive disorder. *J Clin Psychopharmacol* 2005;25:441-7.

4. Brenner R., *et al*. Comparison of an extract of Hypericum (LI 160) and sertraline in the treatment of depression: a double-blind, randomized pilot study. *Clinical Therapeutics* 2000;22:411-19.

5. van Gurp G., *et al*. St. John's wort or sertraline? Randomized controlled trial in primary care. *Canadian Family Physician* 2002;48:905-12; Gastpar M., Singer A., Zeller K. Efficacy and tolerability of hypericum extract STW3 in long-term treatment with a once-daily dosage in comparison with sertraline. *Pharmacopsychiatry* 2005;38:78-86.

6. Szegedi A, *et al*. Acute treatment of moderate to severe depression with hypericum extract WS 5570 (St John's wort): randomized controlled double blind non-inferiority trial versus paroxetine. *BMJ* 2005;330:503.

7. Gastpar M., Singer A., Zeller K. Comparative efficacy and safety of a once-daily dosage of Hypericum extract STW3-VI and citalopram in patients with moderate depression: a double-blind, randomized, multicentre, placebo-controlled study *Pharmacopsychiatry* 2006;39:66-75.

8. Linde K, Berner M. M., Kriston Lm. St John's wort for major depression. *Cochrane Database of Systematic Reviews* 2008; 4. Art. No.: CD000448. DOI: 10.1002/14651858.CD000448.pub3.

9. Rahimi R, Nikfar S., Abdollahi M. Efficacy and tolerability of Hypericum perforatum in major depressive disorder in comparison with selective serotonin reuptake inhibitors: a meta-analysis. *Prog Neuropsychopharmacol Biol Psychiatry* 2009;33:118-127.

10. van Hiele J. J., L-5-hydroxytryptophan in depression: the first substitution therapy in psychiatry? *Neuorpsychobiology* 1980;6:230-40.

11. Poldinger W., Calanchini B, Schwartz W. A functional-dimensional approach to depression: serotonin deficiency as a target syndrome in a comparison of 5-HTP and fluvoxamine. *Psychopathology* 1991;24:53-81.

12. Janicak PG, *et al*. Parenteral S-adenosylmethionine in depression: a literature review and preliminary report. *Psychopharmacol Bull* 1989;25:238-41.

13. Agency for Healthcare and Quality & Agency of U.S. Department of Health and Human Services 2002.

14. Reynolds E., *et al*. Folate deficiency in depressive illness. *Br J Psychiatry* 1970;117:287–92; Carney M. W. P., *et al*. Red cell folate concentrations in psychiatric patients. J Affective Disorders 1990;19:207-13; Crellin R, Bottiglieri T, Reynolds EH. Folates and psychiatric disorders. *Clinical potential. Drugs* 1993;45:623-36.

15. Penninx B. W., *et al*. Vitamin B (12) deficiency and depression in physically disabled older women: epidemiologic evidence from the Women's Health and Aging Study. *Am J Psychiatry* 2000;157:715–21.

16. Hvas AM, *et al*. Vitamin B6 level is associated with symptoms of depression. *Psychother Psychosom* 2004;73:340-3.

17. Levine J, *et al*. Double-blind, controlled trial of inositol treatment of depression. Am J Psychiatry 1995;152:792–4; Levine J, *et al*. Follow-up and relapse analysis of an inositol study of depression. *Isr J Psychiatry Relat Sci* 1995;32:14–21.

18. Hibbeln J. R., Salem N. Dietary polyunsaturated fatty acids and depression: when cholesterol does not satisfy. *Am J Clin Nutr* 1995;62:1-9.

19. Su K. P., *et al*. Omega-3 fatty acids in major depressive disorder. A preliminary double-blind, placebo-controlled trial. *Eur Neuropsychopharmacol* 2003;13:267–71.

20. Nemets H, *et al*. Omega-3 treatment of childhood depression: a controlled, double-blind pilot study. *Am J Psychiatry* 2006;163:1098–100.

21. Nowak G, *et al*. effect of zinc supplementation on antidepressant therapy in unipolar depression: a preliminary placebo-controlled study. *Polish Journal of Pharmacology* 2003;55:1143-7.

22. Darbinyan V., *et al*. Clinical trial of Rhodiola rosea L. extract SHR-5 in the treatment of mild to moderate depression. *Nord J Psychiatry* 2007;61:343-348.

23. Moshiri E., *et al*. Crocus sativus L. (petal) in the treatment of mild-to-moderate depression: a double-blind, randomized and placebo-controlled trial *Phytomea* 2006;13:607-611.

24. Akhondzadeh S., *et al*. Comparison of Crocus sativus L. and imipramine in the treatment of mild to moderate depression: a pilot double-blind randomized trial *BMC Complementary and Alternative Medicine*. 2004;4:12.

25. Akhondzadeh Basti A., *et al*. Comparison of petal of Crocus sativus L. and fluoxetine in the treatment of depressed outpatients: a pilot double-blind randomized trial. *Progr Neuropsychopharmacol Biol Psychiatry* 2007;31:439–42.

26. King D. S., Can allergic exposure provoke psychological symptoms? A double-blind test. Biol Psychiatry 1981;16:3–19; Brown M, *et al*. Food allergy in polysymptomatic patients. *Practitioner* 1981;225:1651–4.

27. Martinsen E. W., Medhus A, Sandivik L. Effects of aerobic exercise on depression a controlled study. BMJ 1985;291:109; Martinsen E. W., Benefits of exercise for the treatment of depression. *Sports Med* 1990;9:380–9.

28. Stress Med 1987; Blumenthal J. A., *et al*. Effects of exercise training on older patients with major depression. *Arch Intern Med* 1999;159:2349–56.

DIVERTICULITIS

Diverticulitis is a disease directly related to what we eat or, in this case, what we don't eat. It is an incredibly common problem that affects millions of North Americans, and yet many do not even know that they have it.

Causes of Diverticulitis

In non-westernized countries, diverticulitis is almost unheard of, and the reason is simple. It is a disease caused mainly by the poor western diet, a diet lacking in fibre. The low fibre diet leads to straining because of constipation, which increases pressure in the colon and causes weak spots to bulge out, forming small sacs in the lining of the colon—diverticula. The resultant condition is known as diverticulosis.

Almost half of Americans between sixty and eighty have diverticulosis, and almost all of them over eighty do. Food and bacteria can get trapped in the diverticula, causing them to become infected, inflamed, perforated or impacted. When this happens, diverticulitis results. Diverticulosis leads to diverticulitis in about 20 per cent of people.

Symptoms of Diverticulitis

The symptoms of diverticulitis include pain in the lower abdomen, cramping, constipation or diarrhoea, feeling of fullness and, if severe or caused by infection, fever, chills, nausea and vomiting. There may be blood in the stool. After an acute attack has passed, many people are lulled into believing that the disease is gone. But, left untreated, it can flare up repeatedly.

Preventing and Treating Diverticulitis with Diet

Since an improper diet is the primary cause of diverticulitis, it makes sense that correcting the diet is the most important step to prevention and recovery. Historically, doctors recommended a low-fibre diet with no fruit or vegetables. This approach is now known to be wrong. Diverticular disease is common in countries where low-fibre diets are the norm, but low or nonexistent in countries with high-fibre diets rich in fruits and vegetables.

So, increasing the fibre in the diet is the most important change to make. This change alone has been shown to prevent or relieve most cases of diverticulitis. A study published in the *British Medical Journal* confirmed that diverticulitis is primarily caused by a low fibre diet. In this study, seventy people with diverticulitis were placed on a high fibre diet of whole wheat bread, high bran cereal and lots of fruits and vegetables. The diet cured or substantially relieved symptoms in a whopping 89 per cent of participants[1].

Several studies show that high fibre diets protect against diverticular disease[2]. They also show that high fibre diets can treat, as well as prevent, diverticular disease[3]. Research has found a 50 per cent increase in diverticular disease in people with diets high in meat and low in vegetables[4].

Not only a high-fibre diet, but also fibre supplements have been shown to help in most, but not quite all[5], studies. One-third to one half of people with diverticular disease reduced their symptoms when supplementing the soluble fibre glucomannan (3 to 4g a day)[6], and psyllium has been shown in a preliminary study to help relieve symptoms[7]. Another study found long-term fibre supplementation protected against complications of the disease [8]. But the key is a high-fibre diet, plenty of fluid, as well as exercise like jogging or running[9]. Obesity may also increase the severity[10].

To help flush the intestines and prevent infection, you should drink at least eight glasses of water a day. Drink the water away from meals.

Find and avoid food allergens, since they can also contribute to the problem. Avoid sugar, processed foods, alcohol and refined grains, such as white bread, white rice and white pasta.

One of the most common dietary recommendations for people with diverticulosis is to avoid tiny, hard foods, such as nuts, seeds, corn and popcorn, that could get stuck in the diverticular sacs and cause infection, leading to the more serious diver-
ticulitis. However, there is very little evidence to support this fear. And a massive study published in the *Journal of the American Medical Association* has now shown that not only is the suspicion untrue, the opposite is true. The study followed 47,228 healthy people for eighteen years and found that, in those who got diverticulosis, there was not only no association between nuts, corn or popcorn and diverticular bleeding, but that people who ate the most nuts were actually 20 per cent less likely to get diverticulitis and those who ate the most popcorn were 28 per cent less likely[11]. So these foods may even help.

If during a severe attack you are having trouble eating anything at all, try eating slippery elm gruel. This herbal porridge has been safely used for centuries for all kinds of digestive problems. And, though "*gruel*" sounds gross, it actually tastes fine. To make slippery elm gruel, simply mix 1 tbsp of slippery elm with warm water to make a paste, as thin or thick as desired, and consume freely. Slippery elm is high in nutrition. It is also healing and soothing to the intestines. If you prefer, it can also be made into a tea. Mix a teaspoon of the powder with one cup of warm water and drink as often as desired throughout the day. If more food is desired and can be tolerated, try eating well-cooked, extra-wet brown rice that has been blended smooth. Consume 1 tbsp or more every hour or so, as can be tolerated.

When things have improved, other food can be

added, starting first with vegetables that have been well-steamed and blended smooth. Or drink juiced vegetables and fruits for easy digestibility and to encourage healing. Carrot juice is especially good. Avoid vegetables that cause gas and bloating at first or take digestive enzymes to help digest them. Open capsules if the enzyme is in a capsule or crush pills if the enzyme is in a pill. Small pills and capsules may get stuck in the pockets, so crush and open everything to be safe.

Treating Diverticulitis with Herbs

The herbal treatment for diverticular disease focuses on antispasmodics to relieve the abdominal pain from the cramping, anti-inflammatories to reduce the general inflammation in the colon, anti-microbials to deal with the infection, carminatives to deal with any gas, and nervines to deal with the stress that may either cause or result from the condition.

Wild yam is a really good choice of herbs because of its antispasmodic and anti-inflammatory actions and because of its specific action in the intestines. Try combining two parts wild yam, one part valerian, one part crampbark and 1 part peppermint into a tincture, and take 5 ml three times a day. A combination of slippery elm powder, marshmallow and cabbage powder, for healing; cranesbill, oak bark, raspberry or nettle to stop bleeding and diarrhea; echinacea, wild indigo, goldenseal or garlic for infection; valerian, pas-

sionflower, hops or skullcap for stress and cramping; and ginger, fennel, anise or peppermint for gas and bloating is very effective.

Other good strategies include sipping an infusion of chamomile slowly throughout the day, eating one clove of fresh garlic or taking a garlic supplement, taking one large teaspoon of slippery elm in water before each meal and taking a flavonoid-rich herb like grape seed extract or hawthorn to strengthen the connective tissue. Make sure you treat any constipation. And avoid smoking and stress, as they are also believed to be causes of the disease.

To prevent the recurrence of acute diverticulitis, herbal authorities Simon Mills and Kerry Bone also say to add immune-enhancing herbs, such as echinacea, and gastrointestinal antiseptics, like goldenseal or grapefruit seed extract. Michael Murray, N.D., also recommends goldenseal.

The high-fibre diet is crucial. During an acute attack, you may have to avoid the high fibre diet and follow a liquid diet. Then gradually increase the fibre again. After six months, Bone and Mills say you can come off the herbal treatment, but continue the high-fibre diet, the slippery elm and the garlic.

More Help

Other useful supplements include 1-3 tbsps of ground flaxseed in plenty of water two to three times a day, a few tablespoons a day of psyllium in lots of water, and wheat bran.

To heal and soothe the intestines, try aloe vera juice or licorice root (the DGL form of licorice may be best). Also try bitters, such as gentian or artichoke, for toning up the intestines, especially if you suffer from constipation. Take vitamin C in the calcium ascorbate form to reduce inflammation and promote healing, a B-complex to help with digestion, and calcium, magnesium and zinc to help heal up the intestines. Also try vitamin A to help heal the lining of the colon and vitamin E to protect the mucous membranes. Flaxseed oil is another important nutrient for healing up the gut. L-glutamine is also important for healing the intestines and providing fuel for the intestinal cells, and for helping to maintain the villi of the intestines, allowing for better absorption of nutrients. Also beneficial are greens such as chlorella, alfalfa, and spirulina, that are high in vitamin K for healing the intestines and chlorophyll for detoxifying and healing.

Since tissue in the intestines may be damaged, preventing the proper absorption of nutrients, it is a good idea to take a multivitamin/mineral for extra nutrients. Probiotics should be used to replenish damaged friendly flora in the intestines. Friendly flora help to digest food and absorb nutrients and are damaged when antibiotics are used.

Chapter Endnotes

1. Painter N. S, et al. "Unprocessed Bran in Treatment of Diverticular Disease of the Colon." *BMJ*, 1972; 2:137.

2. Handler S. Dietary fibre: "Can it prevent certain colonic diseases?" *Postgrad Med* 1983; 73:301–7.

3. Elfrink R. J., Miedema BW. "Colonic diverticula. When complications require surgery and when they don't." *Postgrad Med* 1992; 92:97–8, 101–2, 105, 108.

4. Manousos O., *et al.* "Diet and other factors in the aetiology of diverticulosis: an epidemiological study in Greece." *Gut* 1985; 26:544–9.

5. Ornstein M. H., *et al.* "Are fibre supplements really necessary in diverticular disease of the colon? A controlled clinical trial." *Br Med J (Clin Res Ed)* 1981; 25:1353–6.

6. Papi C., *et al.* "Efficacy of rifaximin in the treatment of symptomatic diverticular disease of the colon. A multicentre double-blind placebo-controlled trial." *Aliment Pharmacol Ther* 1995;9:33–9.

7. Ewerth S., *et al.* "Influence on symptoms and transit-time of Vi-SiblinR in diverticular disease." *Acta Chir Scand Suppl* 1980; 500:49–50.

8. Leahy A. L., et al. "High fibre diet in symptomatic diverticular disease of the colon." A*nn R Coll Surg Engl* 1985; 67:173–4.

9. Aldoori W. H., *et al.* "Prospective study of physical activity and the risk of symptomatic diverticular disease in men." *Gut* 1995; 36:276–82.

10. Ozick L. A., Salazar C. O., "Donelson SS. Pathogenesis, diagnosis, and treatment of diverticular disease of the colon". *Gastroenterologist* 1995; 6:55–63.

11. Strate LL, *et al.* "Nut, corn, and popcorn consumption and the incidence of diverticular disease." *JAMA*, 2008; 300:907-14.

ECZEMA

It strikes more infants than adults, but adults are not immune. Up to 7 per cent of the population suffers from it. Their skin becomes itchy, inflamed, dry, and thickened, and may form small blisters that weep. The skin grows red on the wrists, face, and inside of the elbows and knees. There may even be a family history of asthma. What do these people have? Eczema.

Also called atopic dermatitis, eczema is a chronic problem that can be difficult to get rid of, especially if you decide to try conventional medicine. Antihistamines and cortisone cream are the standard treatments used in conventional medicine. While they may relieve the symptoms in some cases, they do nothing to address the underlying causes of the illness. They are also riddled with side effects, such as fatigue, adrenal burnout, and thinning of the skin.

Can natural medicine help? The answer is yes. But it does take time and commitment. Current research suggests that eczema is an allergic disease. As many as 80 per cent of patients show elevated antibody levels. All eczema patients have positive allergy tests, including food allergy. While the traditional test for allergies, the scratch test, is still performed in Canada, it will only catch 15 per cent of all food and other allergies. The better test is the Eliza test, which can be performed by your doctor in Canada, after he or she orders the Eliza kit from a lab in the States. This test is far more accurate. Or an elimination rotation diet can be used to try and identify and eliminate allergens. Most eczema patients improve on a diet that eliminates common food allergens.

What Are the Most Common Foods to Avoid?

Studies show that the biggest culprit in infants is milk. When milk is eliminated from the infant's diet, and from the mother's if she is breast-feeding, the child tends to get better. If he does not, it is probably because there are still more allergens. The other most common allergens in both children and adults are wheat, citrus, eggs, fish, soy, tomato, and peanuts. Other foods that clearly cause problems include sugar, alcohol, caffeine, refined grains, additives, and chemicals. High consumption of animal proteins is also problematic and should be avoided. It is a good idea to work with a natural healer to determine food allergens and develop a healthy diet that can be maintained. Food allergens, once they have been avoided for a time, can often be reintroduced slowly and consumed occasionally.

What Are the Best Foods to Consume?

The diet should be high in vegetables, whole

grains, fruits, legumes, and seeds and nuts. If any animal protein is consumed, the best choices are fatty fish, such as mackerel, herring, and salmon, since they are high in essential fatty acids and can help to decrease inflammatory prosta-glandins that cause the skin inflammation. Otherwise, animal protein is strongly implicated in eczema. The best EFAs include flaxseed oil and hemp oil. Other good sources of EFAs are borage oil and evening primrose oil. Or use a blend of oils. These oils actually inhibit inflammation and decrease allergic response. People with eczema have an EFA deficiency, or they are deficient in zinc, which helps in the conversion of EFAs. Take 1 to 2 tbsps a day of EFAs.

The Role of Low Stomach Acid

People with eczema often have low stomach acid, as do people with food allergies, so it is not surprising that eczema patients have this problem, since they have both. The best remedy for low stomach acid is to take hydrochloric acid pills. At the same time, herbs or enzymes that help with the digestive system are a good idea. Wide-spectrum plant enzymes are useful, or bitters that tone the entire digestive system and help to increase secretions so that food is properly digested and absorbed. Take HCL or digestive enzymes before each meal.

The Role of Stress

Stress can aggravate eczema. People with eczema tend to have higher levels of anxiety, hostility, and neurosis. So it seems that it is a good idea to take relaxant herbs during an attack to try to decrease stress and reduce the itching. Use herbs such as linden flower, valerian root, scullcap, passionflower, kava, if available, and hops—just keep in mind that any herb can be an allergen and should first be tested in those with eczema.

Candida Connection

Many people with skin problems have an unbalanced gut environment. Overgrowth of yeast, such as candida, and lack of friendly flora lead to decreased absorption of nutrients and inflammatory conditions in the skin, since that can cause leaky gut syndrome. Leaky-gut syndrome occurs when matter that should stay in the intestines passes into the blood-stream, causing allergies, inflammation, skin, and other problems. Anyone who has eczema should try taking probiotics, such as acidophilus and bifidus (between 1 to 20 billion live cells a day) and perhaps something such as grapefruit-seed extract (15 drops three times a day in water) to wipe out harmful microorganisms. This herb is cooling and can help get rid of the damp heat in the intestines that often accompanies eczema.

What are some of the best nutrients for treating eczema?

Bioflavonoids

Bioflavonoids help the activity of vitamin C, increasing its effectiveness. They are also great for inflammatory and allergic conditions. They work by inhibiting the inflammatory process. The dosage will depend on which one you take.

Quercetin

If flavonoids are among the most important anti-inflammatories for eczema, then quercetin is the most important flavonoid for this purpose. It actually stops the release of the inflammation-causing histamine into the body, preventing allergic reactions. Take 400 mg twenty minutes before each meal. Or try using flavonoid-rich herbs, such as blueberry leaf, bilberry, and hawthorn. They contain quercetin as well as other powerful flavonoids. They are extremely powerful inflammatory inhibitors. Because of its flavonoids, and for other reasons, the herb *Ginkgo biloba* may prove helpful.

Vitamins A, E, C

Vitamin A helps develop and maintain skin. It is of particular use to those who suffer from thickening of the skin, commonly seen in eczema patients. Take 5,000 mg a day.

Vitamin C helps the immune system and can be helpful for treating allergies. Take 1 to 10 g of the calcium ascorbate form a day. Both vitamins E and C are involved in skin health. Vitamin E can help to prevent scarring. Take 400 IU of mixed tocopherols a day.

Zinc

Zinc helps an enzyme produce hydrochloric acid in the stomach. It also helps to convert essential fatty acids to anti-inflammatory prostaglandins. Since there is a connection between low stomach acid and eczema, zinc can be of particular help to those with eczema. Take 45 to 60 mg a day, with 3 mg of copper for balance.

Licorice Root and *Coleus Forskolii*

The herbs licorice and *Coleus forskolii* are both extremely valuable in treating eczema. They help to reduce excessive histamine production. Take 1 to 2 gm of licorice, three times a day. Of *Coleus forskolii*, take 50 mg, standardized to contain 18 per cent forskolin, three times a day.

Burdock Root

Burdock root has been used for centuries in the treatment of skin diseases. It is an alterative herb, i.e., a herb that gradually changes the condition of the body to reduce morbid matter, clearing away toxins. It is the seeds and the root of this plant that have been traditionally used to treat skin problems. Burdock is also a blood purifier and a diaphoretic that helps the sweat glands to flush out toxic wastes. Take 40 to 80 drops of a tincture, three times a day.

Traditional Herbal Formula

For skin problems, burdock is often combined with dandelion root, a herb that cleanses and strengthens the liver and kidneys and also aids digestion; sarsaparilla, an anti-inflammatory, alterative, and diaphoretic herb (a herb that induces sweating) that clears heat from the body; sassafras, another alterative herb, diaphoretic, and a blood purifier; yellow dock, an alterative herb and a blood tonic that also clears toxins from the liver; and red clover, an alterative herb that is used for skin diseases. Usually a tea is decocted: 4 tsps of the herbs mixed with 4 cups of cold water, boiled, covered, and then simmered for 40 minutes. Drink three cups a day.

Topical Help

Topical application of chamomile and licorice root is of particular benefit to those with eczema. These two herbs have been shown to work as well or better than cortisone cream when applied topically[1]. And they are without the harmful side effects of cortisone cream; that is, they do not stress the adrenal glands nor do they thin the skin.

Other topical help comes from herbs such as calendula, comfrey, aloe vera, and essential fatty acid. Apply as creams or in poultices three times or more a day.

Final Helpful Touches

Be sure to get all toxins and chemicals out of your environment. Eat organic food and use only personal and household cleaners that are made from natural ingredients. Chemicals increase the load on the immune system, and many people with eczema react to them. Also try to avoid exposure to cardboard and metal against the skin. These two substances seem to aggravate eczema. Linda has seen several clients whose children were reacting to metal jewellery, metal objects that the child played with, and even to a metal headboard. It may seem strange, but sometimes this last step can make all the difference and help to clear up a stubborn case of eczema.

Chapter Endnotes

1. Evans, F. Q. "The rational use of glycyrrhetinic acid in dermatology." Br J Clin Pract, 1958; 12:269'79; Della Loggia, R., et al. "Evaluation of the anti-inflammatory activity of chamomile preparations." Planta Medica, 1990; 56:657'58; Nissen, H. P., H. Blitz, H. W. Kreyel. "Prolifometrie, eine methode zur beurteilung der therapeutischen wirsamkeit kon Kamillosan®-Salbe." Z Hautkr, 1988; 63:184-90; Aergeerts, P., et al. "Vergleichende prüfung von Kamillosan®-creme gegenüber seroidalen (0.25 per cent hydrocortison, 0.75 per cent flucotinbutylester) and nichseroidaseln (5 per cent bufexamac) externa in der erhaltungsterpaie von ekzemerkrankungen." Z Hautkr, 1985; 60:270-77.

HIV/AIDS

The numbers remain staggering. Even with the triple cocktail of antiretroviral drugs, there are an estimated 33.3 million people in the world today with HIV/AIDS, according to the UNAIDS/WHO statistics for 2009. In 2009, there were 2.6 million newly infected people, and 1.8 million people died of AIDS. Those numbers are incomprehensible. Though North America is far from being the continent that is most severely affected, the problem here is severe nonetheless: in 2009, there were 1.5 million people infected with HIV/AIDS on this continent.

Even with the availability of antiretroviral drugs, if natural therapies could help it would be a huge advance for several reasons: resistance to the triple cocktail, expense and availability of the triple cocktail, its side effects and the continuing problem of rebuilding immunity.

This chapter in no way claims that the supplements discussed are cures for HIV/AIDS. But it is a survey of herbs and nutrients that show exciting promise as natural supplements that may be of help to the people behind the staggering numbers above.

Things to watch for to show a supplement may help are studies showing that a supplement can inhibit the progress of HIV to AIDS, that it can increase the number of helper lymphocytes known as CD4 or that it can protect against opportunistic infections.

RESEARCH ON HIV/AIDS: THE PROMISE OF NATURAL HEALTH

SUPPLEMENT	WHAT THE RESEARCH SAYS	SOURCE
Vitamin E	Two articles reviewing the literature on vitamin E and AIDS both conclude that vitamin E may slow the progression of AIDS. It also increases the effectiveness of the AIDS drug AZT.	*Biochem Biophys Res Commun* 1989; *Prog Food Nutr Sci* 1991; *Prog Food Nutr Sci* 1993
	Men with the highest blood levels of vitamin E have a 34 per cent decrease in the risk of progression to AIDS than men with the lowest levels.	*AIDS* 1997
	Antiretroviral therapy for HIV is significantly more effective in reducing viral loads when it is combined with 800mg a day of vitamin E.	*Clin Chem Lab Med* 2002
Multivitamin/ mineral	People with HIV and people with AIDS were given either a high potency multivitamin/mineral or a placebo for 48 weeks. Mortality was significantly lower in the multi group: 6 per cent of the placebo group passed away in that time compared to 3 per cent in the multi group. The benefit was seen only in the AIDS group, not the HIV group.	*AIDS* 2003

	HIV infected pregnant women were given either a multivitamin or a placebo for almost six years. During the first two years, the women on the multi were 59 per cent less likely to progress to the most serious stage four or to die from AIDS than the women on the placebo. The number was still 29 per cent at the end of the study. The women who took the multi had significantly less AIDS symptoms and higher levels of immune cells than the women on the placebo.	*New England Journal of Medicine* 2004
	HIV positive men who were given a multivitamin/mineral had a slower onset of AIDS than men who were not given the multi.	*Med Tribune* 1993
N-Acetylcysteine (NAC)	NAC inhibits replication of HIV in test tubes	*Proc Natl Acad Sci* 1990
	800mg a day of NAC slowed the decline of immune function in people with HIV.	*Proc Natl Acad Sci* 1997
	NAC increased CD4 counts in a double-blind, placebo-controlled study.	*Eur J Clin Pharmacol* 1996
	CD4 cell count increased faster in people given 600mg of NAC per day along with their antiretroviral therapy than in those given a placebo.	*Clin Chem Lab Med* 2002
Selenium	A deficiency of selenium is associated with a high mortality rate in HIV positive people.	*J Acquir Immune Defic Syndr Hum Retroviral* 1997
	HIV positive people who were given selenium had fewer infections and better appetite.	*Biol Trace Elem Res* 1989
	200mcg of selenium a day decreased HIV viral load and increased CD4 counts.	*Arch Intern Med* 2007
Zinc	People with HIV are often low in zinc.	*JAMA* 1988; *J Nutr* 2000
	45mg of zinc per day reduces the number of opportunistic infections in people with AIDS who are taking the AIDS drug AZT.	*Int J Immunopharmacol* 1995
	Zinc increases CD4 counts, reduces viral load and reduces risk of recurrent opportunistic infections in stage IV patients on the AIDS drug AZT.	*J Nutr* 2000
B Vitamins	In people who are HIV positive and who have B vitamin deficiencies, supplementing with a B complex delays progression to, and death from, AIDS.	*J Acquir Immune Defic Syndr* 1999
	B6 improved survival in HIV positive people.	*Am J Epidemiol* 1996

	Niacinamide (B3) inhibits HIV in test tubes. HIV-positive people who consume more than 64mg of B3 per day have a decreased risk of progression to AIDS or AIDS-related deaths.	*Biochem Biophys Res Commun* 1995; *Am J Epidemiol* 1996; *Am J Epidemiol* 1996
Betacarotene & Vitamin A	Vitamin A deficiency is common in people with HIV and is associated with more severe disease.	*Arch Intern Med* 1993
	180mg a day of betacarotene for four weeks increased CD4 counts by 17 per cent in people with HIV.	*J AIDS* 1993
	Natural mixed carotenes significantly prolonged survival time in adults with advanced AIDS who were on conventional therapy and a multivitamin.	*Eur J Clin Nutr* 2006
Coenzyme Q10	CoQ10 is low in people with HIV or AIDS, and preliminary research suggests that 200mg a day of CoQ10 may improve ability to fight infection.	*Biochem Biophys Res Commun* 1988
	100mg a day of CoQ10 increases blood loads of CD4.	*Biochem Biophys Res Commun* 1993
Licorice	Licorice inhibits the reproduction of HIV in test tubes. Preliminary double-blind research suggests that licorice is safe and effective, and better than a placebo, for long term treatment of HIV.	*Antivir Res* 1988 *Int Conf AIDS* 1993
	When 10 people with HIV were given glycyrrhizin from licorice for 1-2 years, none developed AIDS. Of ten people not given glycyrrhizin, three progressed to AIDS and two died.	*5th Int Conf AIDS* 1989
Boxwood	990mg a day of boxwood extract given to people with HIV caused fewer drops in CD4 counts and fewer increases in viral load than a placebo. It also slowed the rate of HIV progression.	*Phytomed* 1998
Cat's Claw	People with AIDS given cat's claw recovered from their opportunistic infections and increased their CD4 counts. CD4 counts remained stable and did not drop for four years.	*Keplinge U,* 1993
Garlic	Garlic reduces the number of infections in people with AIDS.	*Dtsch Zschr Onkol* 1989
Ginseng	A preliminary study found that red Asian ginseng benefitted people with HIV and increased the effectiveness of the AIDS drug AZT.	*Int Conf AIDS* 1994
Echinacea	In a double-blind study, echinacea angustifolia root increased immune activity against HIV.	*Int Conf AIDS* 1998

Other Supplements That May Help
Curcumin, Lipoic Acid, Shiitake Mushroom, Reishi Mushroom, Eleuthero, Bromelain, Vitamin C

INSOMNIA

One of the growing problems that many people are facing in these stressful times is the inability to fall asleep or to stay asleep. Most people would agree that this problem is due to an increased workload, pressure, and stress, which create anxiety, preventing people from relaxing into a deep, natural sleep. Also, diet and lifestyle choices, such as caffeine and alcohol, can contribute to the problem. While taking conventional sleeping pills may give relief for some, they are not without their problems, most notably, many users experience a spaced-out feeling and fatigue the next day. More seriously, they can also be addictive, can cause memory problems, nervousness, confusion, depression, and other undesirable behaviour, as well as inhibiting normal sleep by suppressing REM sleep, leading to the morning hangover feeling. Fortunately, there are a number of natural herbs that create sleep without causing any ill effects the next day. Also, these herbs work to correct the problem, enabling people to achieve a more natural sleep. Let's take a closer look at some of these herbs.

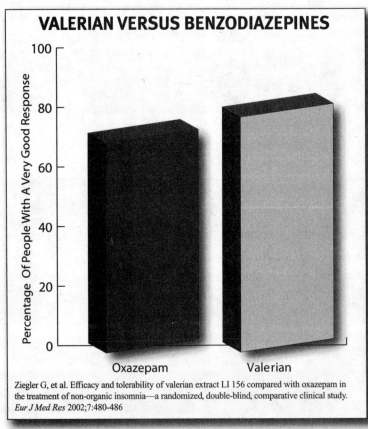

VALERIAN VERSUS BENZODIAZEPINES

Percentage Of People With A Very Good Response

Oxazepam   Valerian

Ziegler G, et al. Efficacy and tolerability of valerian extract LI 156 compared with oxazepam in the treatment of non-organic insomnia—a randomized, double-blind, comparative clinical study. *Eur J Med Res* 2002;7:480-486

St. John's Wort

With this herb making the news lately for its ability to treat depression, most of us have heard of St. John's wort, but this herb is not just for depression; it has many other uses, including the ability to induce a deeper level of sleep. Although it does not directly reduce the time of sleep onset, studies on brain waves have shown that St. John's wort improves the quality of sleep by increasing the intensity of deep sleep. Michael Murray, N.D., cites a study in his book, *The Healing Power of Herbs*, that shows that St. John's wort reduces feelings of anxiety, hypersomnia, and insomnia without side effects. This means that St. John's wort can be helpful both to those who can't sleep well and to those who can't stay awake. Even those suffering from sleep problems due to depression can greatly benefit from this herb.

Valerian

Probably the best-known herb for treating insomnia is valerian. Valerian is a sedative that also helps with anxiety, nervous debility, restlessness, weakness, irritation, and hysteria. Several studies have confirmed valerian's ability to improve sleep quality as well as the time taken to fall asleep, both in people who are suffering from insomnia and in those who are not. And it does so without producing morning sleepiness or impairing mental function. It also does not produce dependency and can, therefore, be used for prolonged periods of time. Recent studies have even found that valerian works better than benzodiazepines, the most commonly used medications for insomnia[1].

Herb expert Steven Foster explains that valerian actually normalizes the central nervous system, acting as a sedative when a person is agitated, but stimulating when there is extreme fatigue. This feature of valerian is very important, since those people who are just too tired to fall asleep can actually be stimulated by valerian just enough to allow a natural sleep to occur. People with chronic fatigue immune dysfunction syndrome often find that a combination of valerian mixed with St. John's wort greatly increases both the quality and duration of sleep, and that it helps them get to sleep faster. Clinically, Linda gets great results when she combines skullcap and passionflower with valerian for people who can't fall asleep because they can't stop thinking.

Skullcap

Another widely used nervine that is useful against depression, anxiety, and insomnia is skullcap. It relaxes nervous tension while at the same time reviving the central nervous system. Herbalist David Hoffman refers to skullcap as the most widely relevant nervine, while herbalist Michael Tierra says that it produces inner calm and counteracts sleeplessness. Old-time herbalists claim that skullcap is extremely useful in restless and wakeful conditions. Its influence extends to the spinal cord and sympathetic nervous system. It even has a place in treating the delirium of fevers, nervous headache, facial neuralgia and in calming patients who are experiencing psychological problems. Herb authority Paul Bergman says that it is great for exhaustion and tension and that it helps you relax throughout the day so that you prepare for sleep at night. It nourishes and energizes the nervous system and calms it.

Kava Kava

One of the best-known herbs for reducing anxiety is kava, and kava can also reduce insomnia. It has been extensively used by the Polynesian people for many years. Visitors to areas where the people regularly consume kava as a tea in their ceremonies claim that these people are the happiest, calmest people in the world. Kava is also not associated with depressed mental function or impairment in driving or in operating heavy machinery. In fact, kava improves mental function.

Kava has been in the news recently because of claims that it is liver-toxic. But the actual evidence against kava is very weak. It turns out that at least eighteen of the twenty-four people who experienced toxicity were using drugs that were liver-toxic at the same time. At least four analyses of the case reports have found no evidence that the liver damage was caused by kava, and that kava is safe. Studies have never found kava to be toxic to the liver. And certainly it has safely been used for thousands of years by people all over the world without anyone ever dying of it before. So what does this mean? Don't use kava if you are on liver toxic drugs, if you have liver disease, if you regularly drink alcohol, or if you are in the 10 per cent of the population whose liver does not detoxify properly.

Having said all of that, why would you want to use kava? Because the anxiety drugs are definitely toxic and because kava is so wonderful for people who are anxious. Kava is one of the best herbs for reducing anxiety, and it has also been shown to reduce insomnia.

Lady's Slipper

This herb is almost a pure nervine and relaxant. Old-time herbalists would use it to calm nervous tension, allowing the patient to sleep calmly and awaken refreshed. In hysteria, headache, sleeplessness, or any irritation arising from weakened nerves, it is of use. Lady's slipper was used traditionally by several of the First Nations of North America as a nervine and sedative. Later it became an accepted home cure for insomnia in American medicine. A nineteenth-century medical botanist named Rafinesque wrote that lady's slipper "produce[s] beneficial effects in all nervous diseases and hysterical affections, by allaying pain, quieting the nerves and promoting sleep."

David Hoffman writes that lady's slipper is one of the most widely applicable nervines that we have. He also says that it is useful for stress, tension, anxiety, and to elevate mood, and that it is at its best when treating anxiety that is associated with insomnia.

Passionflower

Passionflower is very gentle and effective against insomnia, and may be the best tranquillizer yet. Like valerian, it is helpful in both anxiety and insomnia. Recent studies suggest that it may be as effective for anxiety as kava, since it, too, has been shown to be as good as benzodiazepines without the side effects of the drugs[2]. Bergner says it is a reliable herb that induces safe and natural sleep, with no hangover effect. Hoffman says it is one of the best herbs for stubborn insomnia. It helps people to turn off their thoughts and to stop worrying, and it removes tension that prevents people from falling asleep. Clinically, Linda has found passionflower to be an excellent herb for people who are nervous, anxious, and don't sleep because they can't turn off their thoughts. It is also excellent for anxiety when taken throughout the day.

Catnip

For those suffering from built-up emotional tension, try catnip, which, according to Tierra, is extremely helpful for this condition. Although catnip seems to drive cats wild, it is actually a sedative for humans that soothes the nervous system. Use it during the day for relief of nervous tension that prevents you from sleeping at night.

Hops

Hops is a sedative, relaxing nervine that is also able to stimulate. The hops pillow has been a traditional remedy for insomnia for centuries. Hops will soothe and quiet the nervous system. In nervous troubles and delirium, hops has a most soothing effect that will frequently promote sleep in people in an overwrought condition.

Lemon Balm, Linden Flower, Poppy, Lemon Verbena, and Lavender

Lemon balm is a calming herb that is useful for depression and nervous tension. Linden flowers are a nervine, lower blood pressure, and are calming. Poppy is a sedative that is wonderful for insomnia and anxiety and for relieving pain that can stop people from sleeping. Linda gets very good results with California poppy.

Also try lavender and lemon verbena. Lemon verbena is one of our favourite herbs and works well to induce sleep. Inhaling lavender oil can help you sleep as well as sleeping medications[3].

You can frequently combine the properties of several herbs to achieve a deep, lasting sleep. And they come in many forms, too. For those who prefer capsules or tablets, there are several individual herbs as well as combinations, and there are also tinctures, teas, and the loose herbs so that you can create your own combinations in the form best suited to your needs. Important combinations include valerian with lemon balm[4] and valerian with hops[5].

More Help

Probably the best non-herbal nutrient for insomnia is 5-HTP. This amazing nutrient keeps you in REM sleep and deep sleep for a longer portion of your nightly slumber.

Deficiencies in B vitamins, calcium, magnesium, potassium, and essential fatty acids can cause insomnia, too. So take 1200 mg of calcium, 600 mg of magnesium, a B-complex, and a multivitamin/mineral and, if needed, use flaxseed oil. If blood-sugar control problems are present, chromium can help stabilize blood-sugar and help with sleep.

Also try acupuncture. In Linda's clinic, it has been one of the most effective means of relieving tension and anxiety and inducing sleep.

And don't forget exercise, proper diet, full spectrum light sources, and meditation, all of which can greatly aid sleep.

Chapter Endnotes

1. Dorn, M. "Efficacy and tolerability of Baldrian versus oxazepam: efficacy and tolerability in non-organic and non-psychiatric insomniacs: a randomized, double-blind, clinical, comparative study." *Forsch KomplementärmedKlass Naturheilkd*, 2000; 7:79-84; Ziegler, G., *et al*. "Efficacy and tolerability of valerian extract LI 156 compared with oxazepam in the treatment of non-organic insomnia-a randomized, double-blind, comparative clinical study." *Eur J Med Res*, 2002; 7:480-86.

2. Akhondzadeh, S., *et al*. "Passionflower in the treatment of generalized anxiety: a pilot double-blind randomized controlled trial with oxazepam." *J Clin Pharm Ther*, 2001; 26:363-67.

3. Hardy, M., M. D. Kirk-Smith, D.D. Stretch. "Replacement of drug therapy for insomnia by ambient odour." *Lancet*, 1995; 346:701 [letter]; Lewith, G.T., A.D. Godfrey, P. Prescott. "A single-blinded, randomized pilot study evaluating the aroma of Lavandula augustifolia as a treatment for mild insomnia." *J Altern Complement Med*, 2005; 11:631-37.

4. Dressing, H., *et al*. Insomnia: "Are valerian/balm combination of equal value to benzodiazepine?" *Therapiewoche*, 1992; 42:726-36; Dressing, H., S. Köhler, W. E. Müller. "Improvement of sleep quality with a high-dose valerian/lemon balm preparation: A placebo-controlled double-blind study." *Psychopharmakotherapie*, 1996; 6:32-40; Cerny, A., K. Schmid. "Tolerability and efficacy of valerian/lemon balm in healthy volunteers: A double-blind, placebo-controlled, multicentre study." *Fitoterapia*, 1999; 70:321'28.

5. Schmitz, M., M. Jackel. "Comparative study for assessing quality of life of patients with exogenous sleep disorders (temporary sleep onset and sleep interruption disorders) treated with a hops-valerian preparation and a benzodiazepine drug." *Wien Med Wochenschr*, 1998; 148:291'98; Fussel, A., A. Wolf, A. Brattstrom. "Effect of a fixed valerian-hop extract combination (Ze 9109) on sleep polygraphy in patients with non-organic insomnia: A pilot study." *Eur J Med Res*, 2000; 5:385'90.

IRRITABLE BOWEL SYNDROME

Of all the many disorders of the gastrointestinal tract, irritable bowel syndrome is the most common, affecting perhaps as many as 15 per cent of all people. That's a lot of people who need help from this painful and uncomfortable condition. Fortunately, this help is available from nature.

Start with Diet

The pain and bloating is in the digestive system, so it makes sense to start with diet. Two-thirds of IBS sufferers have intolerances to at least one food[1], and many improve when that food is eliminated. The most common culprits are dairy and grains. Refined sugar is also an important contributor[2]. Other sugars can be a big problem too. Some people with IBS have trouble absorbing the lactose in dairy, the concentrated fructose in fruit juice and dried fruit and sorbitol[3]. One double-blind study found that when people who have both IBS and lactose intolerance eliminate lactose from their diet, they relieve the symptoms of their IBS[4]. The lactose-digesting enzyme lactase may also help.

Having identified and gotten rid of the bad foods, now try adding the good ones. And, as long as it does not come in the form of wheat bran, fibre is a good one. Fibre helps IBS[5]. Because grains are a common food sensitivity in people with IBS, try increasing dietary fibre from fruits and vegetables.

So, putting it all together, the IBS diet should eliminate food sensitivities, especially dairy, as well as refined sugar, fructose from juice and dried fruit, sorbitol and caffeine, too. It should limit refined foods and emphasize fibre-rich fruits and vegetables.

Helpful Supplements

Since fibre is so important for IBS, it comes as no surprise that double-blind research identifies psyllium as an effective reliever of symptoms[6].

A number of the supplements and dietary changes that benefit IBS suggest a role for candida and disrupted flora in the colon as underlying factors. Remember that refined and other sugars are an important factor in IBS, and sugar is the primary food of candida. Psyllium and dietary fibre may also help in part because fibre positively affects the bacteria in the colon.

Perhaps it is at least partially for this reason that double-blind research has found that probiotics significantly relieve the symptoms of IBS compared to a placebo[7]. Preliminary research also points to grapefruit-seed extract capsules, another important candida killer, as a potential IBS fighter[8].

The Most Important Help of All

The most important supplement for IBS is peppermint oil. Peppermint oil is effective at killing candida, but peppermint oil's most important contribution to IBS is that it is highly effective at improving the contractions of the intestine and relieving intestinal cramping, while also easing gas and soothing irritation.

All kinds of double-blind research has proven peppermint oil's effectiveness[9]. Peppermint oil reduces abdominal pain, bloating, gas and bowel-movement frequency in about 80 per cent of people, according to one well designed double-blind study[10]. One of the most recent double-blind studies found that there was a greater than 50 per cent improvement in symptoms in 75 per cent of people given peppermint oil compared to only 38 per cent of people given a placebo[11].

Two meta-analyses of controlled studies have concluded that peppermint oil helps relieve the symptoms of IBS[12].

But the most important and exciting peppermint oil study of all found that, when combined with caraway oil, the peppermint oil was even more effective than the drug cisapride[13].

Other double-blind research has also found this combination effective. Peppermint oil combined with caraway oil in both enteric-coated[14] and non-enteric coated[15] capsules has been found to significantly reduce the symptoms of IBS.

Peppermint oil is usually taken in the form of enteric-coated capsules. The non-enteric coated may actually work just as well, but the enteric-coated ones are more studied and may be better tolerated. The usual dose is 2 to 4 ml three times a day.

Double-blind research has also found that half that dose is effective for helping older children with IBS[16].

Still More Help

A little-discussed but amazing herb for digestive problems is artichoke. Several studies have found artichoke has impressive powers to relieve abdominal pain, gas and bloating. And one preliminary study found that artichoke leaf extract improved symptoms in 26 per cent of people with IBS[17].

In an unexpected result, two double-blind studies have found that melatonin helps IBS sufferers[18].

Worrying Just Makes it Worse

Though stress does not cause IBS, once you have IBS, it does make it worse. Two-thirds of people with IBS do better when their conventional treatment is combined with psychotherapy and relaxation than when they have conventional treatment alone. Thus, relaxing herbs may also help.

Herbal Combinations

Approaching IBS from all of its different angles,

herbal authorities Kerry Bone and Simon Mills suggest a formula that includes an antispasmodic herb, such as chamomile, cramp bark or peppermint, a calming herb, such as skullcap or valerian, a liver herb, such as milk thistle (artichoke might be a great alternative here), a soothing herb, such as slippery elm, and a gastrointestinal antiseptic that restores proper flora in the colon, like goldenseal or grapefruit seed extract.

For soothing the digestive system, herbalist Christopher Hobbs suggests combining one part flax seed, one part marshmallow root, and one part fenugreek with a quarter part licorice and a quarter part caraway seed: an excellent formula whenever you need to soothe the digestive tract.

Chapter Endnotes

1. Jones ,A., et al. "Food intolerance: A major factor in the pathogenesis of irritable bowel syndrome." Lancet 1982; ii:1115–7

2. Russo, A, R., M. Fraser, Horowitz, "The effect of acute hyperglycemia on small intestinal motility in normal subjects." Diabetologia, 1996; 39:984-89.

3. Fernandez-Banares, F., et al. "Sugar malabsorption in functional bowel disease: clinical implications." Am J Gastroenterol 1993; 88:2044–50; Choi Y. K., et al. "Fructose intolerance in IBS and utility of fructose-restricted diet." J Clin Gastroenterol 2008; 42:233–38.

4. Bohmer, C. J , H. A. Tuynman, "The clinical relevance of lactose malabsorption in irritable bowel syndrome." Eur J Gastroenterol Hepatol 1996; 8:1013-16.

5. Manning, A. P. et al. "Wheat fibre and irritable bowel syndrome." Lancet 1977; ii:417–8; Hotz J, K. Plein, "Effectiveness of plantago seed husks in comparison with wheat bran no stool frequency and manifestations of irritable colon syndrome with constipation." Med Klin 1994; 89:645–51.

6. Prior A., Whorwell P. J. Double blind study of ispaghula irritable bowel syndrome. Gut 1987; 11:1510-13; Jalihal A., Kurian G., Ispaghula therapy in irritable bowel syndrome: improvement in overall Well-being is related to reduction in bowel dissatisfunction. J Gastroenterol Heputol 1990;5:507-13

7. Kajander, K. et al. "Clinical trial: multispecies probiotic supplementation alleviates the symptoms of irritable bowel syndrome and stabilizes intestinal microbiota." Aliment Pharmacol Ther 2008; 27:48–57.

8. Ionescu, G. et al. "Oral citrus seed extract in atopic eczema: In vitro and in vivo studies on intestinal microflora." J Orthomol Med 1990; 5:155–58.

9. Rees, W. D., B. K. Evans, J. Rhodes, "Treating irritable bowel syndrome with peppermint oil." Br Med J, 1979; 2:835–56; Dew M. J., B. K. Evans, Rhodes J. "Peppermint oil for the irritable bowel syndrome: A multi-center trial." Br J Clin Pract 1984; 38:394–98.

10. Liu, J-H, et al. "Enteric-coated peppermint-oil capsules in the treatment of irritable bowel syndrome: a prospective, randomized trial." J Gastroenterol 1997; 32:765–68.

11. Cappello, G, et al. "Peppermint oil (Mintoil) in the treatment of irritable bowel syndrome: a prospective double-blind placebo-controlled randomized trial." Dig Liver Dis, 2007; 39:530–36.

12. Poynard, T. et al. "Meta-analysis of smooth muscle relaxants in the treatment of irritable bowel syndrome." Aliment Pharmacol Ther 1994; 8:499–510; Pittler, M.H. E. Ernst, "Peppermint oil for irritable bowel syndrome: a critical review and metaanalysis." Am J Gastroenterol, 1998; 93:1131–15.

13. Madisch, A. et al. "Treatment of functional dyspepsia with a fixed peppermint oil and caraway oil combination preparation as compared to cisapride." Arneimittlforschung, 1999; 49:925–32.

14. May, B., H. D. Kuntz, M. Kieser, S. Kohler, "Efficacy of a fixed peppermint/caraway oil combination in non-ulcer dyspepsia." Arzneimittelforschung, 1996;46:1149–53.

15. Friese, J., S. Köhler, "Peppermint/caraway oil-fixed combination in non-ulcer dyspepsia: equivalent efficacy of the drug combination in an enteric coated or enteric soluble formula." Pharmazie 1999; 54:210–15.

16. Kline, R. M., et al. "Enteric-coated, pH-dependent peppermint oil capsules for the treatment of irritable bowel syndrome in children." J Pediatr, 2001; 138:125-8.

17. Bundy, R. et al. "Artichoke leaf extract reduces symptoms of irritable bowel syndrome and improves quality of life in otherwise healthy volunteers suffering from concomitant dyspepsia: a subset analysis." J Altern Complement Med, 2004; 10:667–9.

18. Song, G. H., et al. "Melatonin improves abdominal pain in irritable bowel syndrome patients who have sleep disturbances: a randomised, double-blind, placebo controlled study." Gut, 2005; 54:1402–407; Saha, L. et al. "A preliminary study of melatonin in irritable bowel syndrome." J Clin Gastroenterol, 2007; 41:29–32.

KIDNEY STONES

Ten per cent of all males and 5 per cent of all females will experience one of the most painful things mankind can have: kidney stones. One in one thousand patients who are admitted to the hospital are admitted for kidney stones. Yet, in most cases, kidney stones are preventable.

Some of the factors that can cause kidney stones are urine retention, heavy metals in the body, and a diet that is high in animal foods, low in fibre, high in refined carbohydrates, high in alcohol, high in salt, high in vitamin D, and high in fat. Vegetarians have a reduced risk for kidney stones[1]. Foods that contain oxalic acid, such as rhubarb and spinach, should also be avoided if you have stones or are susceptible, since they are linked to stone formation. It is also a good idea to consume plenty of water to help flush the system out.

Magnesium and B6 are used to treat and prevent kidney stones. Supplementing magnesium has been shown to prevent the recurrences of kidney stones[2], and when B6 is added, it seems to work even better[3]. Use the magnesium citrate form. Vitamin K, which is found in green leafy vegetables, also seems to prevent stones[4]. Potassium citrate is used to prevent stones from recurring, as well.

Madder root and aloe vera, used internally, are especially good at binding to calcium in the urinary tract and reducing the growth rate of crystals in the urinary tract.

According to herbalist David Hoffman, gravel root, hydrangea, parsley piert, stone root, and pellitory of the wall are antilithics— herbs that are used to prevent the formation of and aid in the removal of stones or gravel in the urinary tract system. To protect the urinary tract from cutting from the gravel and to heal it, herbs that contain demulcent properties should be used, such as marshmallow and couch grass. To prevent infection, herbs such as echinacea and/or uva ursi should also be used. Herbalist Michael Tierra gives the following remedy for treating kidney stones: 2 parts of each of gravel root, parsley root, and marshmallow root, and 1/2 parts each of lobelia and ginger root. Simmer two ozs of herbs per quart of water for about one hour. The liquid should be reduced by half. Add an equal volume of vegetable glycerine to preserve it and take 1/2 cup three times a day.

The Egyptian herb khella is very effective at relaxing the ureter so stones can pass through[5]. And, better known as an anticancer nutrient, IP-6 is also helpful in fighting kidney stones[6].

Chapter Endnotes

1. Robertson, W., M. Peacock, D. Marshall. "Prevalence of urinary stone discharge in vegetarians." *Eur Urol*, 1982; 8:334'39.

2. Gershoff, S. N., E. L. Prien. "Effect of daily MgO and vitamin B6 administration to patients with recurring calcium oxalate kidney stones." *Am J Clin Nutr*, 1967; 20(5)393-99; Prien, E.L., S.F. Gershoff. "Magnesium oxide-pyridoxine therapy for recurrent calcium oxalate calculi." *J Urol*, 1974; 112:509-12; Johansson, G., et al. "Magnesium metabolism in renal stone formers. Effect of therapy with magnesium hydroxide." *Scand J Urol Nephrol*, 1980; 53:125'30; Wunderlich, W. "Aspects of the influence of magnesium ions on the formation of calcium oxalate."

Urol Res, 1981; 9:157'60; Johansson, G., *et al*. "Effects of magnesium hydroxide in renal stone disease." *J Am Coll Nutr*, 1982; 1:179-85; Hallson, P., G. Rose, S. M. Sulaiman. "Magnesium reduces calcium oxalate crystal formation in human whole urine." *Clin Sci*, 1982; 62:17'19.

3. Gershoff, S. N., E. L. Prien. "Effect of daily MgO and vitamin B6 administration to patients with recurring calcium oxalate kidney stones." *Am J Clin Nutr*, 1967; 20(5)393-99; Prien, E., S. N. Gershoff. "Magnesium oxide-pyridoxine therapy for recurrent calcium oxalate calculi." *J Urol*, 1974; 112:509'12.

4. Dharmsathaphorn, K., *et al*. "Increased risk of nephrolithiasis in patients with steatorrhea." *Dig Dis Sci*, 1982; 27:401'5.

5. Samaan, K. "The pharmacological basis of drug treatment of spasm of the ureter or bladder and of ureteral stone." *Br J Urol*, 1933; 5:213'24.

6. Grases, F., A. Costa-Bauza. "Phytate (IP6) is a powerful agent for preventing calcifications in biological fluids: usefulness in renal lithiasis treatment." *Anticancer Res*, 1999; 19:3717-22.

MIGRAINE

If you are in severe pain, your head is throbbing, you're sick to your stomach, and every sound and light bothers you, then you are one of the legions of people who suffer the scourge of migraine headaches. That's the bad news. The good news is that there are a number of natural supplements that, when combined with removal of migraine triggers, are effective at fighting off migraines.

Harbingers of Pain: Migraine Triggers

There are many things that can trigger a migraine. The first focus of a comprehensive natural approach to migraines is identification and removal of these triggers. One of those triggers is food allergies. Several double-blind, placebo-controlled studies have shown that eliminating food allergies also eliminates or reduces migraine symptoms in most migraine sufferers. The most implicated aggravators seem to be milk, chocolate, eggs, and wheat.

There are other foods that can trigger a migraine independent of allergies. These foods contain vasoactive amines and include aged cheese, red wine, chocolate, chicken liver, sour cream, and pickled herring. Beer can also be a trigger and for

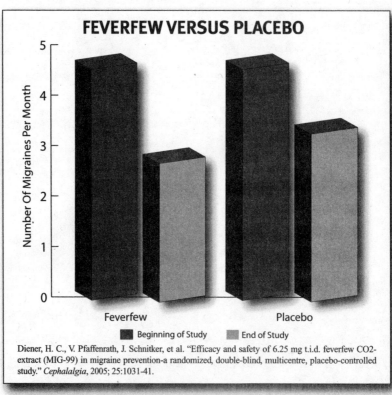

FEVERFEW VERSUS PLACEBO

Number Of Migraines Per Month

Feverfew   Placebo

■ Beginning of Study   ■ End of Study

Diener, H. C., V. Pfaffenrath, J. Schnitker, et al. "Efficacy and safety of 6.25 mg t.i.d. feverfew CO2-extract (MIG-99) in migraine prevention-a randomized, double-blind, multicentre, placebo-controlled study." *Cephalalgia*, 2005; 25:1031-41.

some people, salt. Some migraine sufferers have a low-blood-sugar irregularity called reactive hypoglycaemia in which symptoms of hypoglycaemia appear a few hours after a meal. In these migraine sufferers, making dietary changes to control blood-sugar reduces the frequency and severity of migraines.

Non-food triggers include stress, depression and anxiety, muscle tension, changes in weather, changes in sleep pattern, glaring or flickering lights, odours, smoking, and blood-clotting.

For women, there can also be hormonal triggers. Fluctuations in the menstrual cycle, pregnancy, estrogen-replacement therapy, and birth control pills can all be migraine triggers. This hormonal role is the reason more women suffer from migraines than men. When hormones are involved, you need to go beyond migraine treatments and address the underlying hormonal issues. For this reason, the great women's-hormone-balancing herb chastetree berry makes an unexpected guest appearance as a migraine herb. When hormones are a trigger, herbalist David Hoffmann suggests taking it combined with feverfew every day. It is especially useful for PMS-related headaches.

And here is one last highly ironic trigger of migraine headaches: headache medications. Analgesics increase the tendency to get headaches while they kill the pain of the one you're having. Migraine sufferers who take more than thirty analgesic pills per month suffer twice as many headache days as those who take less than thirty[1].

Flower Power: Feverfew Prevents Migraine Headaches

So, if you can't pop a painkilling pill, what can you pop? Nature's answer is a little flower called feverfew. Feverfew is a common flower that belongs to the daisy family. And it works amazingly well! A small double-blind, placebo-controlled study conducted at the London Migraine Clinic in 1985 was the first study to test people's claims that the herb worked. Researchers took half of a group of people who said that feverfew helped them and let them continue using feverfew, while the other half were unknowingly put on a placebo. The unfortunate ones in the placebo group had an almost 300 per cent increase in migraines. They also had a significant increase in the severity of the headaches and of nausea and vomiting. The ones lucky enough to be put in the feverfew group had no change in their freedom from migraines[2]. A second early double-blind study also found feverfew to reduce both the number and the severity of headaches as well as nausea and vomiting[3].

More recent studies have continued to prove feverfew's power over pain, nausea, vomiting, and sensitivity to noise and light[4]. And, in the largest double-blind, placebo-controlled study of feverfew yet, when 215 migraine sufferers were given either feverfew or a placebo, the ones given the feverfew had a significant reduction in the number of migraine attacks compared to the ones given the placebo[5].

It used to be thought that parthenolide was the ingredient in feverfew that was active against migraines, so dosing information is still often based on parthenolide content. But newer research suggests that it is not the parthenolide that is doing the work. So you should use a feverfew supplement that contains the whole leaf and take 50 to 150 mg a day, every day. Feverfew is not like aspirin: You do not take it only when you need to treat pain. Feverfew needs to be taken on a daily basis to prevent migraines and will take four to six weeks to really start working.

Butterbur: The New Herb for Migraine

One of the best—and also one of the least known—remedies for migraine is a herb called butterbur. Four studies have now proven butterbur's ability to reduce the frequency and intensity of migraines, the number of days suffered, as well as nausea and vomiting[6]. According to the authors of one of the studies, butterbur works as well as migraine drugs, with the advantage of being safer to use. A fifth study found that butterbur also helps children who suffer from migraines, an important finding since children have proven especially difficult to treat[7].

5-HTP: An Amazing New Treatment

for Migraine

5-HTP is getting to be better known, but not for migraine. This nutrient is an incredibly effective way of increasing serotonin and, therefore, of treating serotonin-deficiency states such as depression and insomnia. But 5-HTP also gets great results on migraines because migraine sufferers also have low levels of serotonin, which makes their serotonin receptors overly sensitive. That means that a small amount of serotonin can trigger excessive dilation of the blood vessels, and the result is a migraine headache. Over time, 5-HTP raises serotonin levels back to normal and rebalances the sensitivity of serotonin receptor, thus, controlling migraine.

How well does it work? In a double-blind, placebo-controlled study, 400 mg of 5-HTP a day reduced the frequency, the severity, and the duration of migraines in a full 90 per cent of people[8]. Compared to the most effective migraine drug, 600 mg of 5-HTP a day proved just as effective, but while 12.5 per cent of people taking the drug were forced to drop out of the study because of side effects, none of the 5-HTP group was[9], giving the advantage to the natural remedy. Even better news is that the same impressive results have been achieved in other studies, using the much lower dose of only 200 mg of 5-HTP[10].

To find the dose for you, Michael Murray, N.D., suggests starting with 50 mg three times a day for two weeks, then 100 mg three times a day if there is no improvement, and then up to 150 mg four times a day after two months, if needed.

SAMe, another serotonin-increasing nutrient better known for depression, when used long term can also reduce the symptoms of migraine[11].

Other Supplements for Fighting Migraines: CoQ10, Magnesium and B2

There are several other supplements that can also help you in your fight against migraine headaches. Coenzyme Q10 helped 95 per cent of migraine sufferers in one study. By the second or third month of using coenzyme Q10, people had 60 per cent fewer days with headaches. Nearly two thirds of them reduced their headache days by more than 50 per cent[12]. A second study has confirmed coenzyme Q10's place as a preventer of migraines. In this study, 100 mg of coenzyme Q10 taken twice a day reduced the frequency of headaches significantly better than a placebo. Of the people taking coenzyme Q10, 47.6 per cent had at least 50 per cent fewer attacks, compared to only 14.4 per cent of those taking a placebo[13].

Magnesium also helps because people who get migraines have lower levels of magnesium[14]. When migraine sufferers were given either 600 mg of magnesium a day or a placebo in a double-blind study, magnesium reduced the frequency of the attacks by 41.6 per cent, compared to only 15.8 per cent by the placebo[15].

Like butterbur, magnesium has been shown to help children who suffer from migraines as well. When children between three and seventeen years of age were given 9 mg per kilogram body weight of magnesium in a placebo-controlled study, both the frequency and the severity of their headaches were significantly reduced[16].

As we saw in the migraine trigger section, hormonal changes through the menstrual cycle can be a trigger for migraines. Magnesium can help here, too. One study found that 360 mg a day of magnesium is able to decrease the number of days of premenstrual migraine[17].

At least three studies have also shown vitamin B2's power over migraines. The first two studies used the very large dose of 400 mg. One found a two-thirds reduction in both frequency and severity[18], and the other found that B2 cut the frequency of headaches in half in 59 per cent of people, compared to only 15 per cent of people given a placebo[19]. For such a large dose to be effective, the B2 may need to be taken in several small doses throughout the day. The good news is that a more recent study has found that much smaller doses may do the trick. This preliminary three-month study found that people who took only 25 mg a day was able to reduce the frequency of headaches by a third in chronic migraine sufferers[20].

More Herbal Help

The herbs *Ginkgo biloba* and ginger can also help with migraines. Ginger not only relieves the pain, but also helps with the nausea. Linda loves ginger, and uses it herself, and in the clinic where it works wonders.

Also, don't forget topical help. Rosemary oil and peppermint oil can greatly help with migraines, as can ginger oil and wintergreen oil.

Traditional herbalists believe that headaches are caused by bowel and stomach disorders, tension, stress, weak kidneys, or a sluggish liver, and will flush the system using laxatives and herbs that clear the toxins from the liver. Use herbs like the ones found in Dr. Christopher's lower bowel tonic: cascara sagrada, barberry root, rhubarb root, goldenseal root, raspberry leaves, lobelia, and ginger root. Triphala and fibre, from flax or psyllium, are also good ideas to help keep the bowels moving regularly, and preventing the problem from occurring.

Herbalist Michael Tierra also uses stress herbs for headaches, and they can be helpful for migraines, too. Use herbs such as skullcap, valerian, rosemary, chamomile, and peppermint.

Acupuncture and Migraine

At least two placebo-controlled studies have confirmed what many preliminary reports have shown: Acupuncture relieves migraine headaches and reduces their frequency[21]. And now a study has even found that acupuncture cures migraines at a rate that is far superior to drugs: 75 per cent versus 34 per cent[22]!

Chapter Endnotes

1. Isler, H. "Migraine treatment as a cause of chronic migraine." In F.C. Rose, ed., *Advances in Migraine Research and Therapy.* New York, NY: Raven Press, 1982, pp.159'64.

2. Johnson, E. S., N.P. Kadam, D. M. Hylands, P.J. Hylands. "Efficacy of feverfew as prophylactic treatment of migraine." *Br Med J (Clin Res Ed)*, 1985; 291:569-73.

3. Murphy, J. J., S. Hepinstall, J. R. Mitchell. "Randomized double-blind placebo controlled trial of feverfew in migraine prevention." *Lancet*, 1988; 2:189-92.

4. Palevitch, D., G. Earon, R. Carasso. "Feverfew (Tanacetum parthenium) as a prophylactic treatment for migraine: A double-blind placebo-controlled study." *Phytother Res*, 1997; 11:508-11.

5. Diener, H. C., V. Pfaffenrath, J. Schnitker, et al. "Efficacy and safety of 6.25 mg t.i.d. feverfew CO2-extract (MIG-99) in migraine prevention-a randomized, double-blind, multicentre, placebo-controlled study." *Cephalalgia*, 2005; 25:1031-41.

6. Grossmann, M., H. Schmidramsl. "An extract of *Petasites hybridus* is effective in the prophylaxis of migraine." *Int J Clin Pharmacol Ther*, 2000; 38:430-35; Lipton, R.B., H. Gobel, K. Wilkes, A. Mauskop. "Efficacy of Petasites (an extract from Petasites rhizome) 50 and 75 mg for prophylaxis of migraine: Results of a randomized, double-blind, placebo-controlled study." *Neurology*, 2002; 58(suppl 3):A472; Diener, H.C., V.W. Rahlfs. U. Danesch. "The first placebo-controlled trial of a special butterbur extract for the prevention of migraine: reanalysis of efficacy criteria." *Eur Neurol*, 2004; 51:89-97; Lipton, R.B., H. Gobel, K.M. Einhaupl, et al. "Petasites hybridus root (butterbur) is an effective preventive treatment for migraine." *Neurology*, 2004; 63:2240-44;

7. Pothmann, R., U. Danesch. "Migraine prevention in children and adolescents: results of an open study with a special butterbur root extract." *Headache*, 2005; 45:196-203.

8. De Benedittis, G., R. Massei. "5-HT precursors in migraine prophylaxis: A double-blind cross-over study with L-5-hydroxytryptophan versus placebo." *Clin J Pain*, 1986; 3:123-29.

9. Titus, F., et al. "5-Hydroxytryptophan versus methysergide in the prophylaxis of migraine: randomized clinical trial." *European Neurology*, 1986; 25:327'29.

10. Sciuteri, F. "5-Hydroxytryptophan in the prophylaxis of migraine." *Pharmacological Research Communications*, 1972; 5:213'18; Sciuteri, F. "The ingestion of serotonin precursors (L-5-hydroxytryptophan and L-tryptophan) improves migraine headache." *Headache*, 1973; 13:19-22.

11. Gatto, G., D. Caleri, S. Michelacci, F. Sicuteri. "Analgesizing effect of a methyl donor (S-adenosylmethionine) in migraine: an open clinical trial." *Int J Clin Pharmacol Res*, 1986; 6:15-17.

12. Rozen, T.D., M.L. Oshinsky, C.A. Gebeline, et al. "Open label trial of coenzyme Q10 as a migraine preventive." *Cephalalgia*, 2002; 22:137-41.

13. Sandor, P. S., L. Di Clemente, G. Coppola, et al. "Efficacy of coenzyme Q10 in migraine prophylaxis: a randomized controlled trial." *Neurology*, 2005; 64:713-15.

14. Swanson, D. R.. "Migraine and magnesium: eleven neglected connections." Perpect Biol Med, 1988; 31:526'57; Ramadan, N.M., *et al.* "Low brain magnesium in migraine." Headache, 1989; 29:590'93; Gallai, V., P. Sarchielli, G. Coata, *et al.* "Serum and salivary magnesium levels in migraine. Results in a group of juvenile patients." Headache, 1992; 32:132-35; Baker, B. "New research approach helps clarify magnesium/migraine link." *Family Pract News*, 1993; Aug 15:16; Barbiroli, B., R. Lodi, P. Cortelli, et al. "Low brain free magnesium in migraine and cluster headache: an interictal study by in vivo phosphorus magnetic resonance spectroscopy on 86 patients." *Cephalalgia*, 1997; 17:254; Mazzotta, G., et al. "Intracellular Mg++ concentration and electromyographical ischemic test in juvenile headache." *Cephalalgia*, 1999; 19:802-09.

15. Peikert, A., C. Wilimzig, R. Kohne-Volland. "Prophylaxis of migraine with oral magnesium: results from a prospective, multi-center, placebo-controlled and double-blind randomized study." *Cephalalgia*, 1996; 16:257-63.

16. Wang, F. "Oral magnesium oxide prophylaxis of frequent migrainous headache in children: a randomized, double-blind, placebo-controlled trial." *Headache*, 2003; 43:601'10.

17. Facchinetti, F., G. Sances, P. Borella, et al. "Magnesium prophylaxis of menstrual migraine: effects on intracellular magnesium." *Headache*, 1991; 31:298-301.

18. Schoenen, J., M. Lenaerts, E. Bastings. "High-dose riboflavin as a prophylactic treatment of migraine: results of an open pilot study." *Cephalalgia*, 1994; 14:328-29.

19. Schoenen, J., J. Jacquy, M. Lenaerts. "Effectiveness of high-dose riboflavin in migraine prophylaxis. A randomized controlled trial." *Neurology*, 1998; 50:466-70.

20. Maizels, M., A. Blumenfeld, R. Burchette. "A combination of riboflavin, magnesium, and feverfew for migraine prophylaxis: a randomized trial." *Headache*, 2004; 44:885-90.

21. Lenhard, L., P.M.E. Waite. "Acupuncture in the prophylactic treatment of migraine headaches: pilot study." NZ Med J, 1983; 96:663-66; Vincent, C.A. "A controlled trial of the treatment of migraine by acupuncture." *Clin J Pain*, 1989; 5:305-12.

22. Shuyuan, G., Z. Donglan, X. Yanguang. "A comparative study on the treatment of migraine headache with combined distant and local acupuncture points versus conventional drug therapy." *Am J Acupuncture*, 1999; 27:27-30.

MULTIPLE SCLEROSIS

Want to be let in on a well kept secret? Imagine a disease in which your own immune cells cross the blood-brain barrier into the brain and attack the myelin sheath that surrounds and protects your nerve cells. Without this protective sheath, your nerve function is lost. That's what happens in multiple sclerosis. But that's not the secret. The secret is that there is a treatment. The crime is that no one tells you about it.

A study published in 2000 found that 94 per cent of people with newly diagnosed relapsing-remitting multiple sclerosis stopped the deterioration and actually improved when they were treated with supplements and dietary changes[1].

The real crime is that this treatment wasn't even news: Dr. Roy Swank has been treating people with multiple sclerosis with dietary changes since 1948: you'd think by now the word would be out.

The Swank Diet: Treating Multiple Sclerosis
In 1950, Swank showed that there is a strong association between a diet high in animal and dairy products and multiple sclerosis[2]. And Swank's findings have held up consistently over time. The key is the types of fat in the diet. The saturated fat found in animal products is the problem; the polyunsaturated essential fatty acids found in plants and cold water fish are the solution.

Confirmation came in 1974. A study reported in *Lancet* demonstrated a very high correlation between milk consumption and multiple sclerosis mortality. It also found a positive correlation between multiple sclerosis and total fat, animal protein, butter fat and meat. But the reverse was true for intake of vegetables and fish: they were negatively correlated [3]. In 1986, it was again found that diets high in milk are much more common where there is a lot of multiple sclerosis[4].

DIET AND MULTIPLE SCLEROSIS

Causative	Protective
Meat	Polyunsaturated Fats
Dairy	Vegetables
Saturated Animal Fat	Fruit Juice
Animal Protein	Cold Water Fish
Food Allergies	Foods Rich in Vitamins C, B1, B2, Calcium and Potassium

The support for Swank's diet continued to mount. in 1995 it was again reported that mortality rates from multiple sclerosis correlate with saturated fat and animal fat—except for fish[5]. The same study found that the more polyunsaturated fat and the less saturated fat, the less mortality from multiple sclerosis. A comparison of people with and without multiple sclerosis found that those who ate foods high in saturated animal fat were more likely to develop multiple sclerosis, while those who ate more fish, vegetable protein, fruit juice and foods rich in vitamin C, vitamins B1 and B2, calcium and potassium were less likely to develop multiple sclerosis[6]. A 1997 review of studies showed that MS repeatedly correlates with consumption of animal fat, animal protein and meat and negatively correlates with vegetable and/or fish intake[7].

So Swank put his patients on a diet that banned meat. He encouraged them to eat cold water fish like mackerel, herring and salmon that are rich in omega-3 essential fatty acids. They increased their fruit and vegetable consumption and were banned from eating butter, margarine or other hydrogenated oils. He showed that a diet low in saturated fats was able to reduce the number of attacks and slow down the disease.

In a remarkable thirty-four year study that began in 1949, Swank showed that people who were put on the diet before the development of disabilities suffered little, if any, progress of their disease. In fact, 95 per cent of them suffered no significant increase in their disabilities during the thirty-four years of the study, and only 5 per cent of them were not alive at the end of the thirty-four years. In contrast, of those who were not on the diet, 80 per cent were no longer alive at the study's end. People who were moderately or severely disabled also did far better than the group who were not on Swank's diet[8].

Supplements for Multiple Sclerosis

Since the omega-3 essential fatty acids are crucial for the myelin sheath, protect the blood-brain barrier and modulate the immune system, in addition to the dietary changes—no animal products except for cold water fish and lots of plant foods—they should also be supplemented. One or two tablespoons of flaxseed oil should be taken every day. Adding an omega-6 fatty acid like evening primrose oil may also help, according to a review of three double-blind studies[9].

Other nutrients can be helpful too. Since free radicals are involved in multiple sclerosis, the powerful antioxidant flavonoids from herbs like ginkgo biloba might also help. These flavonoids also protect the blood-brain barrier. The flavonoids from bilberry have also been shown to protect the blood-brain barrier[10]. Other antioxidants, like selenium and vitamin E can also be helpful.

A deficiency of B12 could also make multiple

sclerosis worse. B12 deficiency can cause demyelenation of nerve fibre. Supplementing B12 may help [11].

Vitamin D deficiency could also be involved. People who live in places with a lot of sunlight—and, therefore get a lot of vitamin D—have less multiple sclerosis, and most people with multiple sclerosis are deficient in vitamin D[12]. Putting two massive studies together, researchers found that intake of vitamin D is associated with a lower risk of multiple sclerosis. Women with the most vitamin D had a thirty-three per cent lower risk of multiple sclerosis. Women who supplemented at least 400IU of vitamin D a day were at 41 per cent lower risk than women who took no vitamin D supplements[13]. And a huge study recently concluded that risk of multiple sclerosis decreases as blood level of vitamin D increases. People with the highest blood levels reduced their risk of multiple sclerosis by nearly half[14].

Taking calcium and magnesium may also help.

More Help

At least two small studies have shown that eliminating food allergies leads to improvement. Poor digestion and candida are also common in multiple sclerosis and need to be healed. Enzymes and a candida program complete with acidophilus should be used if necessary.

As with so many other conditions, smoking may aggravate multiple sclerosis[15]. Mercury and organic solvents may also cause multiple sclerosis.

People with multiple sclerosis also benefit from aerobic exercise[16].

Chapter Endnotes

1. Nordvik I., et al. Effect of dietary advice and n-3 supplementation in newly diagnosed multiple sclerosis patients. Acta Neurol Scand 2000;102:143–9.

2. Swank R. L., Multiple sclerosis: a correlation of its incidence with dietary fat. Am J Med Sci 1950;220:421-30; Swank R. L., et al. Multiple sclerosis in rural Norway. N Engl J Med 1952;246:721-728.

3. Agranoff B. W. A., Goldberg D., Diet and the geographical distribution of multiple sclerosis. Lancet 1973;2:1061-1066.

4. Butcher P. J., Milk consumption and multiple sclerosis—an etiological hypothesis Medical Hypothesis 1986;19:169-78.

5. Esparza M. L., Sasahi S., Kesteloot H., Nutrition, latitude, and multiple sclerosis mortality: an ecologic study. Am J Epidem 1995;142:733-7.

6. Ghadirian P., et al. Nutritional factors in the aetiology of multiple sclerosis: a case control study in Montreal, Canada. Int J Epidemiol 1998;5:845–52.

7. Lauer K., Diet and multiple sclerosis. Neurology 1997;49:S55-S61.

8. Swank R. L., Fat-oil relationship. Nutrition 1991;7:368-76.

9. Dworkin R. H., et al. Linoleic acid and multiple sclerosis: a reanalysis of three double-blind trials. Neurology 1984;34:1441–5.

10. Robert A. M., et al. Action of the anthocyanosides of Vaccinium myrtillus on the permeability of the blood brain barrier. J Med 1977;8:321-32.

11. Kira J., Tobimatsu S., Goto I. Vitamin B12 metabolism and massive-dose methyl vitamin B12 therapy in Japanese patients with multiple sclerosis. Int Med 1994;33:82-6.

12. Nieves J., et al. High prevalence of vitamin D deficiency and reduced bone mass in multiple sclerosis. Neurology 1994;44:1687-92.

13. Munger K. L., et al. Vitamin D intake and incidence of multiple sclerosis. Neurology 2004;62:60-5.

14. Munger K. L., et al. Serum 25-hydroxyvitamin D levels and risk of multiple sclerosis. JAMA 2006;296:2832–8.

15. Emre M, de Decker C. Effects of cigarette smoking on motor functions in patient with multiple sclerosis. Arch Neurol 1992;49:1243–7.

16. Petajan J. H., Gappmaier E., White A. T., Impact of aerobic training on fitness and quality of life in multiple sclerosis. Ann Neurol 1996;39:432-41.

NAIL FUNGUS

It is so common: nail fungus. It comes easily and seems to take forever to go away. The most common cause of fungal nail infections is onychomycosis. Nail fungus affects up to 13 per cent of the population. So how do you get rid of it?

Standard treatment includes anti-fungals, both systemic and local, and debridement treatments. The problem is that the rate of recurrence with these kinds of treatments is huge.

The first thing to be aware of is that nail fungus is often a result of systemic fungus and so the suggestions in the Candida section often need to be followed as well.

But what can you do topically to treat nail fungus? Tea tree oil. Tea tree oil is one of the best fungus fighters that there is. You apply it to the nail two times per day. A study looked at the effectiveness of using tee tree oil for nail fungus, and it found that twice-daily application of 100 per cent tea tree oil was as effective as 1 per cent clotrimazole[1].

It is a good idea to take probiotics to help the body rid itself of fungus. Consume 20 billion live cultures a day. Blow-dry nails, as fungus thrives in dampness.

Other possible topical choices include grapefruit seed extract, oregano oil, myrrh, wild indigo, or goldenseal tincture. Also try topical garlic. Lemon juice or apple cider vinegar may also help topically. Hot-water soaks with any of sea salt, eucalyptus, thyme, oregano, tea tree, or lavender oil may also help.

Chapter Endnotes
1. Buc, D.S., D.M. Nidorf, J.G. Addino. "Comparison of two topical preparations for the treatment of onychomycosis: Melaleuca alternifolia (Tee tree oil) and clotrimazole." *J Fam Prac*, 1994; 38: 601'05.

PAIN AND INJURIES

No section in this book will be relevant to more people than this one. Everyone experiences pain. Many people spend their lives in chronic pain. Pain is often a warning that something is wrong, so the cause, as well as the pain, needs to be treated. But even though pain can be a helpful messenger of an underlying condition, it is one time that you *will* want to shoot the messenger. But how?

The Problem with Pain Killers

We are in desperate need of a safe way to kill pain. Why? Because the painkillers we reach for most often, though they work, work at the expense of serious, but little discussed, side effects. Aspirin causes ulcers and gastrointestinal bleeding. Thou-

sands of people die every year from the improper use of aspirin. A meta-analysis of twenty-four controlled studies found that not only is aspirin associated with a significant risk of gastrointestinal bleeding, but that there is no way to get around this problem because even taking a low dose does not reduce the risk[1]. Twenty-eight per cent of people taking low-dose aspirin for the prevention of heart disease develop an ulcer[2]. Aspirin also damages cartilage[3]. Regular use of either aspirin or acetaminophen is toxic to the liver and kidneys. Even short-term use of acetominaphen, if taken at the maximum recommended daily dose, stresses the liver[4]. So significant is the stress on the liver caused by acetominophen, that it has become the most common cause of acute liver failure in the U.S. and U.K., far exceeding other causes. [5] In addition, both Aspirin and acetaminophen suppress the immune system.

A newer class of painkiller called the COX-2 inhibitor was intended to address at least aspirin's biggest problem: ulcers and bleeding. Vioxx® (rofecoxib) and Celebrex® are both COX-2 inhibitors. The idea was a good one. Aspirin, and other nonsteroidal anti-inflammatory drugs (NSAIDs), inhibit both COX-1 and COX-2. It is that inhibiting of COX-1 that causes ulcers. So, the idea was to make a NSAID that inhibits only COX-2: the COX-2 inhibitor. But that solved only

SIDE EFFECTS OF PAIN KILLING DRUGS

DRUG	SIDE EFFECTS
Aspirin	Gastrointestinal bleeding
	Ulcer
	Cartilage damage
	Liver toxicity
	Kidney toxicity
	Immune suppression
Tylenol	Liver toxicity
	Acute liver failure
	Kidney toxicity
	Immune supression
COX-2 Inhibitors	Kidney toxicity
	Ulcer

the ulceration problem. COX-2 inhibitors still have the same kidney toxicity as aspirin. And, it turned out, the studies that showed that COX-2 inhibitors solved the ulceration problem were misleading; they actually cause just as many ulcers[6]. But the big mistake was realized when a 2001 study reported in the Journal of the American Medical Association found that the COX-2 inhibitor Vioxx® (rofecoxib) more than doubled the chance of heart attack, stroke, or angina, compared to the old NSAID naproxen.

And the painkilling news just keeps getting worse. A just-published Canadian study looked at long-acting oxycodone (OxyContin) and opioid related mortality in the province of Ontario. Since Ontario added this painkilling drug to the public drug plan, oxycodone has been associated with a five-fold increase in oxycodone-related deaths and a 41 per cent increase in overall opioid-related deaths[7].

Fortunately, nature offers many very safe herbs that work as COX-2 inhibitors. Some of these herbs are white willow bark, devil's claw, turmeric, ginger, green tea, feverfew, and cayenne.

Aspirin Doesn't Grow on Trees, You Know. Or Does It?

White willow bark is a herbal painkiller. It contains substances that our body turns into salicin and then into salicylic acid. When scientists learned how to turn salicylic acid into acetylsalicylic acid in the laboratory, aspirin was born. But so were its problems. Unlike the synthetic version, the herb does not damage your stomach.

White willow bark is analgesic, anti-inflammatory and anti-fever. It can be used for nearly any kind of pain, including headaches, backaches, toothaches, and arthritis. White willow bark works significantly better than a placebo for osteoarthritis[8] and for back pain[9]. When white willow bark was really put to the test by being compared to Vioxx® (rofecoxib), the herb came out on top by being equally effective but safer[10]. White willow bark also beat the drugs ibuprofen, diclofenac, coxibe and oxicame for people with pain from either chronic wear on their knee cartilage or from noninflammatory degenerative disease of the hip. Of the herb group, 64.4 per cent rated their improvement as very good compared to only 37.5 per cent of people taking one of the drugs. The herb was not only better, but better tolerated[11]. Most of

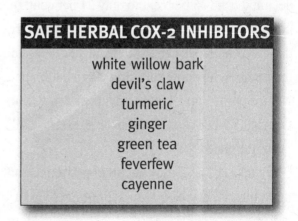

SAFE HERBAL COX-2 INHIBITORS

white willow bark
devil's claw
turmeric
ginger
green tea
feverfew
cayenne

these studies used 240 mg of salicin a day.

A Devil of a Painkiller: Devil's Claw

Out of Africa comes devil's claw. This intriguingly named herb seems to help both rheumatoid and osteoarthritis, but it may be in cases of osteoarthritis that it really shines. Devil's claw has defeated not only placebos, but also pain medications. When people with osteoarthritis were given either devil's claw or the drug diacerhein, 65.3 per cent had good or very good results with the herb, compared to only 60 per cent with the drug. The herb was not only better, but safer, too[12]. Devil's claw is also a great herb for gout, the other major type of arthritis. And it is also emerging recently as an effective painkiller for back pain, for at least some people, whose pain does not radiate to the legs[13]. When people suffering from lower back pain or osteoarthritis were given devil's claw for fifty four weeks, the number of people experiencing no pain increased from just 3 per cent to 31 per cent, the number of people in moderate pain declined from 45 per cent to only 21 per cent, the number of people who were in severe pain went down from 25 per cent to only 11 per cent, and the number of people suffering excruciating pain went down to just 1 per cent from 5 per cent. Overall, 75 per cent of the people given devil's claw responded[14].

Try taking 1 to 2 g of the dried powdered root three times a day or 600 to 1,200 mg a day of a standardized tablet.

Bromelain and Turmeric: Powerful Anti-inflammatories

Two of the most amazing natural anti-inflammatories are bromelain and turmeric. Bromelain comes from pineapple. Its powers as a digestive enzyme when taken with food are well-known. Less well-known is that when taken without food, it is an amazing anti-inflammatory. Bromelain can be used for virtually any inflammatory condition from sprains and strains to back pain and arthritis. It is also a great remedy for bruising and swelling. All kinds of studies show that it helps with postoperative bruising and swelling[15]. In one crazy study, boxers were given either bromelain or a placebo. Within four days, 58 of 74 boxers given bromelain had all their bruises healed, compared to only 10 out of 72 on a placebo[16]. Linda has used bromelain for all kinds of injuries and pain in her clinic, such as tendonitis, bursitis, muscle sprain, strain, ligament problems, arthritis, and trauma, and it has been very effective.

Turmeric, an Ayurvedic herb from India, is a major ingredient in curry. But less well known than its value in cooking is its value as an anti-inflammatory and analgesic. Curcumin, an important component of turmeric, is as effective as the steroidal anti-inflammatory cortisone or the non steroidal anti-inflammatory phenylbutazone in acute inflammation. In chronic inflammation, i is half as effective but safer. Curcumin has been shown to work comparably to the powerful NSAID phenybutazone for rheumatoid arthritis[17]. Turmeric is a member of the ginger family, and ginger is also an anti-inflammatory herb.

Another great anti-inflammatory is the versatile and powerful herb licorice. Licorice has cortisol-like effects and is good for any inflammatory condition, including rheumatoid arthritis, bursitis, and tendonitis.

Antispasmodic Herbs

Antispasmodic herbs are also useful for pain relief. Kava kava, passionflower, butterbur, skullcap, and valerian are some of the best, and, if you can still get it, the best of these is kava kava. This Pacific island herb kills pain by methods unlike any other painkiller, still to be figured out by science. These mysterious painkilling properties coupled with its powerful muscle-relaxing properties make kava kava a great herb for back pain. We like combining it with bromelain. Kava can also be used for headaches. Antispasmodic herbs are also good for cramping pains. Butterbur can be used even for extreme forms of pain, such as in advanced cancer.

California poppy can also help with pain, as can other sedative/nervine herbs such as, hops, vervain, linden, and chamomile, by letting you relax and sleep better.

Topical Painkillers: Killing Pain from the Outside In

If you've ever gotten cayenne in your eyes, you know how much pain it can cause. What you might not know is how much pain it can eliminate. Cayenne cream is one of the most promising topical painkillers. Cayenne seems to block substance P, a neurotransmitter that sends a signal from the site of the injury to the brain, informing it that you are in pain. Cayenne cuts the wire, so you can't get the message. Cayenne cream has helped reduce many different types of pain in many different studies[18]. The usual method for applying cayenne is to use a cream standardized for 0.025 to 0.075 per cent capsaicin, three to four times a day on the painful area. Avoid eyes, mouth, and open cuts-this painkiller can sting!

Topical turmeric can also deplete substance P.

Another good topical painkiller is the homeopathic remedy arnica. Arnica is a very effective treatment for injuries and accidents. Used topically, as either a herb or homeopathic, it is an excellent anti-inflammatory and painkiller. It can be used for sprains, bruises, muscle and joint pain, and more. The herbal form of arnica cannot be used internally, but the homeopathic form can. A double-blind study of homeopathic arnica found that taking it internally led to significantly less bruising after plastic surgery[19].

Another good topical painkiller is the essential oil of peppermint. This essential oil has local anaesthetic and muscle-relaxing effects. It is good for headaches, arthritis, and tendonitis. Or try rosemary essential oil, also good for pain. St. John's wort oil is also good, topically, for pain, where the nerve is involved.

Clinically, Linda has seen combinations used topically that included cayenne, St. John's wort, rue, melilot, arnica, yarrow, and wormwood work very well.

Other combinations of shave grass, ivy, birch, and arnica are also useful.

Bruises, Strains, and Sprains

As the boxing study and many others have already shown, bromelain is a great remedy for bruising. A recent study of fifty-nine people with injuries, including ligament tears, muscle strains, and bruises, showed bromelain's effectiveness for these sorts of injuries. Five hundred milligrams, three times a day, half an hour before meals, quickly improved swelling, inflammation, tenderness, and pain[20].

In addition to bromelain, flavonoids and horse chestnut are great for bruises. A gel made of the herb horse chestnut, standardized for 2 per cent escin, has been shown to heal bruises faster than a placebo[21]. The same gel is also good for treating strains and sprains. Taking horse chestnut tincture internally may also help strains and sprains.

Several studies have shown that a topical application of an ointment made from the herb comfrey is extremely effective for strains and sprains. We found three good studies of comfrey ointment on sprained ankles. The first found that comfrey reduced the pain and increased mobility[22]. The second found that the comfrey ointment, applied four times a day for seven to nine days, reduced pain and sped up improvement in swelling and joint mobility significantly better than a placebo ointment[23]. In the third, the comfrey ointment was compared to diclofenac gel, a topical anti-inflammatory medicine. The herb beat the drug. People using the comfrey ointment had significantly greater improvement in pain and swelling as well as a faster and more complete recovery[24]. That's pretty impressive evidence for comfrey ointment as a remedy for sprains.

Other studies have also found that comfrey ointment may help with muscle pain and swelling[25]. When 120 people with acute pain in the upper or lower back were given either comfrey root-extract ointment or a placebo three times a day for five days, pain intensity on movement plummeted by an average of 95.2 per cent in the comfrey group compared to only 37.8 per cent in the placebo group by the fifth day. Pain was already down by 33 per cent, compared to only 12 per cent in the placebo group, after only one hour. The herbal ointment produced even slightly better results for measures of pain at rest. Eighty per cent of the researchers and 78.4 per cent of the patients rated the comfrey ointment as good or excellent compared to only 18.4 per cent of researchers and patients for the placebo[26].

Other Nutrients for Killing Pain

Methylsulfonylmethane, or MSM, is anti-inflammatory, antispasmodic, and analgesic and has the ability to inhibit the transmission of pain impulses. All of this combines to make a great painkiller that brings about significant relief about 70 per cent of the time, according to MSM specialists Dr. Stanley Jacob and Dr. Ronald Lawrence. They recommend it for arthritis, fibromyalgia, back pain, headache, muscle soreness, strains, sprains, and more.

An excellent serotonin-increasing nutrient is 5-hydroxytryptophan, or 5-HTP for short, which is better known—to the extent it is known at all—for the magic it works on depression and insomnia. Low levels of serotonin lead not only to depression and insomnia, but also to pain. As an added bonus, 5-HTP increases not only serotonin, but endorphins, too. Endorphins are your body's own natural painkillers. Also, 5-HTP is especially good for the pain of migraines and fibromyalgia.

And here's a nutrient that surprised us because we didn't expect it to make it onto the painkiller list: vitamin D. But one study has recently shown that vitamin D can help back pain. The study found that most people suffering from low back pain were low in vitamin D. All of them improved when they were given the vitamin. Strangely, 69 per cent of those without deficiencies of vitamin D also improved. The study suggests, then, that deficiencies in vitamin D may be a surprise cause of back pain and that supplementing it may help[27].

Also consider cat's claw for pain.

The Amazing Painkiller that No One Has Heard of

One of the most researched of all painkillers is a combination of herbs marketed in Europe under the name Phytodolor. Phytodolor does not seem to be available in North America currently, but we hope it soon will be. You could try mixing the herbs yourself. The formula is a combination of three parts of an extract of aspen bark and leaves with one part each of extracts of common ash bark and the aboveground parts of goldenrod. At least seven studies have shown this combination of herbs to be as effective as drugs while also being safer[28]. The recommended dose of this combination is 20 drops three to four times a day. Pain specialist Michael Loes, M.D., says to take forty drops three to four times a day for severe pain.

Acupuncture: Puncturing Pain

Acupuncture is remarkable for pain. Studies have shown it to work for pains as diverse as arthritis, back pain, prostate pain, and the excruciating pain of kidney stones. In fact, after reviewing at least sixty-seven controlled studies, a National Institute of Health consensus statement concluded that acupuncture is good for muscular, skeletal, postoperative, and generalized pain[29].

One interesting study looked at 174 patients, all of whom received conventional treatment. They then were randomly assigned to one of three groups: acupuncture, sham acupuncture, or conventional therapy alone. Each person received twelve sessions over four weeks. At the end of the trial, only 43 per cent of those receiving conventional therapy reported at least 50 per cent reduction in pain, while at least 65 per cent of those getting acupuncture did. At a three-month follow up, only 14 per cent of the people in the conventional therapy group who had had at least a 50 per cent reduction in pain still had a reduction in pain, while the number in the acupuncture group rose to 77 per cent. Among those in the sham group, only 34 per cent reported at least 50 per cent reduction in pain at the end of the trial and 29 per cent at the end of three months. This study proves that acupuncture is effective in immediate reduction of pain and has long-lasting results.

Stay in Shape and Listen to Good Music

Achieving your ideal weight and getting regular exercise can also help manage pain. Though it wouldn't be the first side effect of being overweight that one might think of, overweight people actually may experience pain more quickly and more intensely[30]. And exercise, as long as the condition isn't aggravated by it, can increase tolerance to pain[31].

And now, to end the section with the strangest painkiller of all: When sixty people enduring chronic pain were put into a group that listened to music or a group that didn't, pain dropped by 20 per cent in the music group, compared to only 2 per cent in the non-music group[32].

Chapter Endnotes

1. Derry, S., Y. K. Luke. "Risk of gastrointestinal haemorrhage with long-term use of aspirin: meta-analysis." *BMJ*, 2000; 321:1183'87.

2. Yeomans, N. D., et al. "Prevalence and incidence of gastroduodenal ulcers during treatment with vascular protective doses of aspirin." *Alimentary Pharmacology & Therapeutics*, 2005; 22:795'801.

3. Brooks, P. M., S. R. Potter, W. W. Buchanan. "NSAID and osteoarthritis-help or hindrance." *J Rheumatol*, 1982; 9:3'5; Shield, M.J. "Anti-inflammatory drugs and their effects on cartilage synthesis and renal function." *Eur J Rheum Inflam*, 1993; 13:7'16; Ghosh, P. "Evaluation of disease progression during nonsteroidal anti-inflammatory drug treatment: experimental models." *Osteoarthritis Cartilage*, 1999; 7:340'42; Dingle, J.T. "Cartilage maintenance in osteoarthritis: interaction of cytokines, NSAID and prostaglandins in articular cartilage damage and repair." *J Rheumatol Suppl*, 1991; 28:30'37.

4. Watkins, P. B., et al. "Aminotransferase Elevations in Healthy Adults Receiving 4 Grams of Acetaminophen Daily: A Randomized Controlled Trial." *JAMA*, 2006; 296:87'93.

5. Larson A. M, et al. "Acetaminophen-induced acute liver failure: results of a United States multicenter, prospective study." *Hepatology* 2005;42:1364-72.

6. Hrachovec JB, et al. "Reporting of 6-Month versus 12-Month Data in a Clinical Trial of Celecoxib." *JAMA* 2001;286:2398-2400.

7. Dhalla IA, et al. "Prescribing of opioid analgesics and related mortality before and after the introduction of long-acting oxycodone." *CMAJ* 2009;181.

8. Schmid, B., B. Tschirdewahn, I. Kàtter, et al. "Analgesic effects of willow bark extract in osteoarthritis: results of a clinical double-blind trial." *Fact*, 1998; 3:186.

9. Chrubasik, S., E. Eisenberg, E. Balan, et al. "Treatment of low back pain exacerbations with willow bark extract: A randomized, double-blind study." *Am J Med*, 2000; 109;9'14.

10. Chrubasik, S., et al. "Treatment of low back pain with herbal or synthetic antirheumatic: a randomized controlled study. Willow bark extract for low back pain." *Rheumatology*, 2001; 40:1388'93.

11. Beer A. M., Wegener T. "Willow bark extract (*Salicis cortex*) for gonarthrosis and coxarthrosis - results of a cohort study with a control group." *Phytomed*, 2008: 907-913.

12. Chantre, P., A. Cappelaere, D. Leblan, et al. "Efficacy and tolerance of *Harpagophytum procumbens* versus diacerhein in treatment of osteoarthritis." *Phytomedicine*, 2000; 7:177-83.

13. Chrubasik, S., et al. "Effectiveness of Harpagophytum procumbens in treatment of acute low back pain." *Phytomedicine*, 1996; 3:1'10; Chrubasik, S., J. Junck, H. Breitschwerdt, et al. "Effectiveness of *harpagophytum* extract WS 1531 in the treatment of exacerbation of low back pain: A randomized placebo-controlled double-blind study." *Eur J Anaesthsiol*, 1999; 16:118'29.

14. Chrubasik S., et al. "Patient-perceived benefit during one year of treatment with Doloteffin." *Phytomedicine* 2007; 14:371-76.

15. Tassman, G., et al. "Evaluation of a plant peoteolytic enzyme for the control of inflammation and pain." *J Dent Med*, 1964; 19:73'77; Seltzer, A. P. "A double-blind study of bromelains in the treatment of edema and ecchymoses following surgical and non-surgical trauma to the face." *Eye Ear Nose Throat Monthly*, 1964; 43:54'57; Tassman, G., et al. "A double-blind crossover study of a plant proteolytic enzyme in oral surgery." *J Dent Med*, 1965; 20:51'54; Howat, R., G. Lewis. "The effect of bromelain therapy on episiotomy wounds-a double-blind controlled clinical trial." *J Obstet Gynecol BrCcommon*, 1972; 79:951'53; Zatuchni, G., D. Colombi. "Bromelain therapy for the prevention of episiotomy pain." *Obstet Gynecol*, 1967; 29:275'78.

16. Blonstein, J. "Control of swelling in boxing injuries." *Practitioner*, 1960; 203:206.

17. Deodhar, S. D., R. Sethi, R. C. Srimal. "Preliminary studies on antirheumatic activity of curcumin (diferuloyl methatne)." *Indian J Med Res*, 1980; 71:632'34.

18. Deal, C. L., et al. "Treatment of arthritis with topical capsaicin: A double-blind trial." Clin Ther, 1991; 13:383'95; Hautkappe, M., M. F. Roizen, A. Toledano, et al. "Review of the effectiveness of capsaicin for painful cutaneous disorders and neural dysfunction." *Clin J Pain*, 1998; 14:97-106 [review]; Fusco, B. M., M. Giacovazzo. "Peppers and pain. The promise of capsaicin." *Drugs*, 1997; 53:909-14 [review]; Robbins, W. R., P.S. Staats, J. Levine, et al. "Treatment of intractable pain with topical large-dose capsaicin: preliminary report." *Anesth Analg*, 1998; 86:579-83; Zhang, W. Y., A. Li Wan Po. "The effectiveness of topically applied capsaicin. A meta-analysis." *Eur J Clin Pharmacol*, 1994; 46:517-22 [review]; McCarthy, G. M., D. J. McCarty. "Effect of topical capsaicin in the therapy of painful osteoarthritis of the hands." *J Rheumatol*, 1992; 19:604-07; Altman, R. D., A. Aven, C. E. Holmburg, et al. "Capsaicin cream 0.025 per cent as monotherapy for osteoarthritis: a double-blind study." *Sem Arth Rheum*, 1994; 23(Suppl 3):25-33; Schnitzer, T., C. Morton, S. Coker. "Topical capsaicin therapy for osteoarthritis pain: achieving a maintenance regimen." *Sem Arth Rheum*, 1994; 23(Suppl 3):34-40.

19. *Archives of Facial Plastic Surgery*, 2006; 8:54'59.

20. Masson, M. "Bromelain in blunt injuries of the locomotor system. A study of observed applications in general practice." *Fortschr Med*, 1995; 113:303-06.

21. Calbrese, C, P. Preston. "Reports of double-blind, randomized, single-dose trial of a topical 2 per cent escin gel versus placebo in the acute treatment of experimentally induced hematoma in volunteers." *Planta Med*, 1993; 59:394'97.

22. Koll, R., M. Buhr, R. Dieter, et al. "Efficacy and tolerability of comfrey extract (ectr. Rad. Symphyti) in article distortions: results of a multi-centre, randomized, placebo-controlled double-blind study." *Z Phytother*, 2000; 21:127'34.

23. Koll, R., M. Buhr, R. Dieter, et al. "Efficacy and tolerance of a comfrey root extract (Extr. Rad. Symphyti) in the treatment of ankle distortions: results of a multicenter, randomized, placebo-controlled double-blind study." *Phytomed*, 2004; 11:470'77.

24. Predel, H. G., B. Giannetti, R. Koll, et al. "Efficacy of a comfrey root extract ointment in comparison to a diclofenac gel in the treatment of ankle distortions: results of an observer-blind, randomized, multicenter study." *Phytomedicine*, 2005; 12:707-14.

25. Kucera, M. et al. "Effects of Symphytum ointment on muscular symptoms of functional locomotor disturbances." *Adv Ther*, 2000; 17:204'10.

26. Giannetti, B. M., et al. "Efficacy and safety of a comfrey root extract ointment in the treatment of acute upper or low back pain: results of a double-blind, randomised, placebo-controlled, multi-centre trial." *Br J Sports Med* 2009; [epub ahead of print]. doi:10.1136/bjsm.2009.058677.

27. Al Faraj, S., K. Al Mutairi. "Vitamin D deficiency and chronic low back pain in Saudi Arabia." *Spine*, 2003; 28:177'79.

28. Ernst, E. "The efficacy of Phytodolor for the treatment of musculoskeletal pain-a systematic review of randomized clinical trials." *Natural Medicine Journal*, 1999; 2:14'16.

29. U.S. Department of Health and Human Services. Public Health Service. "Acupuncture. NIH Consensus Statement." 1997; 15:1'34.

30. Pradalier, A., J. C. Willer, J. Dry. "Pain sensitivity in obese individuals." *Ann Med Interne (Paris)*, 1982; 133:528'31.

31. Guieu, R., et al. "Nociceptive threshold and physical activity." *Can J Neurol Sci*, 1992; 19:69'71; Fordyce, W., R. McMahon, G. Rainwater, et al. "Pain complaint-exercise performance relationship in chronic pain." *Pain*, 1981; 10:311'21.

32. Siedliecki, S.L., M. Good. "Effect of music on power, pain, depression and disability." *Journal of Advanced Nursing*, 2006; 54: 553-62

SINUSITIS AND RUNNY NOSE

Many people suffer from recurrent sinus infections or from a frequent runny nose. Sometimes these problems are viral in nature, sometimes they are bacterial or fungal, and sometimes they are from allergens or chronic weakness. Some are chronic and some are acute.

Sinusitis causes a running nose that can have fluid from clear to yellow or even green or brownish. Green, brown, and deep yellow often signify an infection—viral or often bacterial. Clear is usually viral, allergen, chronic weakness, or candida. Yellow can indicate infection of a viral or bacterial nature. Chronic sinusitis may have little discharge but more inflammation and post-nasal drip. Those who have chronic sinusitis are more likely to get recurrent infections.

Symptoms of Sinusitis

Sinusitis can cause a headache, fever, pressure, or pain in the head, ear, face, and throat, cough, toothache, breathing problems, loss of smell and taste, dizziness, ear pain, ringing in the ears, and tenderness over forehead and cheekbones. The post-nasal dripping from the sinuses may cause sore throat, nausea, and bad breath, snoring and loss of sleep. Often, a sinus problem follows a cold virus.

Treatment of Sinusitis

So what can you do to treat sinus problems? If you have candida, see the section on Candida and treat for it. Avoid all known or suspected allergens: environmental allergens such as smoke, dust, mould, and fungus; and food allergens such as milk products, wheat, eggs, corn, soy, beef, tomato, orange, etc. If you are not sure what you are allergic to, work with a healer to find out. Even if you don't have known allergens, try avoiding dairy, sugar, refined grains, and gluten, as these substances can make mucous.

So what can you take to reduce a running and/or stuffy nose? Let's look at bacterial, viral, and fungal infections first. If you have sinusitis caused by one of these problems, try using herbs such as goldenseal root, echinacea, wild indigo, oregano oil, elderberry, bromelain, garlic, fenugreek, licorice, cat's claw, mullein, horehound, cayenne, thyme, sage, or hyssop, and vitamin C, quercetin, and zinc. These herbs and nutrients help to eliminate sinus problems by getting your own immune system to kick in and fight the infection. Some of the herbs also dry up mucous and draw out fluid. Some are antiviral, some are natural antibiotics, and some fight fungus.

Combine several herbs. For example, one combination that Linda finds works very well clinically is to take wild indigo, goldenseal root, bromelain, and licorice together. Herbs are usually used every two to three hours, 40 drops of each in a little water, on an empty stomach, or as teas or pills. Up to 10 g of vitamin C is usually taken with food in divided doses throughout the day. Try mixing it with quercetin. Zinc doses need to be appropriate to age and health, but are usually in lozenge form to be dissolved in the mouth. In one study that looked at bromelain, 87 per cent of patients treated with bromelain obtained good to excellent results in treating sinusitis[1].

One very good remedy is to mix 25 drops of usnea tincture with 1/2 cup saline solution and spray it into the nose four times per day. You can also try eucalyptus packs or ginger packs applied right over the sinuses. Apply a hot cloth with crushed ginger root or eucalyptus oil in it over the sinuses and leave on for at least twenty minutes, replacing it as it cools. You can also try yarrow, white oak bark, and witch hazel bark in the hot cloths. Or try swabbing the nasal passages with bitter orange. Another good remedy is to place hot, steaming water in a large bowl and put drops of eucalyptus or menthol in it then drape a towel around your head and sniff in the steam.

Mary Bove, N.D., suggests the following formula. Mix 1/2 oz of St. John's wort oil with 1 tbsp each of lobelia oil, bayberry root tincture, myrrh tincture, goldenseal tincture, and 1 tsp of cayenne oil or tincture, applied topically with heat one to three times per day.

Postural draining of the nasal passages is also good. Lie face down with your head near the floor and the rest of your body on the bed and expectorate as much as you can into a bowl two times per day. Acupuncture is also excellent for this problem.

Eardrops may be needed to help with ear involvement. They are often made up of garlic, St. John's wort oil, calendula, and mullein in a little olive oil.

If your problem is chronic weakness or allergies, follow the recommendations in the Allergies section. And try taking vitamin C and quercetin and using a saline spray up the nose. You may want to take probiotics, too, especially if you have clear weak discharge or have been on antibiotics at any time in your life and have not replaced the friendly flora. You may need to work to reduce long-time weakness, which is usually systemic. This will rev your immune system and get rid of dampness. Herbs that move dampness, such as gentian, dandelion root, and burdock root, are often added, as are warming herbs such as cayenne and ginger. Herbs that are natural astringents, such as indigo, bayberry, white oak bark, witch hazel, goldenseal, and yarrow, may also be used. Most people who have recurrent sinusitis have deep immune-system problems and need to work on the immune system. Herbs such as astragalus, echinacea, cat's claw, and goldenseal are often used.

Healing Diet

The diet should consist of warm/hot fluids, herbal teas, and soups, and should be free of dairy and sugar. At least 50 to 75 per cent of the diet should be from raw foods, high in fruits and veggies that are rich in vitamin C, flavonoids and carotenes to speed healing. Avoid salt, as it can cause mucous retention. Eat plenty of garlic and onions to speed healing. Spicy foods can also help; use cayenne, ginger, mustard, horseradish, cinnamon, cumin, black pepper, coriander, hot peppers, and turmeric in your food. And drink plenty of liquids. You may need to follow a detox diet. Eat plenty of whole grains such as brown rice, fruits, vegetables, legumes, and nuts and seeds, avoiding known allergens.

H. Pylori bacteria has also been linked to chronic sinusitis. So it is a good idea to get screened for *H. Pylori* and eliminate it if found.

Chapter Endnotes
1. Ryan, R. "A double-blind clinical evaluation of bromelains in the treatment of acute sinusitis." *Headache*, 1967; 7:13'17.

SKIN HEALTH

oils, blisters, and bruises. It almost sounds like a witch's incantation. Yet for many people, these are some of the painful skin problems that just won't go away no matter what they do.

One of the most-asked questions we get is what to do about some kind of skin problem. And there are many: eczema, psoriasis, acne, boils, rashes, infected wounds, warts, stings, or even just discoloration. And we invariably reply with a story we read about a nurse who had a terrible rash on the inside of her leg and who had done everything to get rid of it, to no avail. Fortunately for her, she happened to work for a herbalist, or at that time, a doctor who used herbs, who told her to use chickweed cream. She did, and the rash completely went away; she proclaimed to the herbalist that the stuff he had given her was a miracle cure.

Naturally, any herb with this kind of reputation intrigued us, and we looked into it. We were not surprised to discover that chickweed's reputation is well deserved. We have used it on scores of rashes since then, including a rash that would not go away, just like the nurse's.

Chickweed has anti-inflammatory properties that make it useful for any kind of skin problem, especially rashes—even rashes that you can't see. It works much like cortisone, but is safer and without side effects. Linda even uses it as a base cream for moxibustion, an acupuncture practice that involves burning the herb mugwort, to prevent burning and irritation on the skin. Chickweed is also an emollient that helps to keep surfaces moist, preventing them from drying out. It is most commonly used as an oil or salve, and applied to skin rashes, eczema, psoriasis, and any other kind of skin problem. To make an oil, chop 1 lb of fresh chickweed or use the dried herb and place it in a jar of oil, such as olive oil or almond oil, and leave it for four days. Strain through a cloth and use. Or make a salve: Cut 1 lb of fresh chickweed and place it in a stone baking dish with vegetable shortening and cook, covered, for about 1 hour. Strain if necessary and mix with enough beeswax to make into a salve. Or use chickweed as a poultice for boils and abscesses. Internally, chickweed is valued for treating skin diseases because of its alterative properties, which means it will slowly correct impurities in the bloodstream, and, hence, the whole body.

Licorice and chamomile creams are also especially good topical anti-inflammatories.

While most people want to apply something topically to help clear up skin problems, it is by no means the whole solution. Most skin problems require further care, using herbs such as alteratives that will cleanse the body, including the liver, kidneys, blood, skin, and digestive tract. This method works because skin problems usually originate from the inside.

There are numerous herbs for treating skin problems, our favourites being comfrey, calendula, chickweed, slippery elm, flaxseed, cleavers, burdock, red clover, milk thistle, sassafras, sarsaparilla, blue flag, yellow dock, dandelion root, nettle, echinacea, and aloe. And, although not strictly a herb, essential fatty acids are crucial in treating skin diseases like eczema, psoriasis, and dry skin. Try using flaxseed oil.

Comfrey is used for wound healing, even for healing broken bones. It's known as knit-bone for this reason, and it can be used externally and internally for healing ulcers, sores, wounds, and fractures. It seems to work because of its allantoin content, which increases cell proliferation, allowing for speedy wound healing.

Calendula is also an alterative that can be used internally or externally to treat skin problems. It can be used as an oil, salve, or poultice. Those with burns will find calendula especially useful since it has a well-earned reputation for treating burns, as do St. John's wort oil and cleavers. Calendula can stop bleeding, since it is an astringent and heal wounds, ulcers, and eruptive skin diseases such as rashes. It can even bring relief to those suffering from shingles. Use a strong tea or a poultice or juice from the petals for treating shingles and apply topically.

Slippery elm and flaxseeds make excellent additions to poultices and help to keep surfaces moist, while drawing out infection. Both can be used to treat ulcers, bedsores, and wounds, and are helpful for boils, rashes, and blisters, as well.

Burdock, red clover, sassafras, sarsaparilla, blue flag, yellow dock, dandelion root, nettle, and milk thistle will all help to cleanse the body. Burdock has a reputation for treating skin disorders and is a strong purifier. It works by making the sweat glands eliminate toxic wastes, clearing up carbuncles, canker sores, and infections. Combined with herbs that purify the blood and fight infection, such as dandelion, milk thistle, sassafras, blue flag, yellow dock, nettle, echinacea, wild indigo, Oregon grape root, and sarsaparilla, it can be used to treat skin problems such as eczema, acne, and psoriasis. Milk thistle helps by clearing stored-up toxins from the body, and red clover is wonderful for skin eruptions, psoriasis, and eczema. Echinacea, wild indigo, and Oregon grape root are used for their antibiotic and immune-enhancing properties. Many of the other mentioned herbs cleanse the body and purify the blood, organs, and skin.

Plantain leaves can be used to treat bites, wounds, and stings. Simply crush the leaves and rub onto the affected area. If the sting does not improve, you may need to take some internally as well, in a tea form.

Good wart removers include chapparal, castor oil, tea tree oil, garlic oil, thuja, and celandine.

Aloe is especially good for burns, rashes, acne, or any skin irritation. It has anti-bacterial, anti-viral and anti-fungal properties and aids in healing.

For those with acne, zinc, chromium, the B vitamins, vitamins A, E and C, grapefruit seed extract, and detoxifying can be very helpful. We especially find that when people begin to break out, if they do a juice cleanse with beet, apple, parsley, ginger, greens, and carrot juice, and use acidophilus, grapefruit seed extract, and zinc, their skin usually clears. Fibre is also key: Try using psyllium seeds every day with lots of water to help flush the system. If the skin doesn't clear, there may be an offending food allergy involved or poor diet, or the person may need to take chastetree berry to help balance hormones. Also use those alterative herbs already mentioned. (See Acne section.)

Although many people do not realize it, food allergies cause skin rashes and are found in people with psoriasis and eczema, as well. Also, nutritional deficiencies, low stomach acid, and stress have been found to play a part in skin diseases.

To get rid of bruises, use vitamin C and flavonoids, foods rich in vitamin K, such as dark leafy greens, grapeseed extract and coenzyme Q10, internally; and externally, use poultices with herbs such as rosehips, hyssop, and plantain to draw matter out. Alfalfa is also good for bruises. (See Pain and Injury section.)

And for those who really don't have any skin issues and just wish to have healthy skin, try taking vitamin C with flavonoids such as grape seed extract, vitamin E, B vitamins, a multivitamin/mineral formula, and silica to keep skin healthy. Topically, aloe, vitamins E, C, or CoQ10 creams are excellent choices to keep skin healthy. Brush the skin to get rid of built-up dead, dried skin. And drink lots of water and eat well—lots of fresh foods. What you eat is reflected in your skin. Healthy skin can also benefit from essential fatty acids such as flaxseed oil.

There are numerous herbs that can be used to treat skin disease; we have only mentioned a few. Look for herbs in creams, oils, pills, tinctures, or loose, either together in combinations or alone, in health food stores and other places that sell herbs, or gather them from nature and use.

STRESS

We were travelling in the Mediterranean, talking to a man about our two cultures' lifestyles and our comparative levels of stress, when he said with a smile that left no doubt which one he would choose, "We will always be a third world country, but you will always have high blood pressure."

The alarm clock rips into your sleep, the annoying song on your cell phone means the office is callling, the e-mail catalogues the messages that are waiting for you, the house work is piling up, you're late for work and traffic has you totally stuck. Arggh!

Life has gotten faster and busier, and it seems that you're always on call and can never get caught up. Stress! It's a major problem in our modern North American society. And stress is not only a major health problem itself, it contributes to a whole host of serious problems.

But even if you can't change your life, you can change the way your body deals with stress. And how your body deals with stress, according to Canadian stress research pioneer Hans Selye, may be even more important than how much stress it is under.

How well your body handles stress has a lot to do with how healthy your adrenal glands are. When it comes to stress, the adrenal glands are command central.

Give Your Adrenals the Nutritional Support They Need

If you want your adrenal glands to be up to the modern challenge of the stressful day, then you have to give them plenty of what they need. And what they need, primarily, is lots of vitamins C, B5 and B6 and the minerals zinc, magnesium and potassium.

If you want to study stress, then what better test than math and public speaking? When people were given either 3 grams of vitamin C or a placebo every day for two weeks in a double-blind study, the ones given the vitamin C made it through the math and public speaking with lower levels of stress[1].

Undergoing surgery is also extremely stressful. But when patients were given vitamin C for one week before and after surgery, their stress related hormones went back to normal faster than patients not given vitamin C[2].

You should also supplement B5, B6, zinc and magnesium. Along with vitamin C, these nutrients are crucial for the health of the adrenal gland itself and for its manufacture of adrenal hormones. To boost your potassium, increase the potassium in your diet while decreasing the sodium in your diet. You can accomplish this antistress move by reducing salt and packaged foods and increasing fruits, vegetables, whole grains, nuts, seeds and legumes. You might also want to take extra calcium.

Lifestyle Do's and Don'ts

A number of things we do that we think help us get through a stressful day need to be eliminated, and a number of things we don't think we have time for in a stressful day need to be added. The coffee that you grab to help give you the energy to get through just makes things worse. Try to reduce or eliminate caffeine. Same for junk food. That quick meal or snack you grab because you don't have time for a proper meal is part of the problem. Try to avoid, or at least reduce, refined carbohydrates, sugar, soda, bad fats, and processed and deep fried food: these all put a huge strain on the adrenal glands. The same goes for that drink you may take to help you cope with the stress. It's not helping: it's hurting. Alcohol does not calm you, as people believe. When men were given either alcohol or a placebo, the ones drinking the alcohol suffered significant increases in anxiety[3].

Smoking also contributes to stress. Studies not only show that smoking increases stress[4], but also that quitting smoking reduces stress[5].

You not only need to eliminate things, there are things you need to make time to put back in. Find a fun way to incorporate regular exercise into your day. Relaxation techniques like meditation are also important. And make sure you get enough sleep.

All the Other Nutrients

A high potency, high quality multivitamin helps deal with stress for a number of reasons. The first is that in times of stress, the body is too worried about running away and escaping to bother much about digestion. From an evolutionary viewpoint, this is good: getting away from scary, stressful things is a key to staying alive; from a nutritional viewpoint, this is bad: stress no longer just comes from sabre tooth tigers, and we can't afford to be digesting poorly all the time in this modern world of constant stress. So a good multi will provide all those nutrients that you aren't getting enough of because of stress. It will also help provide the extra punch of B vitamins and vitamin C that your nervous system so desperately needs in order to deal with stress.

Herbal Help for Calming Stress

In addition to vitamins and minerals, there are also a bunch of herbs that are perfect for helping you stay calm and cope with stress.

ESSENTIAL NUTRIENTS FOR THE ADRENAL GLANDS

Vitamin B5
Vitamin B6
Vitamin C
Zinc
Magnesium
Potassium

Ginseng and Eleuthero

First among them is ginseng and its relative Eleuthero, which used to be known as Siberian ginseng (it is not actually a ginseng at all). Both of these herbs support adrenal function and your response to mental and physical stress, improving your level of relaxation, your mood, your quality of work and your overall quality of life.

Licorice

The other great stress herb is licorice. Licorice is a great adrenal tonic. This herb is able to pull off an amazing trick: it fools your body into thinking one of its components is cortisol, the antistress adrenal hormone. It is also able to boost the ability of your body's own cortisol. So licorice is ideal for helping the adrenal gland to deal with stress.

Rhodiola

Rhodiola rosea is one of those herbs bursting with potential that has not really taken off yet. But it should. It helps the body stand up to a huge range of mental and physical stressors. Almost magically, rhodiola can calm you down, but increase your energy at the same time. Students who took Rhodiola rosea during the intense stress of final exams had significantly improved grades, mental fatigue and general well-being compared to students who took a placebo[6]. Other research has also found Rhodiola to decrease mental fatigue and anxiety while increasing work capacity and general well-being.

Ashwagandha

Another great herb that is not nearly well enough known in the west is Ashwagandha. Often referred to as Indian ginseng, this herb is another one that helps the body deal with a wide range of stressors. Ashwagandha is especially good when your nerves are simply exhausted from all the stress. If nervousness from stress and adrenal exhaustion has reduced your libido or affected sexual function, ashwagandha is a great herb to try.

Gotu Kola

Another underutilized herb in the west is gotu kola. Amongst its many uses, gotu kola can soothe stress and anxiety[7].

Green Tea

And a huge study has now discovered that the people who drink less than one cup a day of green tea have the highest rate of stress (8.4 per cent and the ones who drink five or more cups a day have the lowest rate of stress (5.1 per cent)[8]. So try having a relaxing cup of green tea. The more you sip, the less you stress!

An unexpected entry on an antistress list is reishi, the great immunity mushroom. Reishi is another of those incredible herbs that has the duel ability to calm and revitalize the nerves at the same time.

Astragalus

The deep immune tonic, astragalus, is also valuable for stress. According to traditional Chinese medicine, astragalus builds *qi*, the body's vital energy or life force. It builds up both adrenal function and immune function. Both are important during times of stress because adrenal burnout can lead to immune problems.

Nervine Herbs

Rounding out the list of herbs for stress are the nervine, or calming, herbs: valerian, skullcap, lemon balm, chamomile, oats, catnip and hops. Valerian, the great insomnia herb, is also able to calm stress: it has a powerful effect on the nervous system.

Skullcap, though much less known, is one of the most important herbs for toning the nervous system by nourishing and reenergizing it while it calms: it is one of the greatest and most versatile nervine herbs of all. Skullcap is great for exhaustion and tension and helps you to relax throughout the day so that you prepare for sleep at night.

The beautiful smelling lemon balm is one of nature's very best calming herbs. It is the perfect herb for nervous tension or anywhere the word "nervous" shows up: like nervous sleeping disorders and nervous stomach disorders.

Chamomile is another great and gentle calming herb, and so is oats, though it is much less known. Oats is actually one of the very best nervous system tonics, acording to herbalist Rosemary Gladstar. Herbalist David Hoffmann says that it is one of the best herbs for nourishing the nervous system, especially when under stress, and Gladstar says it is a great herb for people who are overworked and stressed: and that's just what we're looking for.

Try catnip if you are suffering from built up emotional tension and need to soothe your nerves. Use it during the day if built up tension is preventing you from sleeping at night. Hops is another good choice for soothing and quieting the nervous system. Hops can promote sleep when you are feeling overwrought.

Chapter Endnotes

1. Brody S., *et al.* A randomized controlled trial of high dose ascorbic acid for reduction of blood pressure, cortisol, and subjective responses to psychological stress. *Psychopharmacology (Berl)* 2002;159:319–24.

2. Gromova E. G., *et al.* Regulation of the indices of neuroendocrine status in surgical patients with lung cancer using optimal doses of ascorbic acid. *Anesteziol Reanimatol* 1990;5:71–4.

3. Montiero M. G., *et al.* Subjective feelings of anxiety in young men anfter ethanol and diazepam infusions. *J Clin Psychiatry* 1990;51:12.

4. Parrott A. C., Cigarette smoking does cause stress. *Am Psychol* 2000;55:1159–60.

5. Long D., Smoking as a coping strategy. *Nurs Times* 2003;99:50,53.

6. Spasov A. A., *et al.* A double-blind, placebo-controlled pilot study of the stimulating and adaptogenic effect of Rhodiola rosea SHR-5 extract on the fatigue of students caused by stress during an examination period with a repeated low-dose regimen. *Phytomedicine* 2000;7:85–9.

7. Ramaswamy A. S., *et al.* Pharmacological studies on Centella asiatica. *Linn. J Res Indian Med* 1970;4:160-75.

8. Hozawa A., *et al.* Green tea consumption is associated withlower psychological distress in a general population: the Ohsaki Cohort 2006 Study. *Am J Clin Nutr* 2009;90:1390-6.

ULCERS

That gnawing, burning pain of an ulcer is something that far too many people are familiar with. About one in ten of us will suffer the pain of ulcers at some time. Ulcer medications have become some of the top selling drugs in the world. These drugs focus on lessening the burning stomach acids. But the stomach acids are crucial for digestion. Besides, they are not really the problem. You are supposed to have stomach acid. The problem occurs when the lining that protects the stomach and duodenum from the acid becomes damaged. The lining can be damaged by many attackers: *H. pylori* bacteria, nonsteroidal anti-inflammatory drugs like aspirin, alocohol, stress and nutritional deficiencies. Of these, the most important are *H. pylori* and aspirin. *H. pylori*

is the main cause of ulcers, and even low doses of aspirin cause gastointestinal bleeding: twenty-eight per cent of people taking low dose aspirin for heart disease get an ulcer[1].

The Natural Approach: Removing the Causes

So what's to be done? There is another approach. Rather than suppress the acid that causes the burning, address the primary cause and heal the lining that protects against it.

The first step in treating an ulcer is to eliminate any factors that are contributing to it. That means no more alcohol[2] or aspirin. It also means no more smoking[3]. Smoking increases the chances of getting an ulcer and decreases the chances of treating it. Stress and nutritional deficiencies can also contribute.

Food allergies are an important cause of ulcers and eliminating them is very effective in treating and preventing ulcers[4]. The common practice of drinking milk to soothe an ulcer is not only a bad idea because milk is so allergenic, but population studies show that the more milk you drink, the greater your chance of getting an ulcer[5].

Eating a lot of sugar[6] or salt[7] may also be linked to ulcers, as can drinking a lot of coffee—caffeinated or decaffeinated[8]—or tea[9].

POSSIBLE CAUSES OF ULCERS

H. Pylori
NSAID's like Aspirin
Alcohol
Smoking
Stress
Nutritional Deficiencies
Food Allergies
Milk
Sugar
Salt
Coffee
Tea

Heal the Ulcer

In addition to eliminating the causes, you can begin to heal the ulcer. The best ulcer healer is licorice. You can use the whole licorice root, but the licorice that is most commonly used for ulcers is a special kind called deglycyrrhizinated licorice, or DGL for short.

Licorice has been proven to be as or more effective than ulcer medications like cimitidine, ranitidine and antacids in head-to-head studies[10]. Unlike the drugs, licorice actually heals the ulcer: it improves the protective lining of the intestines. And once the ulcer has healed, licorice allows fewer relapses than the drugs do[11]. Acid blocking drugs may even make the ulceration process worse while they supress the symptoms, because reducing the acid promotes the growth of *H. pylori*, the bacteria now known to be behind so many ulcers. Licorice, on the other hand, contains several flavonoids which inhibit *H. pylori*[12].

The other great ulcer herb is chamomile. Chamomile protects you against ulcers by soothing and healing the protective lining of the gastrointestinal tract. It also contains a flavonoid called apigenin that inhibits *H. pylori*[13]. Herbal authority Rudolf Fritz Weiss, M.D. says that

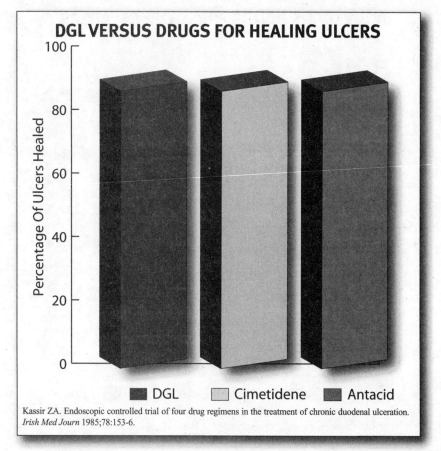

Kassir ZA. Endoscopic controlled trial of four drug regimens in the treatment of chronic duodenal ulceration. *Irish Med Journ* 1985;78:153-6.

chamomile addresses all the hallmarks of an ulcer: spasm, inflammation and ulceration. He says that there is no remedy, including drugs, more tailor-made for ulcers.

Another great treatment for ulcers is cabbage juice. Studies show that one litre of cabbage juice a day can totally heal an ulcer. Cabbage may heal because of its high content of glutamine. One study compared glutamine to conventional therapy: glutamine won. Twenty-two out of twenty-four people on glutamine had their ulcers completely healed in four weeks[14].

Zinc, the great wound healing mineral, can cure an ulcer[15]. Aloe vera gel has also been shown in a study to cure an ulcer[16], and many ulcer sufferers have found that same benefit.

Flavonoids improve your body's defences against ulcers, and, as we have seen from the flavonoids in the great ulcer herbs licorice and chamomile, they inhibit *H. pylori*[17].

Daniel Mowrey, Ph.D., says that peppermint is antiulcer, and James Duke, Ph.D., says that ginger contains an amazing eleven antiulcer compounds. Nettle has also recently been found to have antiulcer activity[18].

Several soothing and healing herbs, like calen-

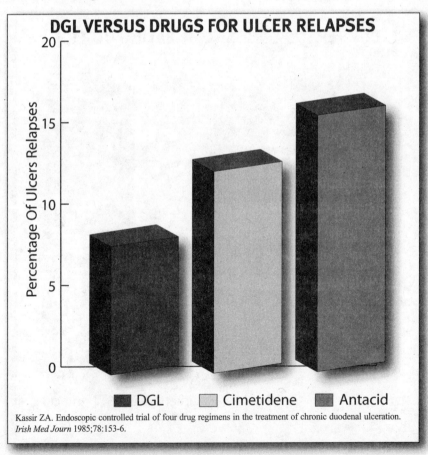

DGL VERSUS DRUGS FOR ULCER RELAPSES

Percentage Of Ulcers Relapses

DGL   Cimetidene   Antacid

Kassir ZA. Endoscopic controlled trial of four drug regimens in the treatment of chronic duodenal ulceration. *Irish Med Journ* 1985;78:153-6.

dula, slippery elm and marshmallow, can also help. Several herbalists suggest combining some of these herbs for treating ulcers. Michael Tierra uses comfrey and marshmallow and adds licorice root and slippery elm.

And finally, make sure your diet is rich in fibre. High fibre diets reduce the rate of ulcers, and, when you heal your ulcer, staying on a high fibre diet reduces the chances of its coming back by 50 per cent[19].

Chapter Endnotes

1. Yeomans N. D., *et al*. Prevalence and incidence of gastroduodenal ulcers during treatment with vascular protective doses of aspirin. *Alimentary Pharmacology & Therapeutics* 2005;22:795-801.

2. Lenz HJ, Ferrari-Taylor J., Isenberg J. I., Wine and five per cent ethanol are potent stimulants of gastric acid secretion in humans. *Gastroenterology* 1983;85:1082-7.

3. Korman MG, *et al*. Influence of cigarette smoking on healing and relapse in duodenal ulcer disease. *Gastroenterology* 1983;85:871-4; Hull DH, Beale PJ. Cigarette smoking and duodenal ulcer. *Gut* 1985;26:1333-7; Chang FY, Lai KH, Lee SD, Effects of cigarette smoking on healing and remission of duodenal ulcer. *Curr Ther Res* 1993;54:313-9.

4. Siegel J., Immunologic approach to the treatment and prevention of gastointestinal ulcers. *Ann Allergy* 1977;38:27-9; Andre C., *et al*. Evidence for anaphylactic reactions in peptic ulcer and varioliform gastritis. *Ann Allergy* 1983;51:325-8.

5. Kumar N., *et al*. Effect of milk on patients with duodenal ulcers. *Brit Med J* 1986;293:666.

6. Yudkin J., Eating and ulcers. BMJ 1980;16:483; Katchinski BD, *et al*. Duodenal ulcer and refined carbohydrate intake: a case-control study assessing dietary fibre and refined sugar intake. *Gut* 1990;31:993-6.

7. Sonnenberg A. Dietary salt and gastric ulcer. *Gut* 1986;27:1138-42.

8. Cohen S, Booth G. H. Jr. Gastric acid secretion and lower-esophageal-sphincter pressure in response to coffee and caffeine. *N Engl J Med* 1975;293:897-9; Feldman E. J., Isenberg J. I., Grossman MI. Gastric acid and gastrin response to decaffeinated coffee and a peptone meal. *JAMA* 1981;246:248-50.

9. Dubey P, Sundram K. R., Nundy S. Effect of tea on gastric acid secretion. *Dig Dis Sci* 1984;29:202-6.

10. Balakrizhnan M., *et al*. Deglycyrrhizinated liquorice in the treatment of chronic duodenal ulcer. *J Assoc Physicians India* 1978;26:811-4; Morgan A. G., *et al*. Comparison between cimetidine and Caved-S in the treatment of gastric ulceration, and subsequent maintenance therapy. *Gut* 1982;23:545-51; Glick L., Deglycyrrhizinated liquorice in peptic ulcer. *Lancet* 1982;2:817.

11. Kassir Z. A., Endoscopic controlled trial of four drug regimens in the treatment of chronic duodenal ulceration. *Irish Med Journ* 1985;78:153-6.

12. Beil W., Birkholz W, Sewing K. F., Effects of flavonoids on parietal cell acid secretion, gastric mucosal prostaglandin production and Helicobacter pylori growth. *Arzneimforsch* 1995;45:697-700; Fukai T., *et al*. Anti-Helicobacter pylori flavonoids from licorice extract. *Life Sci* 2002;71:1449-63.

13. Beil W., Birkholz C, Sewing KF. Effects of flavonoids on parietal cell acid secretion, gastric mucosal prostaglandin production and Helicobacter pylori growth. *Arzneimforsch* 1995;45:697-700.

14. Shive W., *et al*. Glutamine in treatment of peptic ulcer. *Texas State J Med* 1957;53:840-3.

15. Frommer D. J., The healing of gastric ulcers by zinc sulphate. *Med J Aust* 1975;2:793-6.

16. Blitz J. J., Smith J. W., Gerard J. R., Aloe vera gell in peptic ulcer therapy: Preliminary report. *J Am Osteopath Assoc* 1963;62:731-5.

17. Beil W., Birkholz W., Sewing K. F., Effects of flavonoids on parietal cell acid secretion, gastric mucosal prostaglandin production and Helicobacter pylori growth. *Arzneimforsch* 1995;45:697-700.

18. Gülçin I., *et al*. Antioxidant, antimicrobial, antiulcer and analgesic activities of nettle (Urtica dioica L.) *Ethopharmacol* 2004;90:205-15.

19. Rydning A., *et al*. Prophylactic effect of dietary fibre in duodenal ulcer disease. *Lancet* 1982;2:736-9.

URINARY TRACT INFECTIONS

You've just gone to the washroom not five minutes ago, and already you feel like you need to go again. And when you do go, it burns, comes out in spurts, and, no matter how many times you empty your bladder, it still feels full. This is what it can feel like to have a urinary tract infection—one of the most common problems to affect women, often at least once a year.

According to Michael T. Murray, N.D., "10 to 20 per cent of all women have urinary tract discomfort at least once a year, 37.5 per cent of women with no history of urinary tract infections will have one within ten years, and 2-4 per cent of apparently healthy women have elevated levels of bacteria in their urine, indicative of an unrecognized urinary tract infection." Fifty-five per cent of women with recurrent bladder infections will eventually have involvement of the kidneys, which, for some, can mean scarring and even kidney failure. In men, urinary tract infections are less common and often indicate an anatomical abnormality or a prostate infection.

Causes, Diagnosis and Symptoms

The causes of urinary tract infections are many: bacteria entering the urinary tract through the bloodstream, bacteria ascending from the urethra, from faecal contamination or vaginal secretions, or, for men, prostate problems. Those who have what is known as pooling of the urine caused by obstructions or anatomical problems are also at risk, as are those whose immune systems are down.

Adding to the problem, the diagnosis of urinary tract infections can be difficult, since those suffering from symptoms often do not have significant amounts of bacteria in their urine. According to Murray, 40 per cent of women who have typical symptoms of urinary tract infections do not have a significant amount of bacteria in their urine.

Typical symptoms of a urinary tract infection include lower back pain, fever, chills, burning upon urination, urgency of urination, painful urination, odour of the urine, cloudy urine, frequent urination, blood in the urine, nausea, and frequent night-time urination. Although some may have few or no symptoms at all, they may still be infected.

The Problem with Antibiotics

While conventional medicine uses antibiotics to treat urinary tract infections, Balch and Balch say that antibiotics disturb the normal flora and may actually promote recurrent infections by promoting the growth of antibiotic-resistant strains of bacteria[1]. They also report that 50 to 80 per cent of bacteria in our bodies are now resistant to common antibiotics, forcing conventional doctors to prescribe more powerful and dangerous antibiotics that can cause adverse reactions. Antibiotics disturb the friendly flora in the vagina. Since the flora in the vagina protect the bladder from harmful bacteria, this can increase the risk of a urinary tract infection. For the same reason, antibiotic therapy for urinary tract infections in women often triggers vaginal yeast infections.

For most infections, the natural approach is the best route to ensure not only that the infection goes away but also that it does not come back.

The Natural Approach: Support the Immune System

Since for many patients with recurrent bladder infections the immune system is involved, therapy is often also aimed at restoring proper immune function. The diet should consist of fresh whole foods, and you should avoid sugar, caffeine, alcohol, chocolate, carbonated beverages, chemicals in food, and simple carbohydrates, since these substances further weaken the immune system and encourage the growth of bacteria. According to Zoltan Rona, M.D., foods that contribute to allergies should be avoided since these, too, may cause recurrent bladder irritations. Paul Pitchford, author of *Healing with Whole Foods*, suggests using spirulina, marshmallow herb, rehmannia root, asparagus root, and aloe vera gel to strengthen the kidneys and keep them strong. Also, drink plenty of water to help flush out the system.

Sometimes just switching to a healthy diet can strengthen the immune system, but often more help is needed. Perhaps the best herb for enhancing immunity is echinacea. Numerous studies have shown that echinacea has profound effects on the immune system. It is also useful for urinary tract infections, especially when combined with other herbs. Herbalist Michael Tierra recommends taking echinacea every two hours in acute

URINARY TRACT INFECTION: CRANBERRY JUICE

What Cranberry Can Do	Mechanism of Action	Dose
•Treat urinary tract infection •Prevent recurrence of urinary tract infection •Treat antibiotic resistant urinary tract infection	• Cranberry reduces the ability of bacteria to adhere to the walls of the urinary tract	• Dilute pure, unsweetened cranberry juice in water and drink 16 ounces a day or take 10-16 500mg pills or take 400mg of concentrated cranberry extract 2-3 times a day.

infections. If it is specifically the thymus gland, the seat of the immune system, that is affected, licorice and European mistletoe can also be of use, according to Murray. There are many other helpful herbs and nutrients that can help to support the immune system, such as ginseng, goldenseal, boneset, astragalus, ligustrum, vitamin C, B6, beta-carotene, and zinc. It is obviously a good idea to take a multivitamin/mineral daily to help support the immune system and prevent infections from re-occurring. During an infection, it is a good idea to take vitamin C, 500 mg, every two hours, bio-flavonoids, 1g per day, beta-carotene, 200,000 IU per day, and zinc, 30 mg per day. There are also many deep-toning combinations of herbs that can be used to help strengthen a weakened immune system.

Cranberry: Urinary Tract Infection Specialist

For treating a urinary tract infection, one of the best things that you can do is to drink plenty of liquids, including unsweetened cranberry juice. Cranberry juice and cranberry juice supplements have been used to treat urinary tract infections for years. They have been shown in clinical studies to be very effective. In one study, 16 oz of cranberry juice per day was consumed by people with urinary tract infections; 73 per cent of those with active urinary tract infections showed improvement. And when they stopped drinking cranberry juice, 61 per cent of them experienced a recurrence of bladder infections[2]. Cranberry can help you not only to fight off a urinary tract infection, but also to protect you against its coming back. In one study, only 16 per cent of women on cranberry juice who had just recovered from an infection suffered a recurrence, while 39 per cent of those given a placebo did[3].

Although cranberry juice was originally thought to work on infections by acidifying the urine, this may not be the case. According to Murray, one litre of cranberry juice would be needed to acidify the urine, and it doesn't seem to take that much for cranberry juice to be effective. Recent studies indicate that cranberry works by reducing the ability of the bacteria to adhere, or stick, to the lining of the bladder and urethra, allowing the body to fight off the infection[4].

In the book *Beyond Antibiotics*, Dr. Edwin Kass of Harvard is quoted as saying that, "[c]ranberry juice can eliminate bacteria even in those whose bladder infections have been resistant to previous antibiotic therapy." Recent research continues to bear this claim out. When women with urinary tract infections that were, in most cases, antibiotic-resistant were given cranberry juice, the cranberry prevented the bacteria from adhering to the bladder wall in 80 per cent of them[5]. Zoltan Rona suggests juicing fresh, raw cranberries and mixing them with carrot juice and one to two tablespoons of pure ascorbic acid crystals, daily, to fight off infection. Others suggest using 16 to 48 oz a day of cranberry juice or to take capsules of cranberry. Clinically, Linda finds that the juice seems to work better.

Probiotics

To keep the immune system functioning at its peak and to keep infections from coming back, acidophilus and bifidus are also very important. People with low friendly flora from overuse of antibiotics—including antibiotics to treat urinary tract infections—are especially at risk for recurrent urinary tract infections. Take 20 billion live cultures a day to replenish the normal friendly flora and to get rid of the infection and prevent it from coming back.

If an infection is present, wear only underwear made from cotton; use plain, unbleached toilet paper and keep the area clean; women should avoid using tampons and be sure to empty the bladder as soon as the urge to do so is present.

Some of the best herbs for the urinary tract are uva ursi, garlic, goldenseal, buchu, cleavers, marshmallow, goldenrod, and corn silk.

Uva Ursi

Uva ursi is one of the best and most commonly used herbs to treat urinary tract infections. It is effective against *E. coli*, the most common bacteria involved in urinary tract infections, and against other bacterial causes of urinary tract infections, too. Herbalist Michael Tierra says that uva ursi is a diuretic, urinary antiseptic, and an astringent that is useful for urinary tract infections and for blood in the urine. Traditionally it has been used to treat bladder and kidney infections, kidney stones, and edema. A double-blind study using a standardized extract of uva ursi was evaluated on recurrent cystitis, or urinary tract infection. None of the women using uva ursi had a recurrence of cystitis, whereas the placebo group had almost a 20 per cent rate of recurrence[6]. Also, the uva ursi group had no side effects. Uva ursi has also been shown to be extremely effective against acute cystitis.

Garlic

Garlic is effective against several of the bacteria associated with urinary tract infections, including, *E. coli, Proteus spp., Klebsiella pneumonia, and Staphylococus spp*. It is a good idea to consume plenty of fresh garlic, too.

Goldenseal

Goldenseal has a long history of use in the treatment of all infections, including urinary tract infections. Studies have shown it to be effective against *E. coli, Proteus spp., Klebsiella spp., Staphylococcus spp., Enterobacter aerogenes,* and *Pseudomonas spp.*[7]. In addition the direct antibiotic properties of goldenseal, it has also been shown to prevent the adhesion of the bacteria to the urinary tract[8]. It is one of our favourite herbs for treating urinary tract infections because it is effective against such a huge range of bacteria. It also stimulates the immune system, allowing the body to fight off all kinds of infections, and it kills off yeast, one of the causes of infections.

Buchu

Buchu has been used for centuries in South Africa for urinary, kidney, and prostate problems. It is used to relieve inflammation of the kidneys and cramps in the bladder, for gravel and stones in the bladder and to soothe and strengthen the urinary organs. Herbalist David Hoffman says that it can be used for any type of infection of the urinary system, and Michael Tierra calls it one of the best diuretics known, and recommends it for both acute and chronic urinary tract problems.

Cleavers

Cleavers is a diuretic that is useful for all urinary problems, according to Michael Tierra. Old-time herbalists used this herb for scalding urine, dropsy, irritation at the neck of the bladder, and in gravel, especially stones of the bladder.

Corn silk

Corn silk is a demulcent diuretic that is soothing to the urinary tract system. Its antiseptic powers are useful for cleansing the circulation of urea and for cleansing the urinary tract, making it useful for treating urinary tract infections.

Marshmallow Root

Marshmallow root is a great herb for soothing irritation in the urinary tract and is often combined with other herbs to get rid of stones, irritation, blood, and infections.

Goldenrod

Goldenrod is one of the best herbs to use as an anti-inflammatory diuretic and antiseptic. It can be used for cystitis and urethritis.

There are many other useful herbs for the urinary tract, including juniper berries, parsley, plantain, wild carrot, gravel root (especially for stones of the kidney), and white poplar bark (useful for urinary weakness, especially in the elderly, or for anyone who has weak kidneys or incontinence). It is not necessary to use all of them, but rather choose one or a few and combine them either to strengthen the urinary tract, to treat infections or stones, or to clean the urinary system.

Chapter Endnotes

1. Balch, J. F., P. A. Balch. *Prescription for Nutritional Healing*, 2nd ed. Garden City Park, NY: Avery, 1997.

2. Prodromos, P. N., C. A. Brusch, G. C. Ceresia. "Cranberry juice in the treatment of urinary tract infections." *Southwest Med*, 1968; 47:17.

3. Kontiokari, T., *et al*. "Cranberry-Lingonberry juice and Lactobacillus GG drink for the prevention of urinary tract infections in women." *BMJ*, 2001; 322:1'5.

4. Sobota, A. E. "Inhibition of bacteria adherence by cranberry juice: potential use for the treatment of urinary tract infections." *J Urology*, 1984; 131:1,013'16.

5. Howell, A. B., B. Foxman. "Cranberry Juice and Adhesion of Antibiotic-Resistant Uropathogens." *JAMA*, 2002; 287:3082'83.

6. Larsson, B., A. Jonasson, S. Fianu. "Prophylactic effect of UVA-E in women with recurrent cystitis. A preliminary report." *Curr Ther Res*, 1993; 53:441'43.

7. Amin, A. H., T. V. Subbaiah, K.M. Abbasi. "Berberine sulfate: Antimicrobial activity, bioassay, and mode of action." *Can J Microbio*, 1969; 15:1067'76; Johnson, C. C., G. Johnson, C. F. Poe. "Toxicity of alkaloids to certain bacteria." *Acta Pharmacol Toxicol*, 1952; 8:71'78.

8. Sun, D.X., S.N. Abraham, E.H. Beachey. "Influence of berberine sulfate on synthesis and expression of pap fimbrial adhesion in uropathogenic Escherichia coli." *Antimicrob Agents Chemother*, 1988; 32:1274-77.

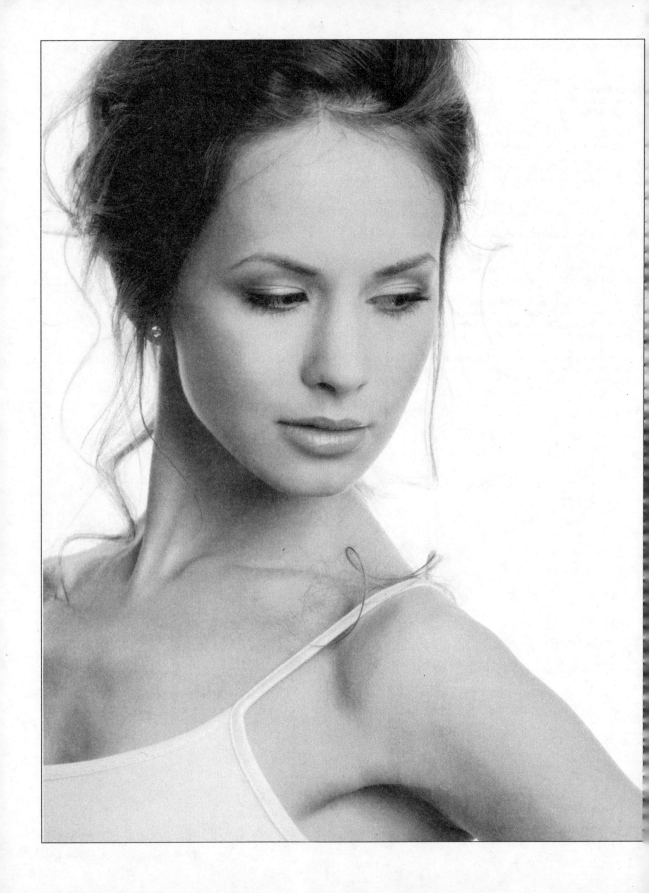

WOMEN'S HEALTH

Women are the most over-drugged population in our society. They are given the pill for just about everything and Prozac, or a similar alternative, for just about everything else. They are often not well listened to by their doctors, and their needs are not met. This is why there is a section in this encyclopedia just for them.

Women's systems are unique and are best treated with an aim to correct the underlying issues, not just covering them up with harmful drugs that often do not correct the underlying problem. Women are the population that uses the most natural health products, and they tend to want to take better care of themselves, and this is where natural medicine can really shine.

Women's health issues are extremely well treated with nutrition, vitamins, herbs and other supplements. And natural health can treat and prevent the whole gamut of women's health problems. Women can finally learn to help themselves and find a sense of empowerment by learning to take care of their own health issues. And they can know that they are doing it the healthy, natural way that works gently with their bodies and leads to better, long term health.

This section will look at some of the extremely common women's health problems and offer safe, effective, easy to use solutions that will actually help to correct these very real and important issues. In this section, we will look at PMS, painful periods, heavy periods, lack of periods, endometriosis, uterine fibroids, ovarian cysts, fibrocystic breast disease, infertility, cervical dysplasia and cervical cancer, breast cancer and menopause: many of the key issues that women of all ages face. And so, it is a section for all women, whether you are young, middle-aged or more mature. You, and all the women you know, can benefit from this section, in this encyclopedia, focused on just women.

AMENORRHOEA
(ABSENCE OF PERIODS)

Some women don't get their period at all and some don't get it for months at a time. Though never getting your period may seem like a blessing, it is a real problem with potentially serious consequences down the road. A stoppage of three months or more is considered amenorrhoea. A woman who does not get her period by age sixteen is also considered to have amenorrhea.

Too Thin to Bleed

Today, the most common cause of lack of menstruation is improper diet, anorexia or bulimia, or overly rigorous exercise. With all the pressure for women to look skinny in today's world, many women are simply not getting the nutrition that they need, especially not good-quality protein and good fats. They are simply starving their bodies to look thin. And one of the many troubling results is lack of menstruation.

HERBAL EMMENAGOGUES

Black cohosh
Blue cohosh
Mugwort
Myrrh
Motherwort
Sqawvine
Pennyroyal oil (externally)
Yarrow
Chastetree berry

Other Causes

Other causes of lack of menstruation include tumours, emotional stress and trauma, hormonal imbalances, obesity, psychological causes, and the birth control pill. The birth control pill is one of the worst culprits. It often takes months or even years for the period to return after coming off the pill. Still other causes include genetics or structural problems, toxins, radiation, autoimmune disease, anemia, low cholesterol, adrenal tumours, thyroid problems, problems of the pituitary and the hypothalamus, and polycystic ovaries. There can also be hormonal imbalances between the hypothalamus, pituitary, ovaries, adrenal glands, and thyroid glands. It is always a good idea to see a practitioner to rule out any underlying causes for the lack of menstruation.

Herbs, vitamins, nutrition, and acupuncture can help correct a woman's cycle and help to reestablish a normal cycle. Talk therapy can also help.

Eating Healthily

Since malnutrition is one of the most frequent causes of amenorrhea, it follows that the very first thing to do is to improve the diet. Eat whole foods with lots of essential fatty acids, such as flaxseed and hemp-seed oils, and other healthy fats. Eat a lot of whole grains, vegetables and fruits, seeds, nuts, legumes, and seaweeds. Ensure ample vegetable protein intake. Contrary to what is always said, nuts and seeds are not fattening at all and provide healthy fats and lots of protein.

Caffeine, chocolate, alcohol, and refined carbohydrates should be avoided. They don't give you anything that you need, and they just make the problem worse.

Women who are underweight should try to gain weight healthily; women who are overweight should try to lose weight healthily. Both are causes of amenorrhea.

Foods rich in bone-building nutrients are also important, since women with amenorrhoea are at greater risk for osteoporosis. Eat deep leafy greens, soy foods, sesame seeds, sea vegetables, and whole grains and legumes. A good bone-building tea is made of chamomile, nettle, alfalfa, and oatstraw.

Herbal Help

According to herbal authority Rudolf Fritz Weiss, M.D., herbs are very effective for bringing on menstruation. Herbs that bring on periods are called emmenagogues.

Black cohosh and blue cohosh are examples of emmenagogues. Often the two are combined with dong quai, cramp bark, and ginger.

Mugwort, myrrh, and motherwort are all helpful. Motherwort is also a relaxant herb, so it helps when the period is stopped due to nervous tension.

Chastetree berry is used to balance hormones when amenorrhoea is caused by a hormonal imbalance. Tori Hudson N.D., says that chastetree berry is an especially good choice if the amenorrhea is caused by lack of ovulation and progesterone, since this herb shifts the hormonal balance from estrogen to progesterone. It is also a good choice when the cause is too much prolactin—a very common cause of amenorrhea[1]. According to Michael Murray, N.D., it takes about three months to work. In one study, ten out of fifteen women with amenorrhea got their periods back when they took 40 drops of chastetree berry extract a day for six months[2]. Chastetree is also used for correcting irregular or absent periods after coming off the birth control pill.

There are many phytoestrogenic herbs. These herbs contain mild estrogens that can balance your own estrogen. When estrogen is too low, they attach to a receptor site and gently raise it; when it is too high, they can lower it by taking a receptor site away from your own more powerful estrogen. This action is useful in treating amenorrhea, since it helps to correct underlying imbalances. Soy, red clover, flaxseed, hops, and alfalfa are all important phytoestrogens.

In addition to being a phytoestrogenic herb, alfalfa is a nutritional powerhouse that can supply the extra vitamins and minerals that may be missing from the diet. Both raspberry leaf and nettle are also often used in suppressed menstruation for their ability to strengthen the system and for their nutritive properties. For women, there are no tonics better than nettle and red raspberry leaf.

Pennyroyal is often used externally as an oil (do not use the oil internally) or in a herbal bath to help bring on absent periods. This herb is an emmenagogue and has a special affinity for the female reproductive organs.

If lack of periods is caused by stress, then anti-stress herbs, such as skullcap, kava, passion-flower, valerian, and linden can be useful, as can herbs that support the adrenal glands, such as ginseng and licorice. The adrenal gland is the headquarters of your body's stress response.

Other useful herbs for bringing on suppressed menstruation include squawvine, dong quai, yarrow, bloodroot, fenugreek, sarsaparilla, wild yam, yucca, and false unicorn, which help to strengthen, nourish, and regulate the reproductive system; liver-supporting herbs such as milk thistle, dandelion root, yellow dock, or fennel; and warming herbs that help to encourage circulation to the pelvic area, such as cinnamon, rosemary, and ginger. Herbalist Rosemary Gladstar uses a combination of these herbs as well as peppermint, lemongrass, and strawberry leaf.

Vitamins and Minerals

Women with absent periods have been found to have B6 and zinc deficiencies[3]. They may also need to supplement iron because women who have not been eating well are often low in this nutrient. A good quality B-complex is also useful, as the B vitamins make blood, detoxify the liver, calm the nerves, help us deal with stress, and aid in hormone production.

Since a lack of nutrition is often the cause of amenorrhoea, it is important to take a high-quality multivitamin/mineral to help supply any nutrients that may be missing from the diet.

Women with prolonged amenorrhea are at serious risk for developing osteoporosis because estrogen deficiency decreases the rate of absorption of calcium[4]. So, women with amenorrhoea need to take in more calcium and other bone nutrients, such as magnesium, manganese, zinc, copper, boron, vitamins K, D, C, and B vitamins to maintain strong and healthy bones. Try taking about 1200 mg calcium, 600 mg magnesium, 25 to 50 mg of zinc balanced with 1 to 2 mg of copper, and 1200 IU of vitamin D a day with food. In addition to calcium, a good bone supplement will also include some level of these other vitamins and minerals (see section on Osteoporosis).

In addition to the vitamins and minerals, Rosemary Gladstar also recommends taking essential fatty acids. So, take flaxseed oil daily.

Other Help

Many natural health practitioners suggest that a woman try to remember when her period used to come and imagine it as still coming at that time.

This helps to reestablish a normal cycle. Women should also spend time with women who are menstruating, as this can also help to bring on menstruation. As bizarre as this may sound, Rosemary Gladstar says she has not only seen this work, but that it has been demonstrated in studies.

Others suggest sleeping in a dark room and going to bed at regular hours to regulate the hypothalamus, cyrcadian rhythms, and hormones. Some suggest exposing yourself to moonlight at the night of the full moon and for two days afterwards.

Also, be sure to treat for underactive thyroid, as this can elevate prolactin levels, which can suppress periods.

The Chinese see amenorrhea as lack of *yin* and dried blood or stagnation of energy and blood. They often use acupuncture to heal this problem. Herbs like ho shou wo and dong quai can be tailored to the specific case.

It can take time, often several months, to reestablish a normal menstrual cycle, so do not expect quick results. But with the right diagnosis and careful attention to a comprehensive program, most women can overcome the problem.

Chapter Endnotes

1. Milewica ,A., *et al.* "*Vitex agnus castus* extract in the treatment of luteal phase defects due to hyperprolactinemia. Results of a randomized placebo-controlled double-blind study." *Arzneim-Forsch Drug Res*, 1993; 43:752'56.

2. Loch, E., *et al.* "Diagnosis and treatment of dyshormonal menstrual periods in the general practice." *Gynakol Praxis*, 1990; 14:489'95.

3. Bove, M., L. Costarella. *Herbs for Women's Health*. New Canaan, CT: Keats Publishing, 1997.

4. Hudson, T. *Women's Encyclopedia of Natural Medicine*. Los Angeles, CA: Keats Publishing, 1999.

BREAST CANCER

We are often told that one in seven or eight women will develop breast cancer. That is very scary. But what we are not often told is that other cultures don't share those numbers. Greek women have much less breast cancer. So do Chinese and Japanese women. Japanese women are only one-fifth as likely to develop breast cancer as North American women are. And genetics has nothing to do with it. When Japanese women move to North America and adopt our diet, their risk of breast cancer climbs until it is the same as ours.

Lowering the Risk of Breast Cancer Through Diet

Diet is the reason that North American women have such high rates of breast cancer. And we can control diet. So the good news is, we can seriously lower those one-in-seven-or-eight numbers.

Good Fats, Bad Fats and Breast Cancer

Let's start with fat. Nowhere has there been more confusion than with fat. That's because many entirely different things—some essential to health and some detrimental to it—have been lumped together under the single name *fat*. The kind of fat you eat is one of the most important determining factors of your health, including your risk of cancer.

The story of good and bad fats is really the story of hydrogen. Fats contain long strings of carbon molecules. If every one of those carbon molecules is bound to as many hydrogen molecules as it can carry, it has been filled, or saturated, with hydro-

---

BREAST CANCER: GOOD AND BAD FOODS

Good Foods:

vegetarian diets	flaxseeds	beans	cruciferous
olive oil and	fibre	lentils	vegetables,
monounsaturated fats	whole grains	nuts	seaweed
omega-3 essential	deep cold water fish	fruit	organic food
fatty acids	soy	vegetables	

Bad Foods:

saturated fat	dairy	refined sugar
meat	trans fatty acids	alcohol

gen. And so it is called a *saturated fat*. If not every carbon molecule has been saturated with hydrogen, the fat is an *unsaturated fat*. Depending on how many carbon molecules are not filled with hydrogen, the fat is either a *monounsaturated* or a *polyunsaturated fat*. *Mono* means one in Greek, and *poly* means many. Simply put, saturated fats are bad for you; monounsaturated fats and poyunsaturated fats, also known as essential fatty acids, are good for you.

Saturated fats are solid at room temperature. They are primarily from animal sources: they are the fats in meat and the dairy fats like butter. Diets that are high in saturated fat, that is, animal fat, increase your risk of breast cancer[1]. In countries where high amounts of meat and dairy are featured in the diet, women have a higher risk of breast cancer[2]. And saturated animal fats not only increase your risk of developing breast cancer, they also decrease your risk of surviving it[3]. So the first message is clear: reduce the amount of saturated animal fat in your diet.

The hydrogenated fats, or trans-fatty acids, that are so much in the news lately are also bad. These fats are often found in margarine and packaged and junk foods. Now that you know that the difference between the bad saturated fats and the good unsaturated fats is the hydrogen, you can easily see why hydrogenating fat is bad for you. Hydrogenated fat is exactly what it sounds like. They take an unsaturated fat and add hydrogen to it: they hydrogen-ate it. In other words, they take a healthy unsaturated vegetable oil and they make it an unhealthy saturated fat, in order to increase the shelf life. Well, they may increase shelf life, but they don't increase yours. Like saturated fats, trans-fats are a significant risk factor for breast cancer[4].

The good fats are the monounsaturated and omega-3 polyunsaturated fats. Preliminary studies suggest that olive oil, which is a monounsaturated fat, reduces the risk of breast cancer[5]. That is probably part of the reason why Greek women have lower rates of breast cancer. Omega-3 essential fatty acids are found abundantly in flaxseeds and cold-water fish. This type of fat is rich in alpha-linolenic acid. Women who have the highest amount of alpha-linolenic acid in their breast tissue have 64 per cent less risk of breast cancer than women who have the lowest amount[6]. That's amazing. But alpha-linolenic acid is not only important in preventing breast cancer, it is also important in preventing its spread if you've already got it. Low levels of alpha-linolenic acid in the breast tissue is the most important determinant of whether the cancer will spread[7]. This facet of alpha-linolenic acid is crucial, since the main cause of death in breast cancer is the spread of the cancer beyond the breast. So when you hear that you should reduce fat to protect against breast cancer, remember that that means reduce saturated fat and trans fats, but not monounsaturated or omega-3 polyunsaturated fats; you should increase those.

Flaxseeds have another benefit in addition to being a good source of omega-3 essential fatty acids: They are also the richest source of lignans. Lignans have many health benefits, and are especially valuable in the fight against breast cancer because they help regulate estrogen and interfere with its cancer-causing effect. So adding flaxseeds to your diet can significantly drop your levels of cancer-related estrogens[8].

In a Canadian study, when flaxseed was added to the diet, the results were amazing. While waiting for surgery, women with breast cancer were given either a muffin with 25 g (about two tbspns) of ground flaxseed or an ordinary muffin every day. At the time of surgery, the flax group had slower-growing tumours and increased apoptosis. Apoptosis is the normal process in which cells are programmed to eventually die. Cancer cells are very adept at avoiding this process. Inducing apoptosis, then, unlike using chemotherapy, is a very safe way of causing the cancer cell to kill itself, without harming the healthy cells surrounding it. The researchers concluded that flaxseeds have the potential to reduce tumour growth in women with breast cancer[9]. Try taking two tablespoons of ground flaxseeds and one tablespoon of flaxseed oil a day. Never cook with flaxseed oil; always use it cold. The best oil to use for cooking is olive oil.

Increasing Fibre

In addition to decreasing the bad fats and increasing the good fats, you should also increase fibre. In one study in China, where breast cancer risk is already low[10] women with the lowest fibre and the highest fat had 2.9 times more risk of breast cancer than women with the highest fibre and the lowest fat.

Several studies show that fibre prevents breast cancer. A meta-analysis of ten good studies found that fibre is protective against breast cancer[1]. How protective is it? A Canadian study of over fifty thousand women found that the ones who had a lot of fibre in their diet had a 30 per cent reduction in the risk of breast cancer, compared to those who had low amounts[11]. Fibre-rich diets may protect against breast cancer by reducing the levels of estrogen[12].

One way of increasing the fibre in your diet is by switching from refined grains to whole grains. It is not surprising that women who eat a lot of whole grains have a low risk of breast cancer[13]. When studies compared women who had breast cancer with women who didn't, the difference in grain consumption was significant: Women with breast cancer ate less grain than women without[14]. Another interesting huge study found that eating a lot of whole grains consistently reduced the risk of virtually every type of cancer, including breast cancer[15].

Vegetarian Diets

Since saturated fat increases the risk of developing breast cancer and fibre decreases the risk, and since saturated fat is found in animal foods and fibre is found only in plant foods, it should come as no surprise that vegetarian women have less breast cancer[16]. Vegetarian women have lower estrogen levels than women who eat meat[17], and they detoxify more estrogen, leaving them with lower levels of the most toxic and dangerous forms of estrogen[18]. Vegetarians also have stronger immune systems than meat-eaters[19].

Most studies have found an association between meat and breast cancer. In an important study of diets from around the world, researchers looked for the factors that increase the risk of breast cancer. They found that the most important things that increased the risk, in order, were: meat, total fat, saturated fat, dairy, refined sugar, calories, and alcohol. On the other hand, fish, whole grains, soy and other legumes, cabbage, vegetables, nuts, and fruits were the most important things that lowered the risk[20]. Meat that is well done may be especially dangerous[21].

Though it is not unanimous, many studies have found that consumption of fruits and vegetables protect against breast cancer[22]. A meta-analysis of twelve high-quality studies found a consistent protective effect from fruits and vegetables[23]. A protective effect has also been found for beans and lentils. Women who eat beans or lentils two or more times a week have a remarkable 34 per cent lower risk of breast cancer than women who eat them once a month or less[24]. Several other specific plant foods have shown special promise for reducing breast cancer.

Broccoli and Cabbage

The American Cancer Society recommends eating cruciferous vegetables to reduce the risk of breast cancer[25]. Cruciferous vegetables include broccoli, cauliflower, cabbage, Brussels sprouts, kale, bok choy, collards, radish, watercress, and others. There is good reason for this recommendation. Many population studies have found that cruciferous vegetables reduce the rates of cancer, especially colon and breast cancer. Women who eat the most cruciferous vegetables have an almost two-fold reduction in risk of breast cancer, compared to women who eat the least[26]. These powerful veggies seem to accomplish this anti-cancer feat largly because of two components found in them: indole-3-carbinol (I3C) and glucoronic acid.

I3C makes a remarkable contribution to the anti-cancer chemistry in your body. It shifts the ratio of estrogen breakdown so that you produce more of the good estrogen and less of the bad, breast cancer-causing estrogen[27]. In addition to increasing your I3C by increasing the cruciferous vegetables in your diet, you can also take it as a supplement. Michael Murray, N.D., recommends that women at high risk of breast cancer include four to five servings a week of cruciferous vegetables in their diet or supplement 200 to 400 mg a day of I3C. When women were given the slightly higher dose of 500 mg of I3C a day, they had a huge increase of the good estrogen after only one week[28].

One of the most important ways your body gets rid of estrogen is by binding it to glucuronic acid and escorting it out, much the same way a policeman handcuffs a criminal and escorts him out of a building. But bad bacteria in the body produce an enzyme called glucuronidase, which cuts the handcuffs, liberating the estrogen and increasing its levels in your body. And that increased estrogen increases your risk of breast cancer. There are four ways to increase your glucuronic acid and decrease the activity of the glucuronidase enzyme. The first two are through diet. Cruciferous vegetables are loaded in glucuronic acid, so eat more of them. Garlic, onion, apples, oranges, grapefruits, and lettuce are also rich sources of glucuronic acid.

Activity of glucuronidase is higher in people whose diets are high in fat and low in fibre. That's the same pattern as has been seen already for breast cancer, so, once again, decrease animal foods and increase plant foods. You can also control the bad bacteria that produce the glucuronidase enzyme by supplementing the good bacteria known as probiotics, including aci-

dophilus and its relatives. And finally, glucuronic acid is available in supplement form as calcium d-glucurate. Preliminary research supports the idea that calcium d-glucurate may be able to reduce the risk of breast cancer by reducing the levels of estrogen[29].

Soy

One of the reasons Asian women have much lower rates of breast cancer than North American women seems to be because they eat much more soy than North American women. Many population studies show that eating lots of soy reduces both risk of and death from breast cancer.

Studies consistently find a benefit for soy in premenopausal women, while some studies in postmenopausal women find a benefit and some don't. Some authors have even suggested concern that soy could increase estrogen and risk in postmenopausal women. Although this concern should not be dismissed, the evidence does not seem very strong. Testing this concern, a study of postmenopausal women found virtually no increase in estrogen when they were given soy[30]. Soy's estrogenic properties are very mild and gentle, while it blocks your body's stronger, harsher estrogens. And while several studies have found benefit for postmenopausal women, we have not found a single study where the soy group had a higher risk of breast cancer. One study even found a greater benefit in postmenopausal women than in premenopausal women. That study found that frequent consumption of miso soup or isoflavones reduced the risk of breast cancer and that the reduction was greater in postmenopausal women[31].

A recent study looked at the question of whether you should eat soy if you have breast cancer. It followed over five thousand breast cancer survivors for an average of four years and found that those who ate the most soy had a significant 29 per cent reduced risk of death and a significant 32 per cent reduced risk of their breast cancer recurring. The benefit held whether the cancer was estrogen receptor-positive or -negative and whether the women were on tamoxifen or not. The researchers concluded that soy "is safe and potentially beneficial for women with breast cancer." Soy's effects on breast cancer seemed comparable to the effects of tamoxifen[32].

A group of flavonoids called isoflavones, one in particular, called genistein, is probably the main reason for soy's impressive effects against breast cancer, although recent research is suggesting that more anti-cancer compounds may secretly be at work in soy. Like all flavonoids, the isoflavones in soy are antioxidants, but these flavonoids have a special affinity for fighting cancer. Soy isoflavones, like genistein, are phyto-estrogens, or plant estrogens (*phyto* is Greek for plant). They have a very mild estrogenic effect. So when they bind to one of your estrogen receptors, they can gently raise estrogen when it is too low, helping in low-estrogen conditions such as menopause, or they can gently lower estrogen when it is too high, helping in excessive estrogen conditions such as breast cancer.

Soy isoflavones' antiestrogenic power is one of the ways it protects against breast cancer[33]. In addition to being antioxidant and anti-estrogen, genistein is also a powerful inhibitor of angiogenesis[34]. Angiogenesis is the formation of the new blood vessels that tumours form in order to get the nutrients they require for growth. Isoflavones also inhibit enzymes that promote cell division and growth. Genistein is also able to induce apoptosis, a natural way in which cells self-destruct without harming the healthy cells around them, and differentiation, which makes the cancer cells less aggressive and less able to proliferate.

Murray recommends eating enough soy to get 25 to 100 mg of isoflavones a day. Some suggest the slightly higher amount of at least 100 mg a day[35]. As a guideline, 40 mg of isoflavones can be found in one cup of soy milk, 4 ozs of tofu, or half a cup of edamame. If you haven't tried edamame, these lightly cooked soy beans are a delicious way of increasing your soy.

Seaweed

Though you don't hear about it much, seaweed is another of the reasons for low breast cancer rates in Japan. Several studies show that the seaweed kombu (*Laminaria*) protects against breast cancer[36]. Try eating kelp, kombu, nori, hijiiki, and dulse as a regular part of your diet.

VITAMINS, MINERALS, AND HERBS: SUPPLEMENTS FOR BREAST CANCER

Vitamin C

In an amazing meta-analysis of dietary factors in breast cancer, vitamin C intake was found to have the single most consistent and statistically significant protective effect against breast cancer[23]. The study concluded that simply consuming at least 380 mg of vitamin C each day could reduce the number of cases of breast cancer by 16 per cent. In addition to preventing breast cancer, vitamin C can increase your chances of surviving with it. Women who consume the most vitamin C have lower breast cancer mortality rates[37].

Vitamin D

The unexpected discovery that breast cancer rates are higher in areas where sun exposure is lower[38] led to the realization that vitamin D could protect against breast cancer. Sunlight produces vitamin D in the body, and vitamin D is activated in the body into a hormone that differentiates cells. Activated vitamin D also fights breast cancer because it has anti-estrogenic properties[39]. And, sure enough, studies have now found that sunlight and vitamin D from the diet correlate with a reduced risk of breast cancer[40]. The most exciting study of

vitamin D and breast cancer has found not only that the higher the level of vitamin D the lower the risk of breast cancer, but that at the highest level, the risk was reduced by a whopping 50 per cent! Not only does vitamin D prevent breast cancer, it also helps you if you have it. Brand-new Canadian research has found that when vitamin D levels are low, breast cancer is 94 per cent more likely to spread and that there is 73 per cent greater chance of death[41].

Carotenes

In addition to the well-known beta-carotene, there is a whole family of lesser-known, but important, carotenes. Several studies have shown that a diet rich in these carotenes is protects against breast cancer. A diet rich in high-carotene foods such as carrots, spinach, and tomatoes has been found to lower the risk of breast cancer[43]. The carotenes in cantaloupe have also been found to be protective. Diets rich in vegetables with the carotenes, lutein and zeaxanthin in them can reduce the risk of breast cancer by 50 per cent[44]. Foods rich in these carotenes include fruit, corn, carrots, potatoes, tomatoes, spinach, and other greens.

Selenium

One of the most amazing anti-cancer nutrients is the mineral selenium. It is not surprising that women with low blood levels of selenium in their blood have a greater risk of developing breast cancer[45]. One researcher has said that the more selenium in the diet, the lower the incidence of breast cancer[46].

Folic Acid

Folic acid protects against breast cancer, as it does against so many other female conditions. Women over fifty who get the most folic acid have 44 per cent less chance of invasive breast cancer than women who get least. Folic acid is especially important if you drink alcohol. Alcohol damages DNA, but folic acid is able to partially reverse this damage. Consuming at least 600 mcg of folic acid a day from food or supplements reduces the risk of breast cancer by 43 per cent in women who have one and half drinks a day or more[47]. New research suggests that alcohol can only cause breast cancer if you are getting less than 300 mcg of folic acid a day[48]. So if you are not getting enough folic acid, don't drink. And if you do drink, make sure you are taking folic acid.

Herbs and Other Nutrients

Women with breast cancer have lower levels of CoQ10 in their blood, and the lower the level, the lower their chance of staying disease-free[49].

Both ginseng and eleuthero, which used to be known as Siberian ginseng, hold promise for breast cancer. Russian research has shown that eleuthero boosts the immune system of women with breast cancer[50]. This herb also reduces the side effects of conventional breast cancer therapy. And, in a massive study of 1,455 women with breast cancer, it was found that those who regularly used ginseng had a significantly reduced risk of death compared to those who didn't use it. Ginseng users also had an improved quality of life[51].

Women's health specialist Tori Hudson, N.D., says that women who regularly drink green tea prior to being diagnosed with breast cancer have increased survival and decreased spread and recurrence of the disease. Green tea also helps with chemotherapy.

Though one study found no benefit for garlic, other studies have found that garlic and onions protect against breast cancer.

Other supplements that may help include bromelain, grapeseed extract, and milk thistle. Grapeseed proanthocyanidins have been shown to kill breast cancer cells in test tubes, and silybin from milk thistle has inhibited the proliferation of breast cancer cells in test tubes. Silybin has also been shown to work synergistically with chemotherapy. Proanthocyanidins and silybin, like soy isoflavones, are both flavonoids.

Some of the most exciting natural anti-cancer agents out there are curcumin, quercetin, maitake mushroom standardised for the MD fraction, and IP6 (Inositol Hexaphosphate). All of these have shown promise against breast cancer. IP6 is also showing itself in studies to be able to prevent the side effects of chemo so effectively that people can finish their course without having their quality of life affected. Another promising natural anti-cancer agent, modified citrus pectin, may help prevent breast cancer from spreading.

Also try traditional anti-cancer herbs such as pau d'arco, cat's claw, suma, the Essiac tea, burdock, and topical poke-root tincture. Traditional herbalists swore they could eliminiate breast tumours by using poke root topically. They also used onion topically.

Or try herbalist Michael Tierra's detox formula that he uses for cancer. It combines echinacea, chapparal, red clover, cascara sagrada, kelp, astragalus, grifola, ginseng, poria cocos, licorice, and cayenne.

Changing Your Risk by Changing Your Lifestyle

There are several important ways of reducing your risk of breast cancer by making changes in your lifestyle. For example, a sedentary lifestyle increases your risk of breast cancer, while physical activity hugely reduces it[52]. Tori Hudson, N.D., says that the results of the research suggest that exercise can prevent breast cancer more effectively than tamoxifen. And you should start early: Girls who get a significant amount of exercise are less likely to develop breast cancer later in life[53]. However, it's never too late to start. One study found that exercise after fifty reduces the risk of post-menopausal hormone

senstitive breast cancer—by far the most common type—by 29 per cent.

Reduce your exposure to environmental chemicals such as pesticides. Higher levels of pesticide residue are found in the fat cells of breasts of women with breast cancer[54]. These increased levels can quadruple the risk of breast cancer. You can reduce your exposure to pesticides by eating more organic food and more plant food; plant food is lower in pesticide.

Two lifestyle factors that won't surprise you are smoking and drinking. What may surprise you is that with all of the links between smoking and cancer, smoking is often not considered a risk factor for breast cancer, and some reports even suggest it has a protective effect. However, cancer specialist Richard Passwater, Ph.D., points to two sophisticated analyses that highlight a very different reality. The Canadian National Breast Screening study, which included over thirty thousand women, found a huge increase in the risk of breast cancer for smokers[55], and a second study found that women who smoke have much greater spreading of their breast cancer[56]. As for alcohol, an analysis of the highest-quality studies has confirmed that women who drink alcohol are at higher risk for breast cancer[57]. And now a landmark study has found that even low to moderate alcohol consumption is associated with a significant increase in risk of breast cancer. As alcohol consumption goes up, so does the risk. There is an increase of eleven cases of breast cancer per one thousand women for each additional glass of alcohol a day[58].

The decision whether to use hormone replacement therapy is another factor. After years of denying the obvious, there is no longer any doubt that taking hormone replacement therapy for menopause increases your risk of breast cancer. Knowledge of this risk is not new. A meta-analysis of fifty-one studies had already found by 1977 that the risk of breast cancer goes up by 2.3 per cent for every year on hormone replacement therapy[59]. A year later, the Harvard Center for Cancer Prevention reviewed every study on hormone replacement therapy and breast cancer that had been published in English, and again concluded that 'postmenopausal hormones cause breast cancer[60].' But despite the evidence, the denial only finally disappeared recently when two landmark studies published their findings that hormone replacement therapy increased the risk of breast cancer, invasive breast cancer, and death from breast cancer[61]. Newly published research has now revealed that as use of hormone replacement therapy has declined in Canada because of awareness of these studies, incidence of breast cancer in postmenopausal women has fallen[62].

Much less known, and much more of a surprise, is that it is now known that antibiotics are associated with increased risk of, and increased death from, breast cancer[63].

And finally, there is an emotional component to fighting breast cancer. Hudson reports that women with breast cancer often tend to be people who hold their anger and other emotions in check. And some studies have found that women with a "fighting spirit" are more likely to survive their breast cancer than women with a hopeless or helpless attitude[64]. Social support is also important. One seven-year study found that women with strong social support and someone to confide in were only half as likely to die from their breast cancer as women who didn't[65]. A second study of women with late-stage breast cancer found the same 50 per cent improvement when the women went to a support group[66]. Though it is, perhaps, chauvanistic that such studies have not been done on prostate cancer, the results are not to be ignored.

Chapter Endnotes

1. Howe, G. R., T. Hirobata, T.G. Hislop. "Dietary factors and the risk of breast cancer: a combined analysis of 12 case-controlled studies." *J Natl Cancer Inst*, 1990; 82:561'69.

2. Armstrong, B., R. Doll. "Environmental factors and cancer incidence and mortality in different countries, with special reference to dietary practices." *Int J Cancer*, 1975; 15:617-31.

3. Holmes, M.D., D. H. Hunter, G.A. Colditz, *et al*. "Association of dietary intake of fat and fatty acids with risk of breast cancer." *JAMA*, 1999; 281:914-20.

4. Enig, M. G. "Dietary fats and cancer trends-A critique." *Fed Proc*, 1978; 37:2215'20.

5. Trichopoulou, A., *et al*. "Consumption of olive and specific food groups in relation to breast cancer risk in Greece." *J Natl Cancer Inst*, 1995; 87:110-16; La Vecchia, C., *et al*. "Olive oil, other dietary fats, and the risk of breast cancer (Italy)." *Cancer Causes Control*, 1995; 6:545-50; Martin-Moreno, J.M., *et al*. "Dietary fat, olive oil intake and breast cancer risk." *Int J Cancer*, 1994; 58:774-80.

6. Klein, V., *et al*. "Low alpha-linolenic acid content of adipose breast tissue is associated with an increased risk of breast cancer." *Eur J Cancer*, 2000; 36:335'40.

7. Bougnoux, P., *et al*. "Alpha-linolenic acid content of adipose breast tissue: a host determinent of the risk of early metastasis in breast cancer." *Br J Cancer*, 1994; 70:330'34.

8. Haggans, C. J., *et al*. "Effect of flaxseed consumption on urinary estrogen metabolites in postmenopausal women." *Nutr Cancer*, 1999; 33:188'95.

9. Goss, P., L. Thompson, *et al*. "Dietary Flaxseed Alters Tumor Biological Markers in Postmenopausal Breast Cancer." *Clinical Cancer Research*, 2005; 11: 3828'35.

10. Yuan, J. M., *et al*. "Diet and Breast Cancer in Shanghai and Tianjin, China." *Br J Cancer*, 1995; 71:1353'58.

11. Rohen, T.E., *et al*. "Dietary fibre, vitamins A, C, and E and the risk of breast cancer: a cohort study." *Cancer Causes Control*, 1993; 4:29'37.

12. Clifford, C., B. Kremer. "Diet as a risk and therapy for cancer." *Clin Nutr*, 1993; 77:725'40.

13. Jacobs, D. R., Jr., *et al*. "Whole-grain intake and cancer: an expanded review and meta-analysis." *Nutr Cancer*, 1998; 30:85-96.

14. Adlercreutz, H., *et al*. "Diet and plasma androgens in postmenopausal vegetarian and omnivorous women and postmenopausal women with breast cancer." *Am J Clin Nutr*, 1989; 49:433'42; Adlercreutz, H., *et al*. "Diet and urinary estrogen profile in premenopausal omnivorous and vegetarian women and in premenopausal women with breast cancer." *J Steroid Biochem*, 1989; 34:527'30.

15. Chatenoud, L., *et al*. "Whole grain food intake and cancer risk." *Int J Canc*, 1998; 77:24'28.

16. Armstrong, B. K., *et al*. "Diet and reproductive hormones: a study of vegetarian and nonvegetarian postmenopausal women." *J Natl Cancer Inst*, 1981: 67:761-67.

17. Armstrong, B. K., *et al*. "Diet and reproductive hormones: a study of vegetarian and nonvegetarian postmenopausal women." *J Natl Cancer Inst*, 1981: 67:761-67; Goldin, B. R., *et al*. "Estrogen excretion patterns and plasma levels in vegetarian and omnivorous women." *N Engl J Med*, 1982; 307:1542'47.

18. Adlercreutz, H., *et al*. "Determination of urinary lignans and phytoestrogen metabolites, potential antiestrogens and anticarcinogens in urine of women in various habitual diets." *J Steroid Biochem*, 1986; 25:791'97; Goldin, B., *et al*. "Effect of diet on excretion of estrogens in pre- and postmenopausal women." *Cancer Res*, 1981; 41:3771'73; Byers, T., S. Graham. "The epidemiology of diet and cancer." *Advances in Cancer Research*, 1984; 41:55'57.

19. Malter, M., G. Schriever, U. Eilber. "Natural killer cells, vitamins, and other blood components of vegetarian and omnivorous men." *Nutr Cancer*, 1989; 32:271-78.

20. Hebert, J., A. Rosen. "Nutritional, socioeconomic, and reproductive factors in relation to female breast cancer mortality: findings from a cross-national study." *Cancer Detection Prevention*, 1996; 20:234'44.

21. Zheng, W., *et al*. "Well-done meat intake and the risk of breast cancer." *J Natl Cancer Inst*, 1998; 90:1724'29.

22. Nutritional Research Council: Diet and Health. *Implications for reducing chronic disease risk*. National Academy Press, Washington, DC, 1989; Rogers, A.E., M.P. Longnecker. "Biology of Disease: Dietary and nutritional influences on cancer: a review of epidemiological and experimental data." *Lab Invest*, 1998; 59:729'59; Steinmetz, K. A., J. D. Potter. "Vegetables, fruit and cancer I and II." *Cancer Causes Control*, 1991; 2:325'57,427'42.

23. Howe, G. R., *et al*. "Dietary factors and risk of breast cancer: combined analysis of 12 case-control studies." *J Natl Cancer Inst*, 1990; 82:561'69.

24. *International Journal of Cancer*, 2005; 114:628'33.

25. American Cancer Society. Nutrition and cancer: cause and prevention. *American Cancer Society*, NY, 1984.

26. Terry, P., *et al*. "Brassica vegetables and breast cancer risk." *JAMA*, 2001; 285:2975'77.

27 Michnovicz, J. J., H. L. Bradlow. "Altered estrogen metabolism and excretion in humans following consumption of indole-3-carbinol." *Nutr Cancer*, 1991; 16:59-66; Wong, G. Y., *et al*. "Dose-ranging study of indole-3-carbinol for breast cancer prevention." *J Cell Biochem Suppl*, 1997(28-29):111'16; Michnovicz, J. J. "Increased estrogen 2-hydroxylation in obese women using oral indole-3-carbinol." *Int J Obes Relat Metab Disord*, 1998; 22:227'29; Shertzer, H. G., A. P. Senft. "The micronutrient indole-3-carbinol: implications for disease and chemoprevention." *Drug Metab Drug Interact*, 2000; 17:159'88; Reed, G. A., *et al*. "A phase I study of indole-3-carbinol in women: tolerability and effects." *Cancer Epidemiol Biomarkers Prev*, 2005; 14:1953'60.

28. Michnovicz, J. J. "Induction of estradiol metabolism by dietary indole-3-carbinol in humans." *J Natl Cancer Inst*, 1990; 82:947'49.

29. Heerdt, A. S., C. W. Young, P.I. Borgen. "Calcium glucarate as a chemopreventive agent in breast cancer." *Isr J Med Sci*, 1995; 31:101-05.

30. Baird, D., *et al*. "Dietary intervention study to assess estrogenicity of dietary soy among postmenopausal women." *J Clin Endocrin Metab*, 1995; 80:1685'90.

31. Yamamoto, S., *et al*. "Soy, isoflavones, and breast cancer risk in Japan." *J Natl Cancer Inst*, 2003; 95:906'15. Shu XO, *et al*. "Soy food intake and breast cancer survival." *JAMA* 2009;302:2437-43.

32. Shu XO, *et al*. Soy food intake and breast cancer survival. *JANA* 2009; 302:2473-43.

33. Rose, D. "Diet, hormones, and cancer." *Annu Rev·Publ Health*, 1993; 14:1'17.

34. Fotsis, T., *et al*. "Genistein, a dietary-derived inhibitor of in vitro angiogenesis." *Proc Natl Acad Sci USA*, 1993; 90:2690'94.

35. Stoll, B. "Eating to beat breast cancer: potential role for soy supplements." *Ann Onc*, 1997; 8:323'25.

36. Kagawa, T. "Impact of westernization on the Japanese. Changes in physique, can-

cer longevity and centenarians." *Preventative Medicine*, 1978; 7:205'17; Hirayama, T. "Epidemiology of breast cancer with special reference to the role of diet." *Preventative Medicine*, 1978; 7:173'95; Wynder, E.L. "Dietary habits and cancer epidemiology." *Cancer, Supplement*, 1979; 43:1955'61; Fujimoto, I., *et al.* "Descriptive epidemiology of cancer in Japan: current cancer incidence and survival data." *National Cancer Institute Monographs*, 1979; 53:5'15; Nomura, A., *et al.* "Breast cancer and diet among the Japanese in Hawaii." *Am J Clin Nutr*, 1978; 31:2020'25; Teas, J. "The dietary intake of Laminaria, a brown seaweed, and breast cancer prevention." *Nutrition and Cancer*, 1983; 4:217'23.

37. Jain, M., *et al.* "Premorbid diet and the prognosis of women with breast cancer." *J Natl Cancer Inst*, 1994; 86:1390'97.

38. Gorham, E. D., F. C. Garland, C. F. Garland. "Sunlight and breast cancer incidence in the USSR." *Int J Epidemiol*, 1990; 19:820-24.

39. Demdirpence, E., *et al.* "Antiestrogenic effects of all-trans-retinoic acid and 1,25-dihydroxyvitamin D3 in breast cancer cells occur at the estrogen response element level but through different molecular mechanisms." *Cancer Res*, 1994; 54:1458-64.

40. John ,E.M., *et al.* "Vitamin D and breast cancer risk: the NHANES I Epidemiologic follow-up study, 1971-1975 to 1992." *Cancer Epidemiol Biomarkers Prev*, 1999; 8:399-406.

41. Annual Meeting of the American Association for Cancer Research 2006 (not yet published). Goodwin P, *et al.* "Study sees link between vitamin D, breat cancer prognosis." *CA Cancer J Clin* 2008;58:264-5.

42. Goodwin P., *et al.* Study sees link between vitamin D, breast cancer prognosis. *CA Cancer J Chin* 2008; 58:264-5

43. Hunter, D. J., *et al.* "A prospective study of the intake of vitamins C, E, and A and the risk of breast cancer." *N Engl J Med*, 1993; 329:234'40.

44. Freudenheim, J. L., *et al.* "Premenopausal breast cancer risk and intake of vegetables, fruits, and related nutrients." *J Natl Cancer Inst*, 1996; 88:340'48.

45. Schrauzer, G. N., *et al.* "Selenium in the blood of Japanese and American women with and without breast cancer and fibrocystic disease." *Japanese Journal of Cancer Research*, 1985; 76:374'77; Krsnjavi, J., D. Beker. "Selenium in serum as a possible parameter for assessment of breast disease." *Breast Cancer Research and Treatment*, 1990; 16:57'61.

46. Ladas, H. S. "The potential of selenium in the treatment of cancer." *Holistic Medicine*, 1989; 4:145'56.

47. Rohan, T. E., *et al.* "Dietary folate consumption and breast cancer risk." *J Natl Cancer Inst*, 2000; 92:266-69; Zhang, S., *et al.* "A prospective study of folate intake and the risk of breast cancer." *JAMA*, 1999; 281:1632-37.

48. Tjonneland, A. "Folate intake, alcohol and risk of breast cancer among postmenopausal women in Denmark." *Eur J Clin Nutr*, 2006; 60:280'86.

49. Jolliet, P., *et al.* "Plasma coenzyme Q10 concentrations in breast cancer: prognosis and therapeutic consequences." *Int J Clin Pharmacol Ther*, 1998; 36:506-09.

50. Gvamichava, A. R., *et al.* "First results of the use of Eleutherococcus in the combined treatment of breast carcinoma." *Lek Sredestva Dal'nego Vostoka*, 1966; 7:231-35; Kupin, V.I., YeB. Polevaia, A. M. Sorokin. "Stimulation of the immunological reactivity of cancer patients by Eleutherococcus extract." *Vopr Onkol*, 1986; 32:21-26.

51. Yong, Cui., *et al.* "Association of ginseng use with survival and quality of life among breast cancer patients." *Am J Epidemiol*, 2006; 163:645'53.

52. Thune, I., *et al.* "Physical activity and the risk of breast cancer." *N Engl J Med*, 1997; 336:1269.

53. Marcus, P. M., *et al.* "Physical activity at age 12 and adult breast cancer risk (United States)." *Cancer Causes Control*, 1999; 10:293-302.

54. Falck, F., *et al.* "Pesticide and polychlorinated biphenyl residues in human breast lipids and their relation to breast cancer." *Arch Environ Health*, 1992; 47:143'46.

55. Schechter, M., *et al.* "The relationship of cigarette smoking and breast cancer in the Canadian National Breast Screening Study." *Am J Epidemiol*, 1985; 121:479'87.

56. Hager, J. C., *et al.* "Cancer recurrence after mastectomy." *Medical World News*, April 22, 1985: 13'14.

57. Smith-Warner, S. A., *et al.* "Alcohol and breast cancer in women. A pooled analysis of cohort studies." *JAMA*, 1998; 279:535-40.

58. Allen N. E., *et al.* Moderate alchol intake and cancer incidence in women. *JNCI* 2009; 101:296-305.

59. Collaborative Group on Hormonal Factors in Breast Cancer. "Breast cancer and hormone replacement therapy. Combined reanalysis of data from 51 epidemiological studies involving 52,705 women with breast cancer and 108,411 women without breast cancer." *Lancet*, 1997; 350:1047'59.

60. Colditz, G. "Relationship between estrogen levels, use of hormone replacement therapy, and breast cancer." *J Natl Cancer Inst*, 1998; 90:814'23.

61. Fletcher, S.W., G.A. Colditz. "Failure of Estrogen Plus Progestin Therapy for Prevention." *JAMA*, 2002; 288:366'68; Beral, V. "Million Women Study Collaboration. Breast cancer and hormone-replacement therapy in the Million Women Study." *Lancet*, 2003; 362:419'27. Allen NE, *et al.* "Moderate alcohol intake and cancer incidence in women." *JNCI* 2009;101:296-305.

62. Mayor S., "Incidence of breast cancer falls with less HRT, Canadian study confirms." *BMJ* 2010;341:c5307.

63. Velicer, C.M., *et al.* "Antibiotic use in relation to the risk of breast cancer." *JAMA*, 2004; 291:827'35.

64. Pettingall, K. W., *et al.* "Mental attitudes to cancer: an additional prognostic factor." *Lancet*, 1985; i:750; Greer, S., *et al.* "Psychological response to breast cancer and 15-year outcome." *Lancet*, 1990; 335:49-50 [letter].

65. Mausell, E., J. Brisson, L. Deschênes. "Social support and survival among women with breast cancer." *Cancer*, 1995; 76:631-37.

66. Spiegel, D., *et al.* "Effect of psychosocial treatment on survival of patients with metastatic breast cancer." *Lancet*, 1989; ii:888-91.

CERVICAL DYSPLASIA AND CERVICAL CANCER

Cervical dysplasia, also known as cervical in-traepithelial neoplasia, is a precancerous condition. It is diagnosed by an abnormal PAP smear. If left untreated, cervical dysplasia can progress to cervical cancer. Most types of cervical dysplasia progress very slowly, usually taking ten to fifteen years to progress to cancer if left un-treated. There is no need for this progression to happen, though, since PAP smears can detect cer-vical dysplasia early and since cervical dysplasia is treatable.

CERVICAL DYSPLASIA & CERVICAL CANCER:

Rate of Progression of Cervical Dysplasia in 4 Months: Untreated Versus Folic Acid

Butterworth, C. E., Jr., K. Hatch, M. Macaluso. "Folate deficiency and cervical dysplasia." *JAMA*, 1992; 267:528'33

Causes and Risk Factors

Cervical dysplasia/cancer is a sexually transmit-ted disease that in about 90 per cent of cases is caused by the human papillomavirus (HPV)[1]. Herpes simplex type II can also cause it. Risk fac-tors for cervical dysplasia/cancer include multiple partners or a partner who has had multiple part-ners, early age of first intercourse, giving birth be-fore twenty-two, smoking, oral contraceptives, and nutritional and dietary factors. The biggest risk factor of all seems to be smoking, which can triple your risk of cervical dysplasia/cancer[2] and increase the chance that a mild form of dysplasia will progress to a more severe form[3].

Your Diet Can Protect You

Treating this condition mostly involves healthy di-etary changes that all of us should be making any-way and taking supplements that most women should already be on, though at higher doses.

The dietary changes involve a shift toward a vegetarian diet. A huge number of studies show that diets high in fat increase your risk of cervical dysplasia/cancer, while diets rich in fruits and vegetables significantly decrease it[4]. Dark yellow and orange vegetables[5] and tomatoes[6] may be es-pecially protective. Deep leafy greens, rich in folic acid, are also crucial.

The Importance of Antioxidants

The most promising nutrients for cervical dysplasia/cancer are folic acid and antioxidants. Though there is no evidence yet that taking vitamin C can help in the treatment of cervical dysplasia, antioxidant expert Richard Passwater, Ph.D., says that it can help return the cells to normal, preventing the progression to cancer[7]. What there is evidence of is that not getting enough vitamin C is a risk factor, increasing your odds of getting cervical dysplasia/cancer by as much as 6.7 times[8].

Women with cervical dysplasia also seem to have lower levels of the antioxidant vitamins E and beta-carotene[9]. Not getting enough beta-carotene triples the risk of cervical dysplasia[10]. The important cancer-fighting antioxidant, selenium, is also significantly lower in women with cervical dysplasia[11].

Supplementing antioxidants is important. Beta-carotene should be taken in the form of a natural-source supplement offering a mix of carotenes at a dose of around 200,000 IU a day. Recommendations for vitamin C range from 1 to 11 g. Vitamin C is safe and is a very important antioxidant and anti-cancer nutrient. A buffered form is best. Vitamin E must be taken in its natural form and

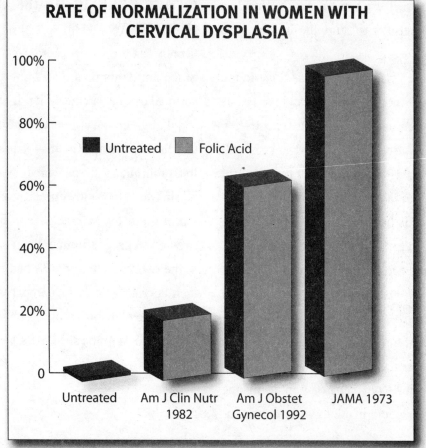

RATE OF NORMALIZATION IN WOMEN WITH CERVICAL DYSPLASIA

can be used at a dose of 200 IU four times a day. A mixed source is best. Selenium can be used at a dose of 400 mcg a day.

Folic Acid: The Greatest Promise of All

Perhaps the most important nutrient for those with cervical dysplasia/cancer is folic acid. Not getting enough folic acid increases the risk of cervical dysplasia and increases the effect of other risk factors, while supplementing folic acid can reverse it[12]. The reason is that a deficiency of folic acid helps the HPV to get into the DNA of the cells of the cervix[13]. So folic acid is like the front line of defence for the cervix. When it is absent, invaders get in; when it returns to duty, the invaders are kicked out.

And that's just what folic acid has done in the research. Though not every folic acid study has been positive, a number of them have been very positive. If left untreated, cervical dysplasia will progress by about 16 per cent in four months. But when treated with folic acid, there is no progression after four months[14]. So folic acid can stop the progression of cervical dysplasia. But that's not all. Folic acid can also improve the cells and even return them to normal. Left untreated, cervical dysplasia normalizes in about 0 to 1.3 per cent of people. But when treated with a high dose of (10 mg), folic acid turned the cells back into healthy cervical cells in 20 per cent of people in one study[15], in 63.7 per cent in another[16] and in an in-credible 100 per cent in a third[17]. So folic acid can stop the progress of, improve, and even normalize cervical dysplasia. Though the high dose of 10 mg a day is necessary to treat the dysplasia, after about three months, the dose can be reduced to 2.5 mg a day.

Folic acid is one of the family of B vitamins. Other B vitamins might help as well. B6 is low in one-third of women with cervical cancer[18], and one study found that women who have a higher intake of vitamins B1, B2, B12, and folic acid have a lower risk of cervical dysplasia[19].

OTHER HELPFUL HERBS AND NUTRITENTS

Green Tea

Since antioxidants are so important in cases of cervical dysplasia/cancer, it might not be surprising that green tea—a very rich source of important flavonoid antioxidants—has shown promise. In a preliminary study, women with cervical dysplasia were given either green-tea flavonoids, 200 mg of green tea extract, or a placebo for eight to twelve weeks. Sixty-nine per cent of the women in the two green tea groups had improvement in their cervical dysplasia, compared to only 10 per cent in the placebo group[20]. Other flavonoid-rich herbs such as grape seed extract can also be useful.

Indole-3-Carbinol

Another nutrient showing promise is the exciting anti-cancer nutrient indole-3-carbinol (I3C), a component of cruciferous vegetables. The cruciferous family includes vegetables such as broccoli, cauliflower, Brussels sprouts, cabbage, and kale. When thirty women with cervical dysplasia were given either 200 mg of I3C, 400 mg of I3C, or a placebo for twelve weeks, 50 per cent in the 200 mg I3C and 44 per cent of the women in the 400 mg I3C group had a complete regression of their cervical dysplasia, compared to none of the women in the placebo group[21].

Coenzyme Q10

Coenzyme Q10 is another important antioxidant and immune-system booster. One study found that levels of CoQ10 and vitamin E were significantly lower in women with cervical dysplasia/ cancer[22].

Feverfew

Feverfew is a herb best known for fighting migraines, but a test-tube study has found that parthenolides from feverfew reduce the proliferation of cervical-cancer cells. This study was done just in test tubes and not on humans, but John Boik, an expert on natural supplements for cancer, tells us that this study is worthy of further investigation. Boik also pointed us to a more recent test-tube study that found a feverfew extract to inhibit the growth of cervical cancer cells. Once again, it was the parthenolides in the feverfew that were the most active[23].

Other Herbs

Other herbs that herbalists mention frequently include red clover, dandelion root, licorice, echinacea, thuja, and especially, goldenseal. Goldenseal can be used both orally and topically and may be helpful in a number of ways. Since a thriving immune system can often stop HPV from causing cervical dysplasia and is capable of reversing cervical dysplasia, strengthening the immune system with herbs is important.

For the same reason, other general cancer fighters may be useful, such as shiitake, reishi, miatake, pau d'arco, and Essiac tea.

Flaxseeds and probiotics also may be useful.

Chapter Endnotes

1. Syrjanen, K. "Spontaneous evolution of intraepithelial lesions according to the grade and type of the implicated human papillomavirus (HPV)." *Eur J Obstet Gyn Reprod Biol*, 1996; 65:45.

2. Lyon, J., et al. "Smoking and carcinoma in situ of the uterine cervix." *Am J Pub Health*, 1983; 73:558'62; Clarke, E., et al. "Cervical dysplasia: associaton with sexual behaviour, smoking, and oral contraceptive use." *Am J Ob Gyn*, 1985; 151:612'16; de Vet, H. C., F. Sturmans. "Risk factors for cervical dysplasia: implications for prevention." *Public Health*, 1994; 108:241'49; Becker, T. M., et al. "Cigarette smoking and other risk factors for cervical dysplasia in southwestern Hispanic and non-Hispanic white women." *Cancer Epidemiol Biomarkers Prev*, 1994; 3:113'19; Kanetsky, P. A., et al. "Cigarette smoking and cervical dysplasia among non-Hispanic black women." *Cancer Detect Prev*, 1998; 22:109'19.

3. Daly, S. F., et al. "Can the number of cigarettes smoked predict high-grade cervical intraepithelial neoplasia among women with mildly abnormal cervical smears?" *Am J Obstet Gynecol*, 1998; 179:399'402; Cerqueira, E.M., et al. "Genetic damage in exfoliated cells of the uterine cervix: Association and interaction between cigarette smoking and progression to malignant transformation?" *Acta Cytol*, 1998 ;42:639'49.

4. Marshall, J., et al. "Diet and smoking in the epidemiology of cancer of the cervix." *J Natl Cancer Instit*, 1983; 70:847'51; Kwasniewska, A., et al. "Dietary factors in women with dysplasia colli uteri associated with human papillomavirus infection." *Nutr Cancer*, 1998; 30:39'45; Romnev, S. L., et al. "Nutrient antioxidants in the pathogenesis and prevention of cervical dysplasia and cancer." *J Cell Biochem Suppl*, 1995; 23:96'103[review]; Herrero, R., et al. "A case control study of nutrient status and invasive cervical cancer." *Am J Epid*, 1991; 134:1335'46; Slattery, M., et al. "Dietary vitamins A, C, and E and selenium as risk factors for cervical cancer." *Epid*, 1990; 1:8'15; Brock, K., G. Berry, et al. "Nutrients in diet and plasma and risk of in situ cervical cancer." *J Natl Cancer Inst*, 1988; 80:580'85; and many others.

5. Ziegler, R.G., et al. "Diet and the risk of in situ cervical cancer among white women in the United States." *Cancer Causes Control*, 1991; 2:17'19.

6. Kantesky, P. A., et al. "Dietary intake and blood levels of lycopene: associaton with cervical dysplasia among non-Hispanic black women." *Nutr Cancer*, 1998; 31:31'40; Van Eenwyk, J., F. G. Davis, P. R. Bown. "Dietary and serum carotenoids and cervical intraepithelial neoplasia." *Int J Cancer*, 1991; 48:34'38.

7. Passwater, R. A. *Cancer Prevention and Nutritional Therapies.* (New Canaan, CT: Keats Publishing, 1978), p.179.

8. Wassertheil-Smoller, S., et al. "Dietrary vitamin C and uterine cervical dysplasia." *Am J Epid*, 1981; 114:714'24; Dawson, E., J. Nosovitch, E. Hannigan. "Serum vitamin and selenium changes in cervical dysplasia." *Fed Proc*, 1984; 43:612; Romney, S., et al. "Plasma vitamin C and uterine cervical dysplasia." *Am J Ob Gyn*, 1985; 151:978'80.

9. Palan, P.R., et al. "Plasma levels of antioxidant beta-carotene and alpha-tocopherol in uterine cervix dysplasias and cancer." *Nutr Cancer*, 1991; 15:13'20; Ho, G.Y., et al. "Viral characteristics of human papillomavirus infection and antioxidant levels as risk factors for cervical dysplasia." *Int J Cancer*, 1998; 78:594'99.

10. Wylie-Rosett, J., et al. "Influence of vitamin A on cervical dysplasia and carcinoma in situ." *Nutr Cancer*, 1984; 6:49'57.

11. Dawson, E., J. Nosovitch, E. Hannigan. "Serum vitamin and selenium changes in cervical dysplasia." *Fed Proc*, 1984; 43:612.

12. Butterworth, C. E., Jr., et al. "Folate-induced regression of cervical intraepithelial neoplasia in users of oral contraceptive agents." *Am J Clinl Nutr*, 1980; 33:926; Butterworth, C. E., Jr., K. Hatch, S. J. Soong. "Oral folic acid supplementation for cervical dysplasia. A clinical intervention trial." *Am J Obstet Gynecol*, 1992; 166:803'09; Butterworth, C. E., Jr., et al. "Improvement in cervical dysplasia associated with folic acid therapy in users of oral contraception." *Am J Clin Nutr*, 1982; 35:73'82.

13. Fekete, P., A. Hammani. "Folic acid-like deficiency in cervicovaginal smears: a possible manifestation of papillomavirus infection." *Acta Cytologica*, 1987; 31:697; Butterworth, C. E., Jr. "Effect of folate on cervical cancer: synergism among risk factors." *Annals of the New York Academy of Science*, (Sept. 30,1992) 669:293'99.

14. Butterworth, C. E., Jr., K. Hatch, M. Macaluso. "Folate deficiency and cervical dysplasia." *JAMA*, 1992; 267:528'33

15. Butterworth, C. E., Jr., et al. "Improvement in cervical dysplasia associated with folic acid therapy in users of oral contraceptives." *Am J Clin Nutr*, 1982; 35:73'82.

16. Butterworth, C. E., Jr., K. Hatch, S. J. Soong. "Oral folic acid supplementation for cervical dysplasia. A clinical intervention trial." *Am J Obstet Gynecol*, 1992; 166:803'09.

17. Whitehead, N., F. Reyner, J. Lindenbaum. "Megaloblastic changes in the cervical epithelium association with oral contraceptive therapy and reversal with folic acid." *JAMA*, 1973; 226:1421'24.

18. Ramaswamy, P., R. Natarajan. "Vitamin B6 status in patients with cancer of the uterine cervix." *Nutr Cancer*, 1984; 6:176'80.

19. Hernandez, B.Y., et al. "Diet and premalignant lesions of the cervix: evidence of a protective role for folate, riboflavin, thiamine, and vitamin B12." *Cancer Causes and Control*, 2003; 14:859'70.

20. Ahn, W.S., et al. "Protective effects of green tea extracts (polyphenon E and EGCG) on human cervical lesions." *Eur J Cancer Prev*, 2003; 12:383'90.

21. Bell, M.C., et al. "Placebo-controlled trial on indole-3-carbinol in the treatment of CIN." *Gynecologic Oncol*, 2000; 78:123'29.

22. Mikhail, M. S., P. R. Palan, S. L. Romney. "Coenzyme Q10 and alpha tocopherol concentrations in cervical intraepithelial neoplasia and cervix cancer." *Obstet Gynecol*, 2001; 97:35.

23. Wu, C., et al. "Antiproliferative activities of parthenolide and golden feverfew extract against three human cancer cell lines." *J Med Food*, 2006, spring; 9(1):55'61. Thanks to John Boik for pointing this study out to us.

DYSMENORRHOEA (PAINFUL PERIODS)

It's that time of the month again, dreaded by so many women because of the painful cramps their period will bring. But periods don't need to mean pain. By rebalancing the underlying problem, soon you may not even know your period has started; the cramping will be gone.

As many as 60 per cent of women suffer from painful periods. For 10 per cent of them, the pain is so severe that it is incapacitating. So, as you can see, this is a very serious health problem that needs to be more seriously addressed.

Period pain is caused by cramping in the uterus that is often also felt in the lower back. The pain is usually felt before or at the beginning of the period, easing off when the main part of the blood has flowed. Sometimes there are bowel disturbances and reduced pain tolerance. Nausea, vomiting, fatigue, diarrhoea, headache, lower backache, dizziness, and fainting can also accompany the cramps. Bloating, breast tenderness, weight gain, and irritability round out this disturbing set of symptoms.

What Causes Dysmenorrhoea?

It is possible that your pain is being caused by a more basic underlying problem, such as endometriosis, fibroids, infection, or cysts. If that is the case, though the suggestions given in this section will still be helpful, you will also need to ad-

dress the underlying condition.

If there is no structural problem, then the pain could be a result of abnormal prostaglandin production, which causes the painful muscle and uterine contractions as well as inflammation. Women with cramping have high levels of the hormone prostaglandin F2 alpha in the menstrual blood. This hormone sends the uterus into spasm, and you start to feel the cramping.

A sluggish liver, or *qi* blockage in the liver, or blood stagnation, or heat, can also cause dysmenorrhoea. Not surprisingly, so can hormonal imbalances. Less obvious causes include bad diet, stress, poor fitness, poor blood flow, candida, bowel toxicity and behavioural and psychological factors.

Fix the Diet, Fix the Pain

As always, the place to start is diet. And the focus is eliminating arachidonic acid. Found in

---

CAUSES OF PAINFUL AND BENEFICIAL PROSTAGLANDINS

Causes of Painful Prostaglandins:
arachidonic acid found in meat, chicken, turkey and dairy

Causes of Beneficial Prostaglandins:
essential fatty acids

meat, chicken, turkey, and dairy, arachidonic acid produces those painful prostaglandins that cause the muscle and uterine cramping. So while saturated animal fats and animal protein will cause an increase in the pain-producing prostaglandins, unsaturated essential fatty acids found in plants actually help reduce the inflammation and pain. According to Tori Hudson, N.D., dietary improvements alone can relieve cramps. Simply reducing or eliminating dairy may significantly help a third of all women suffering through painful periods.

For this central reason, the diet should be primarily or totally vegetarian. It should focus on whole foods, vegetables, grains, legumes, nuts, and seeds, and be low in hydrogenated and saturated fats. It should have plenty of fibre to keep stool soft and moving to prevent constipation, which makes the problem worse. Use castor oil packs frequently to keep the bowels moving and reduce the stagnation in the abdomen, which makes the condition worse. Use psyllium or flaxseed to keep the bowels moving and free from toxins.

There are some other things that it is helpful to avoid in order to eliminate their contribution to the problem. Coffee, alcohol, chocolate, pop, sugar, and refined carbohydrates all leach out the essential fatty acids and minerals that help to promote a strong reproductive system. Salt can also contribute to dysmenorrhoea. Since an underac-tive thyroid can also be involved, sea vegetables should be included in the diet for their wealth of minerals—especially iodine—which help to regulate an underactive thyroid.

HELPFUL HERBS
Black Haw
There are also several herbs that are very helpful. The perfectly named cramp bark and its close relative, black haw, just might be the best herbs for painful periods. They work by relaxing the smooth muscle of the uterus. Cramp bark also helps to decrease the spasming of the cervical neck. Try combining them, as First Nations healers did.

Donq quai is one of the best herbs for relieving painful cramping. It works by bringing warmth into the pelvic region and encouraging blood flow. Stop taking dong quai a week before you start bleeding and start it again only once the bleeding has stopped.

Black and Blue Cohosh
Black cohosh and blue cohosh are also used to relieve menstrual pains. Though better known as the single greatest treatment for menopause, black cohosh is actually a powerful antispasmodic that helps to relax the body and ease cramping. Blue cohosh helps bring blood into the abdomen, easing congestion and pain. The two cohoshes are often combined for painful periods, along with

chamomile, raspberry leaves, and cayenne.

Ginger

Ginger brings warmth to the abdomen and can help to relieve the pain. It is an antispasmodic and anti-inflammatory herb that can help to relieve the cramping. When 150 women with moderate to severe dysmenorrhoea were given either 250mg of ginger four times a day or the anti-inflammatory drugs ibuprofen or mefenamic acid for three days, beginning on the first day of their periods, the improvement in pain relief and satisfaction with the treatment was equally good in the ginger group as in the drug groups. The study's authors concluded that ginger is as effective as the drugs[1]. Ginger is also the best herb for nausea, so, for those who suffer from nausea during their periods, ginger is an ideal herb to include. It can also get rid of intestinal gas and help to correct bowel functions.

Motherwort

Motherwort is a powerful antispasmodic and nervine that is excellent for women who experience cramping. It is often combined with donq quai and cramp bark.

Chamomile

Chamomile is one of the best and easiest herbs to take to prevent and to treat cramping. Simply drink properly infused chamomile tea all day long during pain to get relief. Chamomile is a relaxant, and it is high in easily assimilated calcium that helps to prevent cramping.

Passionflower

Passionflower acts as a painkiller and an antispasmodic and is wonderful for painful periods.

Mugwort

The Chinese herb mugwort is used as a tea to reduce cramping in women with dysmenorrhoea. It can also be used in moxibustion by a trained acupuncturist to reduce cramping. In moxibustion, mugwort is burnt on or over meridians on the body to alleviate stagnation and to bring energy and warmth to the area.

Chastetree Berry

Taken over time, the excellent female herb, chastetree berry, will correct an underlying hormonal imbalance and help to reduce cramping. Chastetree berry is perhaps the best herb for correcting any underlying period-related problems.

Liver Herbs

Liver herbs such as milk thistle, Oregon grape root, blessed thistle, yellow dock, and dandelion root are used to clear out a clogged and sluggish liver. The liver is almost always involved in menstrual irregularities. Traditional Chinese medicine attributes many menstrual problems to blocked liver *qi* (energy) and blood.

Turmeric is an effective liver herb that also relieves pain and inflammation and can greatly help to reduce dysmenorrhoea.

An old recipe from India combines turmeric with aloe. If you take 1/4 oz or more of aloe juice with 1 to 2 tsps or more of turmeric each day, you will clear out the problems that cause period pain.

Rosemary

Rosemary improves circulation, liver function, and the metabolism of estrogen, helping to reduce period pain. Rosemary is also a natural painkiller.

Herbs that Relax You and Your Cramps

Stress also causes cramping. Many natural-health practitioners believe that women who lead unbalanced lives are prime candidates for cramping. Unresolved anger, frustration, and resentment can also contribute, as they can stagnate *qi* and blood, making the problem worse.

One of the beautiful things about the herbs that help relax us is that they also help relax spasming and cramping muscles. Valerian, passionflower, hops, and linden flower are just some of these wonderful herbs. Linden flower can also help to relieve headaches that are associated with menstrual problems, including migraine headaches.

Other useful herbs include raspberry leaf, yarrow, squaw vine, nettle, wild yam, catnip, false unicorn root, and prickly ash.

Essential Fatty Acids

Essential fatty acids are crucial to preventing the inflammation that can cause cramping. Try using hemp or flaxseed oil as these oils are high in omega-3s, which are best for relieving inflammation. Some women do find that evening primrose oil, high in omega-6, helps, too. Just be sure to keep the oils in balance.

Helpful nutrients for converting these good oils into powerful antispasmodics and anti-inflammatories include B6, zinc, magnesium, vitamin C, and niacin.

VITAMINS, MINERALS, AND OTHER SUPPLEMENTS

Calcium and Magnesium

Many women are low in calcium and magnesium, and these deficiencies tend to be found in women with dysmenorrhoea. And, just to make matters worse, blood calcium levels begin to drop prior to menstruation. A low level of blood calcium manifests itself by muscle cramps, water retention, and achiness, among other problems. In other words, low calcium levels cause dysmenorrhoea. Supplementing calcium can reduce the pain[2]. Magnesium helps to reduce sensitivity to pain and improves symptoms[3].

B Vitamins

The B vitamins are crucial for relieving dysmenorrhoea. B6 when taken together with a B-complex has been found to reduce both the intensity and the duration of cramping, according to research cited by Christiane Northrup, M.D., in her book *Women's Bodies, Women's Wisdom*. And B6 also helps to reduce water retention and moodiness, so is doubly useful for period imbalances. So take a B-complex and extra B6. Perhaps the most important B vitamin for painful periods is B3. This B vitamin has been shown in clinical studies to be over 87 per cent effective in relieving menstrual cramps[4]. That is a very high precentage. B3 may be acting as a vasodilator in the uterus, reducing the pain. Adding vitamin C and flavonoids such as rutin make the B3 work even better[5].

Vitamin E

The simple step of taking 200 to 800 IU of vitamin E can help relieve dysmenorrhoea. Early research showed that about 70 per cent of women experience relief using vitamin E[6]. Two impressive recent studies have confirmed this exciting result. In a double-blind study, teenage girls with dysmenorrhoea were given either 500 IU of vitamin E or a placebo for five days, beginning two days before menstruation. The girls taking the vitamin E had a significantly greater improvement in menstrual pain[7]. In a second study that worked the same way but gave only 400 IU of vitamin E, the girls on the vitamin E not only had less pain, but the pain didn't last as long and they lost less blood[8].

SAMe and 5-HTP

Both SAMe and 5-HTP can also help. Their powerful ability to increase serotonin will make you less sensitive to pain.

MSM

Although MSM is not usually thought of as a treatment for dysmenorrhoea, Linda has found clinically that it really helps relieve cramping. MSM is an anti-inflammatory and painkiller that is more typically used for joint problems. It helps to stop spasming muscles.

Bromelain

Bromelain has been used to reduce inflammation, pain and reduce cramping. It is one of the best natural anti-inflammatories and can be extremely effective.

Essential Oils

Try rubbing pennyroyal oil on the lower abdomen to ease painful periods. It helps to bring blood flow into the area. Don't take pennyroyal oil internally.

A new use for essential oils was recently found when an aromatherapy study showed reduced menstrual cramping. A group of women who suffered from dysmenorrhoea were given an abdominal massage using lavender, clary sage, and rose essential oils in an almond oil carrier or just the almond oil. The women who got the essential oil massage had significantly less cramping[9].

If candida is involved as a cause of your dysmenorrhoea, then treat the candida (see section on Candida).

Still More Help

Sitz baths and castor-oil packs can also help. For the sitz bath, you alternate between sitting in hot- and cold-water baths. For the castor-oil packs, the castor oil is heated and applied as a foment to the abdomen. Progesterone cream may also be helpful.

Further help comes from acupuncture[10], avoidance of food allergies, improving digestive function, avoiding tampons and IUDs, and increasing exercise. Exercise is key to avoiding stagnation of blood and *qi*, which can contribute to the problem.

Given a little time and effort, painful periods can be stopped, and you will wonder why you waited so long to deal with the problem.

Chapter Endnotes

1. Ozgoli G, Goli M, "Moattar F. Comparison of effects of ginger, mefenamic acid, and ibuprofen on pain in women with primary dysmenorrhea." *J Altern Complement Med* 2009;15:129-32.

2. Penland, J., P. Johnson. "Dietary calcium and manganese effects on menstrual cycle symptoms." *Am J Obstet Gynecol*, 1993; 168:1417'23.

3. Fontana-Klaiber, H., B. Hogg. "Therapeutic effects of magnesium in dysmenorrhea." *Schweiz Rundsch Med Prax*, 1990; 79:491-94.

4. Hudgins, A. P., "Niacin for dysmenorrhea." *Am Practice Digest Treat*, 1952; 3:892-93.

5. Hudgins, A.P. "Vitamins P, C and niacin for dysmenorrhea therapy." *West J Surg*, 1954; 62:610-11.

6. Butler, E., E. Mcknight. "Vitamin E in the treatment of primary dysmenorrhoea." *Lancet*; 1955:1:844'47.

7. Ziaei, S., *et al*. "A randomised placebo-controlled trial to determine the effect of vitamin E in treatment of primary dysmenorrhoea." *Br J Obstet Gynaecol*, 2001; 108:1181-83.

8. Ziaei, S., M. Zakeri, A. Kazemnejad. "A randomised controlled trial of vitamin E in the treatment of primary dysmenorrhoea." *Br J Obstet Gynaecol*, 2005; 112:466-69.

9. Han, S. H., *et al*. "Effect of aromatherapy on symptoms of dysmenorrhea in college students: A randomized placebo-controlled clinical trial." *J Altern Complement Med*, 2006; 12:535'41.

10. Helms, J. M. "Acupuncture for the management of primary dysmenorrhea." *Obstet Gynecol*, 1987; 69:51-56.

ENDOMETRIOSIS

Almost half a million Canadian women suffer from endometriosis, yet it is only now that we are beginning to hear of it. Why?

Endometriosis was rarely recognized because of the difficulty of diagnosis and how long diagnosis could take, since other illnesses had to be ruled out first. But this is changing. More and more women are being told they have endometriosis.

Endometriosis occurs when bits of the uterus lining grow outside the uterus, causing pelvic pain, painful periods, painful intercourse, painful bowel movements, intestinal discomfort, bleeding between periods or irregular menstrual flow, and infertility.

According to Christiane Northrup, M.D., the infertility is not caused by the endometriosis. Whatever is causing endometriosis may also cause

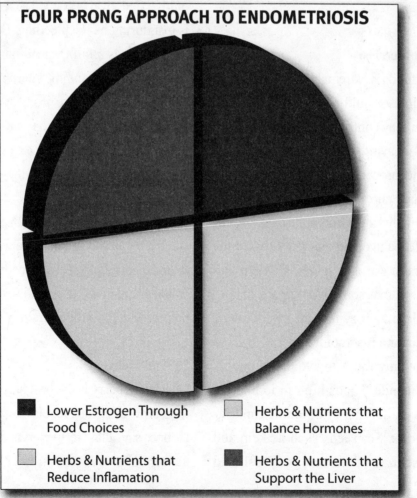

FOUR PRONG APPROACH TO ENDOMETRIOSIS

- ◼ Lower Estrogen Through Food Choices
- ◻ Herbs & Nutrients that Balance Hormones
- ◻ Herbs & Nutrients that Reduce Inflamation
- ◼ Herbs & Nutrients that Support the Liver

infertility, but one does not cause the other.

Endometriosis is an estrogen-sensitive disease, so estrogen levels must be lowered through food choices, herbs, and nutrients that balance hormones, reduce inflammation, and support the liver. The liver is addressed because it not only excretes estrogen but also breaks down the harmful estradiol into estriol, a safer form of estrogen. Herbalist Rosemary Gladstar says that a high ratio of estriol to estradiol limits the amount of endometrial tissue that is produced and also reduces the pain.

Diet and Endometriosis

Your choice of foods is extremely important. Meat and dairy products should be avoided, since the excess estrogen may contribute to endometriosis. You should also avoid chocolate, coffee, salt, sugar, fried and processed foods. Women who drink more than a cup and a half of coffee a day may be more likely to get endometriosis[1]. Alcohol, too, should be avoided since it stresses the liver and can raise estrogen levels. Carolyn Demarco, M.D., says that some women are able to completely relieve their symptoms by following a vegetarian diet or a macrobiotic diet.

There are not only foods to avoid, but important foods to include. Foods high in iodine are important, since a deficiency of iodine can trigger endometriosis. Seaweeds such as kelp and dulse are rich sources of iodine. The diet should also be rich in vegetables, whole grains, legumes, nuts, and seeds.

To help reduce inflammation, include essential fatty acids, such as flaxseed oil, in your diet.

Vitamins and Minerals

Many vitamins and minerals can help treat endometriosis. B vitamins help the liver to break down and excrete estrogen. Since free-radical damage may be involved in endometriosis, antioxidants such as vitamins A, E, and C are recommended. Iron is needed to replace the iron that is lost during heavy bleeding. Sea vegetables and herbs such as alfalfa, spirulina, and chlorella are also rich in iron. Taking vitamin C will help your body to absorb more iron, and vitamin C and bioflavonoids will help to reduce the heavy bleeding. Flavonoids have the extra benefit of being weakly estrogenic. Because they are much weaker estrogens than your body's, they can actually lower the excessive estrogen by stealing a receptor site from your body's stronger estrogen. Vitamins A and E are helpful for bleeding and hormone balance. Calcium, magnesium, and potassium can help prevent painful cramping.

Herbal Help

Chastetree berry is the best herb for balancing estrogen/progesterone levels. Herbalist Christopher Hobbes says that German gynaecologists are having remarkable success using chastetree berry to treat endometriosis. Chastetree berry can also be combined with other herbs for maximum benefits.

Gladstar recommends this combination: dandelion root, wild yam, burdock root, pau d'arco, Oregon grape root, chastetree berry, and donq quai. These herbs are used for their ability to balance hormones, to aid the liver and the digestive system, for their antispasmodic and anti-inflammatory properties, and to shrink growths.

If heavy bleeding is a problem, try astringent herbs such as shepherd's purse. Other good herbs to try for heavy bleeding include yarrow, nettle, raspberry leaf, and oak bark.

Herbs that stimulate circulation to the pelvic region are also used in treating endometriosis. Try black cohosh, ginger, witch hazel, and castor oil packs.

More Help

Or try foot baths. Use very hot water on your feet for half an hour a day while putting a cold pack on your abdomen to draw away inflammation and to stimulate the immune system.

Since many women who suffer from endometriosis develop anemia, strengthening herbs such as eleuthero (formerly Siberian ginseng) are used for energy, and nettle tea, which aids digestion and supplies iron to replace lost iron stores. A liquid iron supplement is also recommended.

Candida expert Dr. Orion Truss says that there is a very high association between endometriosis and candida and says you can get dramatic relief of endometriosis symptoms by treating candida (see section on Candida).

Demarco also points out that there is a connection between pesticides and endometriosis. She explains that many industrial chemicals mimic estrogen in the body, which can lead to an excessive estrogen-to-progesterone balance, which can lead to endometriosis.

Another excellent choice for helping with endometriosis is acupuncture. Acupuncture can stimulate the immune system, shrink growths, reduce pain and inflammation, and clear out congestion.

Chapter Endnotes
1. Grodstein, F., *et al.* "Relation of female infertility to consumption of caffeinated beverages." *Am J Epidemiol*, 1993; 137:1353-60.

FIBROCYSTIC BREAST DISEASE

Finding a lump in her breast is one of a woman's worst fears. It simply terrifies most women. Before deciding to treat the lump, it is always wise to get it checked first to know exactly what the problem is. For many women, the lump turns out to be fibrocystic breast disease and is not cancerous. This condition is so common that up to 40 per cent of premenopausal women get it. Not only is the condition treatable, many women are able to completely reverse the problem by using dietary and lifestyle changes and some supplements.

The Many Causes of Fibrocystic Breast Disease

Fibrocystic breast disease can be a very painful problem. There are many causes of fibrocystic breast disease. The most common being excess estrogen. This excess can be the result of too much red meat and dairy—which are high in estrogen—plastics, birth control pills, or environmental sources. Other causes include stress, poor diet, candida, sluggish liver, metals, toxins, low thyroid, and caffeine. Caffeine is such a culprit that when women eliminated caffeine, 97.5 per cent of them improved in one study. Of the women who, though they didn't eliminate caffeine, cut it way down, 75 per cent improved[1].

Because fibrocystic breast disease is an estro-gen-sensitive condition, the focus of the natural treatment is to reduce estrogen. The subduing of estrogen has three prongs: diet, liver support, and hormone-balancing herbs.

Diet and Fibrocystic Breast Disease

The most important dietary change for fibrocystic breast disease is the change to a more plant-based vegetarian diet. This helps because animal-based foods are too high in estrogen and too low in fibre. Excessive estrogen caused the problem in the first place, and when the saturated fat found in animal products is reduced, estrogen goes down and the pain and lumpiness of fibrocystic breast disease improves[2]. Fibre is found only in plant food, and studies have linked a low-fibre diet to fibrocystic breast disease. Insufficient fibre also causes constipation, and women who have fewer than three bowel movements a week are four and half times more likely to suffer from fibrocystic breast disease than women who have daily bowel movements. A lack of dietary fibre encourages improper bacterial flora. These bad bacteria produce an enzyme that frees estrogen from the glucoronic acid that captures it and escorts it out of the body. Vegetarian women have 55 per cent less unbound estrogen in their blood because they excrete so much more estrogen than women who eat meat. For this reason, acidophilus, which is usually thought of for candida, can also help women with fibrocystic breast disease, because these good bacteria overwhelm the bad bacteria that release estrogen back into circulation. Dr. Christiane Northrup recommends that women with fibrocystic breast disease cut out all dairy products for three months. Clinically, Linda has seen even better results when the dairy products are left out even longer to prevent recurrence. Also, try taking fibres such as flaxseed or psyllium.

Look to the Liver

To get rid of fibrocystic breast disease, you must help the liver. How does the liver fit in with all of this? Well, as the chief organ of detoxification, it falls to the liver to clear excess estrogen from the body by binding it to glucoronic acid and taking it out. This job requires B6, folic acid, and the other B vitamins. A deficiency of any of these B vitamins can cause fibrocystic breast disease.

Dr. Carolyn Demarco suggests taking 100 to 200 mg of vitamin B6 a day throughout the cycle, along with the other B vitamins, to relieve breast pain.

You should also use supporting and detoxifying liver herbs such as milk thistle, dandelion root, ginger, artichoke, and Oregon grape root. Milk thistle is the king of the liver detoxifiers.

Reinforcing the glucoronic acid with supplements in the form of calcium D-glucorate can also help.

Supplements for Balancing Hormones

Since excess estrogen can cause fibrocystic breast disease, it is crucial to take advantage of herbs that balance hormones. Wild yam cream is used to help increase progesterone levels safely and naturally. Because of the excessive ratio of estrogen to progesterone, Dr. Mauvais-Jarvis has found that 95 per cent of fibrocystic breast disease patients have their breast pain relieved when a natural progesterone cream is rubbed into the breasts. John Lee, M.D., the progesterone doctor, has had similar positive results. Since the herb chastetree berry works by balancing estrogen/progesterone levels, slightly favouring progesterone, and by reducing excess prolactin, it is a perfect herb for treating fibrocystic breast disease.

Women with fibrocystic breast disease often have problems with their prolactin levels, too. Taking evening primrose oil, borage oil, or flaxseed oil will all help normalize the level of this hormone. Several studies have found some relief from fibrocystic breast disease with evening primrose oil[3].

Clinical studies have shown that people with fibrocystic breast disease can recover using iodine[4]. Supplementing with iodine reduces breast tenderness, prolactin levels, and breast lumps, even in patients with so-called normal thyroid function. Most people do not get enough iodine, because soil is so often depleted of iodine, and, therefore, the food that grows in it is low in iodine as well. Kelp and other sea vegetables provide a good source of iodine and can be used in soups, salads, stews, pastas, or wherever you like, or can be taken in convenient tablet form.

More Natural Help

Several, but not all, double-blind studies have shown vitamin E to be very useful in treating fibrocystic breast disease[5].

Coenzyme Q10 can also be helpful. It can help to shrink growths and improve the cellular oxygenation. Also try indole-3-carbinol to help shrink growths. The mushrooms reishi, shiitake, and maitake can also shrink growths.

Other useful supplements for treating fibrocystic breast disease include immune-supporting herbs such as shiitake and reishi mushroom, astragalus, and antioxidants such as vitamin C and selenium, nutrient-rich foods such as spirulina, liver-supporting herbs such as dandelion and milk thistle, fat-dissolving nutrients such as lecithin, and mass-shrinking herbs such as pau d'arco and poke root. Some have found lymph-supporting herbs such as red root, echinacea, calendula, and cleavers to be of aid, as well.

A good formula to shrink breast lumps is to combine red clover, burdock root, dandelion root, Oregon grape root, rosemary, cleavers, calendula, and European mistletoe as tinctures, and consume 40 drops three to four times daily. These herbs help to shrink growths, cleanse the liver, balance hormones, and drain lymph nodes.

Also try topical oils of poke root, calendula, lemon, dandelion, lavender, rosemary, juniper, and red clover. These oils also help to shrink growths. Topically, many women have also found success using castor-oil packs on the breast for an hour or more, four times a week. Castor-oil packs help alleviate the pain and inflammation and can be used for detoxifying purposes. Other useful topical agents include green-clay packs, four times a week for detoxifying, and poke root applied topically daily. Poke-root has been used traditionally for years to help get rid of all kinds of lumps, including breast lumps.

You can also try acupuncture, which is great to relieve stagnation and break up lumps.

Or try hydrotherapy. Put your feet in very hot water and place cold packs on the breasts. This will bring blood circulation to the area and help to break up lumps. Do this for twenty minutes at a time, two times per day, four times or more per week.

You can also try upper-body exercises that get the blood moving in the chest area to help move stagnation out.

Taking Care of Yourself Helps Take Care of the Fibrocystic Breast Disease

It is vitally important that some method be used to reduce stress in women with fibrocystic breast disease. Herbalist Rosemary Gladstar, author of *Herbal Healing for Women*, talks in her book about how she developed fibrocystic breast disease after going through a great deal of stress, which she had ignored for some time, and how she was only able to achieve healing after she completely re-examined her life, making changes that led her to take care of herself, allowing her to recover. After several months on a regimen that included supplements as well as rest and stress reduction, her lumps had completely disappeared. So, try yoga, meditation, acupuncture—whatever works for you to reduce stress.

Chapter Endnotes

1. Minton, J. P., *et al*. "Clinical and biochemical studies on methylxanthine-related fibrocystic breast disease." *Surgery*, 1981; 90:229-'304.

2. Rose, D. P., *et al*. "Low fat diet in fibrocystic disease of the breast with cyclic mastalgia: a feasibility study." *Am J Clin Nutr*, 1985; 41(4):856; Rose, D. P., *et al*. "Effect of a low-fat diet on hormone levels in women with cystic breast disease. I. Serum steroids and gonadotropins." *J Natl Cancer Inst*, 1987; 78:623-26; Boyd, N. F., *et al*. "Effect of a low-fat high-carbohydrate diet on symptoms of cyclical mastopathy." *Lancet*, 1988; ii:128-32; Woods, M. N., et al. "Low-fat, high-fibre diet and serum estrone sulfate in premenopausal women." *Am J Clin Nutr*, 1989; 49:1179-83.

3. Pye, J. K., R. E. Mansel, L. E. Hughes. "Clinical experience of drug treatments for mastalgia." *Lancet*, 1985; ii:373-77; Harding, C., *et al*. "Hormone replacement therapy-induced mastalgia responds to evening primrose oil." Br J Surg, 1996; 83(Suppl 1):24; Preece, P.E., *et al*. "Evening primrose oil (EFAMOL) for mastalgia." In: *Clinical Uses of Essential Fatty Acids*, ed. DF Horrobin, Montreal: Eden Press, 1982, 147-54; Pashby, N., *et al*. "A clinical trial of evening primrose oil in mastalgia." *Br J Surg*, 1981; 68:801'24.

4. Ghent, W.R., *et al*. "Iodine replacement in fibrocystic disease of the breast." *Can J Surg*, 1993; 36:453'60.

5. Abrams, A. A.. "Use of vitamin E in chronic cystic mastitis." *N Engl J Med*, 1965; 272:1080-81; London, R.S., *et al*. "Endocrine parameters and alpha-tocopherol therapy of patients with mammary dysplasia." *Cancer Res*, 1981; 41:3811-13; London, R.S., *et al*. "The effect of alpha-tocopherol on premenstrual symptomatology: a double-blind study. II. Endocrine correlates." *J Am Col Nutr*, 1984; 3:351'56.

INFERTILITY

There was a time when fertility, and not infertility, was the problem, when couples couldn't help but have huge families. Today the modern problem is quite the opposite. Couples are frustrated by infertility, and fertility clinics—a ridiculous idea a couple of generations ago—have become common. Though in different times in history either the male or the female has been held responsible for fertility and infertility, we now know that successful conception is a shared responsibility: 40% of the time the female is infertile, 40% of the time the male is, and 20% of the time either they both are or the cause is unknown.

The Many Causes of Infertility

When women are having trouble with fertility, the possible causes are many. It can be caused by uterine fibroids, ovarian cysts, endometriosis, irregular ovulation, hormonal imbalances, being excessively under- or overweight, past birth-control use, pelvic inflammatory disease, infection, low thyroid, tilted uterus, chemicals, radiation, scar tissue, allergies, eating disorders, stress and exhaustion, strenuous exercise, nutritional problems, and even antibodies to sperm or fertilized eggs. Studies have even shown that being excessively focused on having a baby, ironically, can interfere with having a baby. For many of these causes, the underlying problem will need to be addressed.

Chastetree Berry: The Most Important Way to Correct Infertility

The most important thing to take for infertility is the women's hormone-balancing herb chastetree berry. Although most chastetree berry studies have focused on women's health issues other than infertility, several of them have been struck by the power of that herb to help infertile women conceive[1]. In the most recent study, sixty-six women who had been unsuccessful in becoming pregnant for one to three years were given either a combination formula featuring chastetree berry or a placebo. Ten became pregnant while using the chastetree berry, compared to half as many using the placebo[2]. Chastetree berry may be especially effective when the infertility is related to a luteal phase defect and elevated prolactin.

Luteal-phase defect can cause infertility because a lack of the hormone progesterone prevents the uterine lining from developing properly. In addition to chastetree berry, vitamin C can also help women with this condition become pregnant. Taking 750 mg of vitamin C a day helped 25 per cent of women with luteal phase defect become pregnant, compared to only 11 per cent of women who did not take vitamin C[3].

More Herbal Help

Though chastetree berry is the most important single herb for infertility, there are several other herbs, often taken in combinations that include chastetree berry, that can gently ease a woman's body back to fertility.

When the origins of infertility are hormonal, dong quai, red clover, and squaw vine are helpful, along with the chastetree berry. If you are using dong quai, don't use it while you are menstruating. Herbalist Amanda McQuade Crawford says that skullcap is a reproductive relaxant that is very good for enhancing fertility. She also recommends using red raspberry and alfalfa as nourishing tonics, and yarrow as an antimicrobial herb with affinity to the reproductive tract when infection is involved.

Traditional herbalists usually use combinations of herbs instead of single herbs so that the different actions of the herbs can act synergistically. One of our favourite herbalists, Rosemary Gladstar, recommends the following two formulae for female infertility:

Fertility Tonic

4 parts rehmania
1 part astragalus
1 part dong quai
2 parts false unicorn root
3 parts wild yam
1 part chastetree berry

This formula is taken as a capsule or tincture three times a day. If you've never heard of rehmania before, you're not alone, but this little-known herb is also referred to by another of our favourite herbalists, Michael Tierra, as an important herb that Chinese herbalists use for female infertility. False unicorn root, another strange-sounding herb in this formula, has a long tradition of use as a herb for the female reproductive system, including being used by early North American medical healers for infertility.

Female Fertility Tea

3 parts wild yam
2 parts licorice
4 parts sassafras bark or root
1 part chastetree berry
1/2 part dong quai
1 part ginger
1 part cinnamon
1/2 part false unicorn root
1/4 part orange peel
pinch of stevia

This formula should be taken as a tea three to four times a day.

Gladstar also says that ginseng helps with infertility.

Other useful herbs include motherwort, astragalus, marigold, dandelion leaf and root, basil, suma, horsetail, blue and black cohosh, rosemary, damiana, sarsaparilla, uva ursi, ground ivy, and blessed thistle. Some of these herbs can be used to prepare you to get pregnant, but should not be used when you are pregnant.

Vitamins for Infertility

Nutritional deficiencies can be a cause of infertility, and double-blind research has shown that taking a multivitamin/mineral increases female fertility. Giving 200 IU of vitamin E to the woman and 100 IU to the man significantly increases fertility in infertile couples[4]. Though the hint has never been picked up by modern research, one very early study found that 100 mg of PABA—a distant relative of the B vitamins—taken four times a day helped twelve out of sixteen infertile women to become pregnant[5]. And when women suffering from infertility and endometriosis were given either a placebo or 500 mg of propolis twice a day, pregnancies went up from 20 per cent in the placebo group to 60 per cent in the propolis group[6].

Zinc can also be key. Other useful nutrients include vitamin C, bioflavonoids, flaxseed oil, beta-carotene, magnesium, selenium, B12, and B6.

Ancient Help: Acupuncture

Acupuncture can help when the infertility is caused by problems of ovulation; it has been shown to improve ovulation in 83 per cent of women who are not ovulating[7]. Ear acupuncture has actually been shown to work as well as hormone therapy. Fifteen out of forty-five women in one study became pregnant in both the acupuncture and the hormone group, but unwanted side effects only occurred in the hormone group[8]. In another study, acupuncture outperformed the fertility drug clomiphene with a pregnancy rate of 65 per cent to 45 per cent for the drug.

Diet and Lifestyle

As always, the things you do and the things you eat can have an effect. And, as always, caffeine, smoking, and drinking are among those things you might want to avoid. Coffee and caffeine reduce fertility[9]. Smoking can also lessen your chances of becoming pregnant[10], perhaps by as much as three times. And, though not all the studies agree, the research suggests that if you want to become pregnant, eliminating alcohol will increase your chances[11]. Also avoid sugar and refined grains, and get plenty of sunlight, whole grains, vegetables, fruits, raw seeds, raw nuts, and legumes.

And, as we have already seen, weight problems, whether the problem is being excessively underweight or excessively overweight, can contribute to infertility[12].

Chapter Endnotes

1. Loch, E-G., H. Selle, N. Boblitz. "Treatment of premenstrual syndrome with a phytopharmaceutical formulation containing *Vitex agnus castus.*" *Journal of Women's Health & Gender-Based Medicine*, 2000; 9:315'20; Propping, D., T. Katzorke. "Treatment of corpus luteum insufficiency." *Z Allg Med*, 1987; 63:932-33; *Gynakol*, 1994; *Therapiewoche*, 1993; *Therapeutikon*, 1991.

2. Gerhard, I., *et al.* "Mastodynon® for female infertility. Randomized, placebo-controlled, clinical double-blind study." *Forsch Komplementärmed*, 1998; 5:272-78.

3. Henmi, H., *et al.* "Effects of ascorbic acid supplementation on serum progesterone levels in patients with a luteal phase defect." *Fertil Steril*, 2003; 80:459-61.

4. Bayer, R. "Treatment of infertility with vitamin E." *Int J Fertil*, 1960; 5:70-78.

5. Sieve, B. F. "The clinical effects of a new B-complex factor, para-aminobenzoic acid, on pigmentation and fertility." *South Med Surg*, 1942; 104:135-39.

6. Ali, A. F. M., A. Awadallah. "Bee propolis versus placebo in the treatment of infertility associated with minimal or mild endometriosis: a pilot randomized controlled trial. A modern trend." *Fertil Steril*, 2003; 80(Suppl 3):S32 [abstract].

7. Mo, X., *et al.* Clinical studies on the mechanism for acupuncture stimulation of ovulation. *J Tradit Chin Med*, 1993; 13:115-19.

8. Gerhard, I., Postneek, F. "Auricular acupuncture in the treatment of female infertility." *Gynecol Endocrinol*, 1992; 6:171-81.

9. Wilcox, A., C. Weinberg, D. Baird. "Caffeinated beverages and decreased fertility." *Lancet*, 1988; 2:1453-56; Williams, M.A., *et al.* "Coffee and delayed conception." *Lancet*, 1990; 335:1603 [letter]; Hatch, E. E., M.B. Bracken. "Association of delayed conception with caffeine consumption." *Am J Epidemiol*, 1993; 138:1082-92; Grodstein, F., *et al.* "Relation of female infertility to consumption of caffeinated beverages." *Am J Epidemiol*, 1993; 137:1353-60; Stanton, C.K., R.H. Gray. "Effects of caffeine consumption on delayed conception." *Am J Epidemiol*, 1995; 142:1322-29.

10. Howe, G., *et al.* "Effects of age, cigarette smoking, and other factors on fertility: findings in a large prospective study." *BMJ*, 1985; 290:1697-99.

11. Grodstein, F., M. B. Goldman, D. W. Cramer. "Infertility in women and moderate alcohol use." *Am J Public Health*, 1994; 84:1429-32; Hakim, R. B., R. H. Gray, H. Zacur. "Alcohol and caffeine consumption and decreased fertility." *Fertil Steril*, 1998; 70:632-37.

12. Green, B. B., N. S. Weiss, J. R. Daling. "Risk of ovulatory infertility in relation to body weight." *Fertil Steril*, 1988; 50:621-26.

MENOPAUSE

Menopause is not a disease. It is a natural progression in a woman's life. For many women, it is even a time of spiritual growth and creativity, and a time, finally, for themselves. But this natural stage is usually treated in a most unnatural way: Women are aggressively drugged on synthetic hormones.

The discomfort of menopause is real. In western culture, most menopausal women suffer through hot flashes, night sweats, palpitations, and vaginal dryness and thinning. Depression, anxiety, decreased mental sharpness, weight gain, and other problems are also common.

But there are natural solutions to these natural problems. Women neither have to suffer through menopause, nor do they need to go on dangerous hormones to get relief.

The Problem with Hormones

The problem with hormones is that, while they do stop hot flashes, they also cause cancer and heart disease. As early as 1997, a meta-analysis of fifty-one studies had already found that the risk of breast cancer goes up by 2.3 per cent for every year on hormone replacement therapy[1]. Now it is known that hormone replacement therapy increases the risk of breast cancer, invasive breast cancer and death from breast cancer[2]. New research has added ovarian cancer to that list[3]. In fact, the British researchers of the ovarian cancer study have said that while ovarian, breast, and endometrial cancer account for 40 per cent of all female cancers in the U.K., the incidence of these three cancers combined is 63 per cent higher in women who are currently using hormone replacement therapy.

Less well-known than the cancer-causing risk of hormone replacement therapy is the increased risk of heart disease. Hormone replacement therapy increases your risk of heart attack, stroke, and blood clots[4]. Even less well known is that HRT also increases your risk of Alzheimer's disease[5].

Black Cohosh: The Answer to Hormones

Now what would you say if you knew that there was a perfectly safe herb that has been shown in head-to-head studies to work better than hormone replacement therapy?

The herb is black cohosh. Originally, black cohosh was believed to be a phytoestrogenic herb, i.e., a herb that contains mild plant estrogens that can lower or raise your body's estrogen as needed. It is now known that it is not estrogenic[6]; yet this herb continues to outperform estrogen therapy in the treatment of menopause.

Black cohosh is extremely effective for hot flashes, sweating, and heart palpitations. It even works on the vaginal thinning and drying that hormone therapy hardly helps[7]. And studies have also shown black cohosh to be extremely effective in treating the nervousness, irritability, depression, anxiety, and sleep disturbances that can also accompany menopause[8].

There have been several interesting studies on black cohosh. In one, 80 per cent of the women experienced an improvement of symptoms. Many of them had tried hormone replacement therapy before, and for 72 per cent of them, the herb had advantages over the hormone. The herb helped both the physical and the psychological symptoms of menopause. Hot flashes improved in 86.6 per cent of the women, sweats in 88.5 per cent, heart palpitations in 90.4 per cent, and there was improvement in depression in 82.5 per cent, and of nervousness and irritability in 85.6 per cent[9].

When black cohosh was compared directly to estrogen and valium, the herb beat both drugs. Again, black cohosh also beat both drugs for helping with the psychological symptoms of depression and anxiety[10].

When black cohosh again went head to head with estrogen in a double-blind study, the herb was again better than the hormone on menopause and anxiety scales. In the black cohosh group, hot

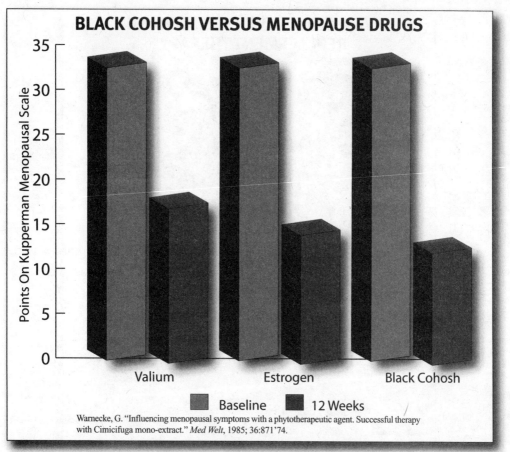

BLACK COHOSH VERSUS MENOPAUSE DRUGS

Points On Kupperman Menopausal Scale

Valium   Estrogen   Black Cohosh

Baseline   12 Weeks

Warnecke, G. "Influencing menopausal symptoms with a phytotherapeutic agent. Successful therapy with Cimicifuga mono-extract." *Med Welt*, 1985; 36:871'74.

flashes dropped from five a day to only one, while the estrogen dropped them to only 3.5 from the original five. While estrogen provided little help for the vaginal lining, black cohosh dramatically improved it[11]. This last advantage is important because the thinning and drying of the vaginal lining that can occur with the drop in estrogen at menopause can make intercourse painful and can also increase the susceptibility to infection, itching, and burning.

A 1991 double-blind study that demonstrated the ability of black cohosh to significantly improve menopausal symptoms, including hot flashes, also demonstrated significant improvement in the vaginal lining[12].

The black cohosh used in these studies was standardized to 1mg triterpenes calculated as 27-deoxyacteine. Four pills a day were given.

New research shows that black cohosh even builds bone—an important bonus for menopausal women. A double-blind study looked at this issue. Women were given either estrogen or 40 mg of standardized black cohosh for twelve weeks. The black cohosh was shown to be as effective as HRT without the dangerous estrogenic effect. But what's even more impressive is that markers for

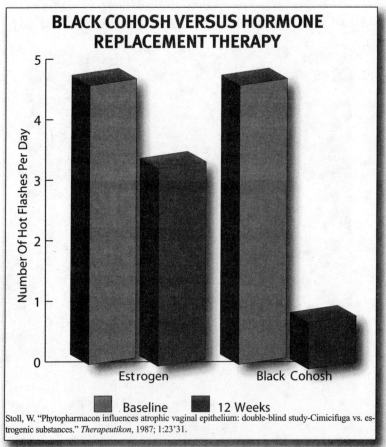

BLACK COHOSH VERSUS HORMONE REPLACEMENT THERAPY

Number Of Hot Flashes Per Day

Estrogen   Black Cohosh

Baseline   12 Weeks

Stoll, W. "Phytopharmacon influences atrophic vaginal epithelium: double-blind study-Cimicifuga vs. estrogenic substances." *Therapeutikon*, 1987; 1:23'31.

bone degeneration decreased in both groups, and markers for bone formation increased only in the black cohosh group[13].

Because black cohosh is not estrogenic, it has the advantage over estrogen therapy of not stimulating breast tumours—quite the opposite; it markedly inhibits them[14]. It is even safe for women with who are at high risk for breast cancer[15]. The most recent research even suggests that black cohosh may help prevent breast cancer[16].

Despite some recent claims, black cohosh is perfectly safe on the liver, producing no elevations in liver enzymes[17] and, perhaps, even a slight decrease[18]. Most recently, a one-year study has found that black cohosh significantly decreases the frequency and severity of hot flashes with no significant changes in tests of liver function[19].

Other Supplements for Menopause:
Isoflavones

Isoflavones are nutrients found in soy and red clover that are weakly estrogenic, giving them an incredible ability. If your estrogen levels are low, as in menopause, they gently raise them, but if they are too high, as in breast cancer, they lower them by stealing receptor sites from your own more powerful estrogen. Studies have shown soy isoflavones help not only with hot flashes, but also with vaginal dryness and thinning[20] and breast cancer (see Breast Cancer section). A very recent study has also found that the isoflavones found in red clover may have cardiovascular benefits for menopausal women[21]. Other foods that contain phytoestrogens include fennel and parsley.

Chastetree Berry

This amazing women's herb is the great hormone balancer: It balances the ratio of estrogen to progesterone and so helps treat some of the underlying causes of many of the uncomfortable symptoms of menopause. It slightly favours progesterone over estrogen. Progesterone's role in relieving menopause is often overlooked. This incredible herb helps with vaginal dryness, hot flashes, dizziness, and the depression of menopause. Herbalist David Hoffmann says that chastetree berry is effective for hot flashes, and Christopher Hobbs agrees, adding that it helps reduce vaginal dryness and depression, as well.

Dong Quai

Dong quai has a long history in China as a herb for women. Because it is a cardiovascular and hormonal tonic as well as a nervine, dong quai is a useful herb in any menopause formula. Dong quai is a strengthening and nourishing herb that is good for easing into menopause

In a recent study, fifty-five menopausal women were given either the unusual combination of dong quai and chamomile or a placebo for twelve weeks. While there was no change in hormones in the herb group, there was a major change in the frequency of hot flashes and night sweats. The women on the herbal combination had a 90 per cent decrease in daytime hot flashes and a 96 per cent decrease at night. The placebo group had only a 15 to 25 per cent decrease. All the women on the herbs said they had a moderate to maximum decrease in the intensity of their hot flashes, with 75 per cent of them reporting a decrease in intensity of 80 to 100 per cent[22].

Licorice

Licorice is an ancient and versatile herb. Licorice possesses estrogen-like activity, making it a wonderful herb for menopause. However, it is also believed to balance estrogen and progesterone, increasing estrogen when it is too low and lowering it when it is too high. It is another effective herb for getting rid of hot flashes and depression. Murray and Pizzorno, N.D.s, agree, saying that licorice is helpful because of its beneficial effects on both estrogen and progesterone. Herbalist Amanda Crawford adds that licorice, as well as ginseng, also contributes by supporting the adrenals. The adrenals are able to produce a little estrogen when the ovaries call it quits. Other useful herbs for supporting the adrenal glands are rhodiola, suma, and ashwagandha. The adrenals are often in need of support in menopause (see Stress section for more on adrenal support).

Wild Yam

Wild yam regulates the balance of estrogen and progesterone, making it a useful herb for menopause. It also helps detoxify the liver, making it especially useful when liver problems are also behind the hormone imbalance. Wild yam contains steroidal precursors that your body may use in a similar manner to its own hormones.

Sage and Other Useful Herbs

For hot flashes and night sweats, the herb sage is a specialist. Because of its astringent properties, sage is often considered the best herb for drying up menopausal sweats. Many sources agree, and Bone and Mill add that motherwort and hawthorn are also useful here. Amanda McQuade Crawford says that motherwort actually addresses many of the unpleasant aspects of menopause, saying it is excellent for hot flashes and palpitations, as well as sweats. Linden and yarrow are other herbs that she says can address many aspects of menopause. Yarrow is an astringent to dry up sweats, and linden helps to calm the system.

St. John's wort is not only good for menopausal depression, as might be expected, but also brings another surprising contribution. According to Tori Hudson, N.D., 86 per cent of postmenopausal women will suffer from reduced libido, but in a recent study, St. John's wort was not only able to significantly reduce symptoms including sweating, irritability, and palpitations, but it also reversed loss of libido. It significantly reduced feelings of unattractiveness in 77 out of 82 women. Women on St. John's wort were more likely to initiate sex, and, although at the beginning of the study, many regarded sexuality as not as important as it once was, 80 per cent said their sexuality had been "substantially enhanced" by the herb[23].

Other good choices for the depression, sleep disturbances, and anxiety that accompany menopause are 5-HTP and SAMe, two nutrients that help to raise serotonin levels, and get rid of anxiety, depression, and sleep problems. Other good antianxiety/sleep herbs include passionflower, kava kava, skullcap, hops, valerian, and verbena.

You may also want to try schizandra, a herb that tones the adrenals, liver, and kidneys, and can stop sweating and improve memory and sleep.

Also, try astragalus while perimenopausal to improve *qi* (energy). It can also help stop sweating.

Liver Herbs: Dandelion Root and Milk Thistle

The liver is an important organ for the production, regulation, and detoxification of hormones, thus herbs that work on the liver, such as dandelion and milk thistle, are excellent herbs for menopause. Other good liver herbs include Oregon grape root, turmeric, artichoke, and boldo.

Eating for a Healthy Menopause

Women who have lived their lives consuming a diet that is rich in whole foods, such as fresh vegetables, whole grains, and fruits, and who avoid alcohol, caffeine, simple carbs, and sugar will have an easier time in menopause. Consuming a vegetarian diet that is high in fibre, antioxidants and essential fatty acids and low in unhealthy animal fats and trans fats will also help. Try to eat more phtyoestrogenic foods such as soy, fennel, celery, parsley, flaxseeds, and other raw seeds and nuts. And eat bone-building foods such as deep leafy greens, tahini, and herbs such as chamomile, nettle, alfalfa, and oatstraw. Also, try eating sea vegetables, such as kelp, nori, and dulse for thyroid health, since the thyroid often becomes under-active in menopause. For under-active thyroid, as well as seaweed try using nutrients such as L-tyrosine and selenium.

Soy

It is well known that soy helps with such menopausal symptoms as hot flashes. But a new study has found that it can also help fight osteoporosis in menopausal women. This study watched 24,403 women for four and a half years and found that the more soy foods they ate, the less chance of bone fracture they had. Soy was able to reduce the risk of fracture significantly[24].

To help reduce menopausal symptoms, the diet

should be high in soy. The isoflavones in soy are estrogenic. Studies have found that soy isoflavones reduce hot flashes[25]. According to Hudson, they also help vaginal atrophy, cholesterol, bones, and prevention of breast and uterine cancers. So, eat lots of soy or supplement to get about 50 to 150 mg of isoflavones, the amount that would be found in a traditional diet.

Other Help

Regular exercise throughout a woman's life can also case menopausal symptoms, as can taking supplements and herbs to keep the body healthy. Also, regular internal cleansing of the body throughout life can aid at menopause. And don't forget to do something to relieve stress and fulfill your dreams.

Supplementing the diet with a good quality multivitamin/mineral complex can also be of help, as can a B-complex, calcium, magnesium, and vitamin C, especially for stress. Acupuncture also helps.

And for hot flashes, try adding natural-source, mixed tocopherol vitamin E, up to 1200 mg, and vitamin C, up to 1 to 3 g a day with bioflavonoids.

Also, don't forget bone-building nutrients, such as calcium, magnesium, vitamins D, C, B6, B12, and folic acid, manganese, boron and zinc (see Osteoporosis section).

For vaginal dryness, try using vitamins E and A, zinc, flaxseed oil, soy, nettle, saw palmetto, black cohosh, and topical applications of vitamin E, almond oil, and calendula cream. Mixed probiotics are also helpful, internally and topically.

Menopause does not have to be spent in pain, discomfort, and depression. Often women find menopause to be a time of great liberation, freedom, and growth, a time to find themselves and truly be all that they can be.

So spend some good quality time on yourself, and get some exercise and maybe do a little meditation or yoga, or take up some other kind of physical exercise program.

Tuning in to your body and supplying it with what it needs to make the transition can make this important time of your life a healthy, joyful, and productive one.

Chapter Endnotes

1. Collaborative Group on Hormonal Factors in Breast Cancer. "Breast cancer and hormone replacement therapy. Combined reanalysis of data from 51 epidemiological studies involving 52,705 women with breast cancer and 108,411 without breast cancer." *Lancet*, 1997; 350:1047'59.

2. Fletcher, S. W., *et al*. "Failure of Estrogen Plus Progestin Therapy for Prevention." JAMA, 2002; 288:366'368; Beral, V. "Million Women Study Collaborators. Breast cancer and hormone-replacement therapy in the Million Women Study." *Lancet*, 2003; 362:419'27.

3. Beral, V. "Ovarian cancer and hormone replacement therapy in the million women study." *Lancet* (online), April 19, 2007.

4. Fletcher, S. W., G. A. Colditz. "Failure of Estrogen Plus Progestin Therapy for Prevention." *JAMA*, 2002; 288:366'68; Wassertheil-Smoller, W., *et al*. "Effect of Estrogen Plus Progestin on Stroke in Postmenopausal Women. The Women's Health Initiative: A Randomized Trial." *JAMA*, 2003; 289:2673'84; Viscoli, C. M., *et al*. "A clinical trial of estrogen-replacement therapy after ischemic stroke." N Engl J Med, 2001; 345:1243-49; Mitka, M. "New advice for women patients about hormone therapy and the heart." *JAMA*, 2001; 286:907.

5. Shumaker, S.A., *et al*. "Estrogen Plus Progestin and the Incidence of Dementia and Mild Cognitive Impairment in Postmenopausal Women. The Women's Health Initiative Memory Study: A Randomized Controlled Trial." *JAMA*, 2003; 289:2651'62.

6. Liske, E., P. Wustenberg. "Therapy of climacteric complaints with Cimicifuga racemosa: a herbal medicine with clinically proven evidence." *Menopause*, 1998; 5:250; Liske, E., *et al*. "Physiological investigation of a unique extract of black cohosh (Cimicifuga racemosa rhizoma): a 6-month clinical study demonstrates no systemic estrogenic effect." *J Women's Health Gend Based Med*, 2002; 11:163'74.

7. Stoll, W. "Phytopharmacon influences atrophic vaginal epithelium: double-blind study-Cimicifuga vs. estrogenic substances." *Therapeutikon*, 1987; 1:23'31; Duker, E., *et al*. "Effects of extracts from Cimicifuga racemosa on gonadotropin release in menopausal women and ovariectomized rats." *Planta Med*, 1991; 57:420'24.

8. Stoltz, H. "An alternative to treat menopausal complaints." *Gynecology*, 1982; 1:14'16; Warnecke, G. "Influencing menopausal symptoms with a phytotherapeutic agent. Successful therapy with Cimicifuga mono-extract." *Med Welt*, 1985; 36:871'74.

9. Stoltz, H. "An alternative to treat menopausal complaints." *Gynecology*, 1982; 1:14'16.

10. Warnecke, G. "Influencing menopausal symptoms with a phytotherapeutic agent. Successful therapy with Cimicifuga mono-extract." *Med Welt*, 1985; 36:871'74.

11. Stoll, W. "Phytopharmacon influences atrophic vaginal epithelium: double-blind study-Cimicifuga vs. estrogenic substances." *Therapeutikon*, 1987; 1:23'31.

12. Duker, E., *et al*. "Effects of extracts from Cimicifuga racemosa on gonadotropin release in menopausal women and ovariectomized rats." *Planta Med*, 1991; 57:420'24.

13. Wuttke, W., D. Seidlova-Wuttke, C. Gorkow. "The Cimicifuga preparation BNO 1055 vs. conjugated estrogens in a double-blind placebo-controlled study: effects on menopause symptoms and bone markers." *Maturitas*, 2003; 44:S67'S77.

14. Nesselhut, T., *et al*. "Studies of the proliferative potency of phytodrugs with estrogen-like effect in breast cancer cells." *Arch Gyneco Obstet*, 1993; 817'18; Hostanska, K., *et al*. "Cimicifuga racemosa extract inhibits proliferation of estrogen receptor-positive and negative human breast carcinoma cell lines by induction of apoptosis." *Breast Cancer Res Treat*, March 2004; 84:151'60.

15. Pockaj, B., *et al*. "Pilot evaluation of black cohosh for the treatment of hot flashes in women." *Cancer Invest*, 2004; 22:515'21.

16. Rebbeck, T. R. "A retrospective case-control study of the use of hormone-related supplements and association with breast cancer." *Int J Cancer*, 2007; 120:1523-28.

17 Osmers, R., *et al*. "Efficacy and Safety of Isopropanolic Black Cohosh Extract for Climacteric Symptoms." *Obstet Gynecol*, 2005; 105:1074'83; Nappi, R., *et al*. "Efficacy of Cimicifuga racemosa on climacteric complaints: a randomized study versus low dose transdermal estradiol." *Gyneological Endocronology*, 2005; 20:30'35.

18 Wuttke, W., C. Gorkow, D. Seildova-Wuttke. "Effects of black cohosh (Cimicifuga racemosa) on bone turnover, vaginal mucosa, and various blood parameters in postmenopausal women: a double-blind, placebo-controlled, and conjugated estrogens-controlled study." *Menopause*, 2006; 13:85'196.

19. Nasr A, Nafeh H. "Influence of black cohosh (Cimicifuga racemosa) use by postmenopausal women on total hepatic perfusion and liver functions." *Fertil Steril* 2009;92:1780-2.

20. Messina, M., S. Barnes. "The roles of soy products in reducing risk of cancer." *J Natl Cancer Inst*, 1991; 83:541'46.

21. Nestel, P.J., *et al*. "Isoflavones from red clover improve systemic arterial compliance but not plasma lipids in menopausal women." *J Clin Endocrinol Metab*, 1999; 84:895-98.

22. Kupfersztain, C., *et al*. "The immediate effect of natural plant extract, Angelica sinensis and Matricaria chamomilla (Climex) for the treatment of hot flushes during menopause. A preliminary report." *Clin Exp Obstet Gyneco*, 2003; 30:203'06.

23. Grube, B., A. Walper, D. Wheately. "St. John's Wort extract: efficacy for menopausal symptoms of psychological origin." *Adv Ther*, 1999; 16:177'86.

24. Zhang, X., *et al*. "Prospective cohort study of soy food consumption and risk of bone fracture among postmenopausal women." *Arch Intern Med*, 2005; 165:1890'95.

25. Albertazzi, P., F. Pansini. "The effect of dietary soy supplementation on hot flashes." *Obstet Gynecol*, 1998;.91:6'11; Han, K.K., *et al*. "Benefits of soy isoflavone therapeutic regimen on menopausal symptoms." *Obstet Gynecol*, 2002; 99:389-94; Faure, E.D., *et al*. "Effects of a standardized soy extract on hot flushes: a multicenter, double-blind, randomized, placebo-controlled study." *Menopause*, 2002; 9:329'34.

MENORRHAGIA (EXCESSIVE BLOOD FLOW)

It is becoming epidemic. With the increase in fibroids, hypothyroidism, ovarian cysts, and endometriosis, many women are suffering from extremely heavy periods that are making their lives increasingly difficult. Others have heavy bleeding with no known cause. Some women suffer from such heavy bleeding that they feel drained and lethargic from the blood loss. The heavy blood loss can lead to anemia. If left untreated, it can lead to general weakening of the body from lack of vitamins and minerals. As many as 60 per cent of all women over thirty-five suffer from heavy periods.

Causes

There are many causes of heavy bleeding: fibroids, cysts, tumours, hormonal imbalances, miscarriage, von Willebrand's disease, polyps, chronic illness, infection, fragile blood vessels, circulatory problems, stress, smoking, toxins, food sensitivities, endometrial hyperplasia, and endometriosis. It can also be caused by deficiencies of iron, calcium, or vitamins A and K. These causes should first be ruled out and addressed if they are found, although many of the suggestions given can still be of aid in the presence of these problems.

Heavy bleeding is often the result of imbalances of various organ systems of the body, especially the thyroid and liver. So supporting and nourishing the thyroid and liver can help return the flow to normal.

Traditional Chinese medicine considers menorrhagia to be related to a spleen deficiency, and /or lack of kidney and liver yin, and/or liver heat.

Diet, herbs, vitamins, and minerals are crucial in correcting these imbalances.

Diet

The key to the diet is shifting your fat intake from animal source to plant source so that you can eliminate the arachidonic acid that leads to the bad prostaglandins that contribute to the problem, and replace it with the essential fatty acids that lead to the good prostaglandins that will help solve the problem.

Eat plenty of deep leafy greens, such as kale, chard, broccoli, collard greens, mustard greens, beet greens, and bok choy. These greens are loaded with iron and vitamin K that will help stop bleeding, and with calcium and other important vitamins and minerals.

Try to eat more seaweed. Seaweed is loaded with many minerals and vitamins that help support bodily functions. It also helps to support the endocrine system, especially, and importantly for menorrhagia, the thyroid glands. Try kelp, nori, dulse, hijiki, and kombu.

Eat whole grains, legumes, seeds, nuts, and high-quality vegetable protein. Try using flaxseed oil and hempseed oil to boost your intake of essential fatty acids. Flaxseed oil can be taken as a supplement, but it is also great in salad dressing or drizzled over steamed vegetables. You can also sprinkle ground flax seeds over your food.

Avoid refined foods, excess salt, aspirin (since it thins the blood and increases bleeding), simple carbohydrates (but not complex carbohydrates), sweets, alcohol, caffeine, and junk food.

HERBAL HELP
Shepherd's Purse
Of all the many herbs that are recommended for menorrhagia, the one that most consistently gets mentioned is shepherd's purse. Shepherd's purse is an astringent herb that helps to dry up excess fluids and is perfect for women who are suffering from heavy bleeding. It is often used every half-hour during an attack or until the bleeding has subsided, but it can also be used from ovulation on to stop heavy bleeding before it starts. Shepherd's purse should be used fresh or as a tincture of the fresh herb.

Nettle
Nettle is another astringent herb that helps to dry up bleeding. This herb is a nutritional powerhouse that is loaded in vitamins and minerals, including the iron, calcium, and vitamins C and K that are so crucial for menorrhagia. For uterine bleeding, including endometriosis, it is often combined in equal parts with agrimony, bayberry, and cinnamon bark. Drink a cupful every hour until the bleeding subsides. Nettle is a great tonic for the female reproductive system that is often used throughout the month.

Yarrow
Yarrow is another astringent herb that is excellent for stopping bleeding. It is frequently used in excessive uterine bleeding or other bleeding from the reproductive tract. Herbalist Rosemary Gladstar recommends that you start taking it preventatively several days before the menstrual cycle begins.

Cinnamon
Cinnamon is also extremely valuable in treating uterine bleeding. Some of Linda's clients have had very good success using cinnamon with other astringent herbs. This great-tasting herb is also valuable for its ability to cover the taste of the other unpleasant-tasting herbs. Cinnamon is a heating herb and should be used with caution by those who have internal heat conditions.

Red Raspberry Leaf
Red raspberry leaf has been used for centuries for all kinds of women's disorders. It is a great tonic for the female reproductive system and is another

astringent herb that is particularly useful for frequent or excessive bleeding.

Other Astringent Herbs

Other good astringent herbs include witch hazel, cransebill, and oakbark. Red root may also be used. Goldenseal may prove useful as well, since it is an astringent that can also clear up an infection, if you have one. Other good herbs for infections, a possible cause of heavy bleeding, include garlic, licorice, wild indigo, and echinacea.

Chastetree Berry

Perhaps the most important women's herb of all, chastetree berry, normalizes hormones by balancing estrogen and progesterone. Balancing the hormones, and thereby normalizing the cycle, can help to reduce bleeding, including bleeding that is caused by fibroids and endometriosis. You can use chastetree berry on a daily basis by itself or with liver herbs and, sometimes, also with licorice (to strengthen the adrenal glands) to rebalance the system. One study found that chastetree berry statistically shortened time of bleeding in women with menorrhagia[1].

Herbs such as squaw vine, mugwort, lady's mantle, and blue cohosh are also useful.

Putting all of this together, a good herbal combination is two parts each of yarrow, shepherd's purse, nettle, and raspberry leaf, and one part cinnamon bark. Use 1 tsp to 1 tbsp per cup of water, decoct hard parts of the plant for forty minutes, then add and infuse soft parts for twenty minutes. Drink every half-hour if bleeding is present. It can also be consumed on a daily basis to strengthen the system. Drink three times a day.

Liver Herbs

Liver herbs help the liver detoxify and eliminate excess harmful estrogen. Eliminating excess estrogen helps to correct the hormonal imbalance that may lead to excess or prolonged bleeding. Some examples of liver herbs include milk thistle, dandelion root, yellow dock, artichoke, and boldo. Liver herbs also help the body eliminate toxins.

Iron

You would expect iron deficiency to be an effect of heavy bleeding, but one of the really strange things about anemia is that it can be a cause of heavy bleeding as well as an effect. So supplementing the diet with iron may be vital. Murray and Pizzorno, N.D.s, cite a study in which 75 per cent of women given iron improved, compared to only 32.5 per cent given a placebo.

There are many forms of iron. The forms that are best absorbed and that do not cause constipation are ferrous succinate and fumerate.

To help absorb the iron, take it with vitamin C-rich foods or vitamin C supplements. In addition to helping you absorb iron, vitamin C seems to help in its own right by mending the capillary fragility that may be involved in heavy bleeding. When women with menorrhagia were given vitamin C with bioflavonoids, 88 per cent of them improved[2]. The bioflavonoids also help mend the capillary fragility as well as correcting prostaglandins. Grape seed extract is a great supplement for getting more flavonoids. The B vitamins are also needed for proper absorption and utilization of iron.

You can also use herbs rich in iron, such as yellow dock, parsley, alfalfa, raspberry, and nettle.

Also try vitamin A, which can help to stop bleeding. When women with heavy bleeding were given vitamin A, 92.5 per cent of them improved significantly[3].

Vitamin E also decreases capillary fragility and corrects prostaglandins.

Getting rid of heavy bleeding can often take time. Don't expect to see immediate results. The body needs time to rebalance itself and regain strength. Expect it to take three to six months for the system to correct itself, or even longer if you have had the menorrhagia for a very long time. Be patient and stick to your program, and, almost always, results will come. In the meantime, the astringent herbs can greatly lessen the symptoms, while you work to correct the underlying problems.

Chapter Endnotes

1. Bleier, W. "Phytotherapy in irregular menstrual cycle or bleeding periods and the gynecological disorders of endocrine origin." *Zentrlbl Gynakol*, 1959; 18:701'09.

2. Cohen, J. D., H. W. Rubin. "Functional menorrhagia: treatment with bioflavonoids and vitamin C." *Curr Ther Res*, 1960; 2:539'42.

3. Lithgow, D. M., W.M. Politzer. "Vitamin A in the treatment of menorrhagia." *S Afr Med J*, 1977; 51:191-93.

OVARIAN CYSTS

It is estimated that one out of every five women will have an ovarian cyst at some point in their lives.

When a follicle fails to rupture or release an egg during the cycle, fills up with fluid and becomes semi-solid, a little sac forms and becomes an ovarian cyst. Ovarian cysts can also form during the formation of the corpus luteum in the hormone cycle. Low adrenal function and under-active thyroid are also thought to be causes.

Early symptoms include excessive menstrual bleeding, painful periods, and pain in the pelvic region. Later, the abdomen may become distended, mirroring the early stages of pregnancy. Some women get no symptoms at all.

Ovarian cysts respond well to natural treatments and can often be completely taken care of without surgery.

Eliminating Cysts Naturally

The natural treatment focuses on detoxifying the liver, balancing hormones, shrinking growths, decreasing inflammation in the pelvis, and promoting lymph drainage. Herbs such as milk thistle, dandelion root, black radish, turmeric, artichoke, burdock, yellow dock, wild yam, Oregon grape root, and nettle cleanse and detoxify, Red root, echinacea, and cleavers are great lymph drainers; Chaparral, shiitake and reishi mushrooms, pau d'arco, and indoles shrink growths.

Diet

As with every condition, diet is crucial. The diet should be rich in foods that prevent estrogen levels from climbing and that are cleansing. Eat lots of whole grains, fruits, vegetables, seeds, raw nuts, and legumes. Eat lots of dark-green leafy vegetables. Avoid dairy, eggs, red meat, sugar, white flour, refined foods, and caffeine. Avoid the bad fats, such as saturated fat and trans-fats; eat good fats, such as essential fatty acids, flaxseed, or hempseed oil. Eat foods high in antioxidants, such as vitamins C, E, and selenium, as they help to detoxify estrogen. Also eat foods such as garlic, onions, and beans that are rich in sulphur-containing amino acids. Avoid storing foods in or eating foods from plastic, as this has been shown to increase estrogen in the body

Detoxifying the Liver

Since cysts are estrogen sensitive, the natural treatment focuses on detoxifying the liver because the liver is the main way that excess estrogen is eliminated from the body. Glutathione is one of the most important things the liver uses to detoxify our bodies. Vitamin C is one very effective way to raise glutathione in the liver. The other is the great liver detoxifying herb, milk thistle. SAMe is an excellent nutrient for helping a sluggish liver. A safe and reliable detoxifier for the body is a combination of the herbs burdock, slippery elm, rhubarb, and sheep sorrel. This formula detoxifies the body and is used for everything from fibroids to cysts to cancer. You can also try taking an old-time liver detoxifier from India: drink 2 to 4 ozs of aloe juice daily with 2 tsps of turmeric powder in it. Detoxifying the liver with lipotropic factors is also a good idea. Try choline and inositol. These nutrients help to detoxify and eliminate waste and fat from the liver.

You can also cleanse the system and eliminate toxins from your body by taking flax-seeds and psyllium.

Balancing Hormones

Chastetree berry is an excellent herb to use to reduce the excess estrogen and rebalance the hormones.

Herbs that contain phytoestrogens or that act as tonics to the reproductive system should also be used. Phytoestrogenic herbs help to balance the hormones by nudging your hormones in the direction your body needs them to go, whether up or down. In the case of ovarian cysts, they help lower estrogen by stealing a receptor site from your body's own estrogen, and binding a weaker estrogen to it. Herbs such as red clover, soy, fennel, licorice, and alfalfa can act as phytoestrogens in your body. Good reproductive tonics include red raspberry leaf, black cohosh, motherwort, lady's mantle, blue vervain, and blue cohosh.

As part of her program, herbalist Rosemary Gladstar recommends using a vaginal bolus that is inserted five nights in a row, then rest for two nights and repeat for several weeks. The bolus is:

1 part yellow dock root powder

1 part chaparral leaf powder

1 part goldenseal powder

3 parts slippery elm powder

1 part witch hazel bark powder

1/2 part black walnut hull powder

1 to 2 drops of essential oil of myrrh and/or tea tree oil

Topical Applications: Working from the Outside

There are also excellent ways to shrink growths topically. Linda has seen pokeroot work wonders for shrinking growths. Apply the tincture to the area and leave it on overnight. Repeat every day until the growth has shrunk. Give yourself a day or two of rest every week if you need to.

You can also try the old-time castor oil pack remedy to help you detoxify. Warm castor oil and place it on the whole lower abdomen. Cover the liver area, too. Then cover with a soft cotton cloth, or use the traditional red flannel, and a hot-water bottle. Keep it on for one hour or more. Do this for five days in a row and rest for two. Repeat for several weeks or months, if needed.

You can also try applying wet clay that has been made into a paste. Use about 1/2 to 1 cup of clay. First, apply a few drops of olive oil to the lower abdomen and then apply the clay. Cover with a piece of gauze. Leave on for one to two hours or overnight, then wash off. Green clay has a strong ability to draw toxins out of the body and will increase blood circulation to the area, helping to reduce stagnation and congestion and break up the cyst.

Acupuncture is also excellent for the same reason. It helps to detoxify the liver, breaks up stagnation and congestion, rebalances the body, and shrinks cysts.

The old hydrotherapy remedy known as the sitz bath is another option you can try. It also helps to remove stagnation and congestion and will help to break up the cyst. You will need two large basins that you can sit in. Fill one with the hottest water you can stand without burning yourself and one with the coldest water you can stand. Start with the hot one. Sit in it for a few minutes and then switch to the cold one and sit in it for a few minutes. Go back and forth four times. Finish with the cold one. Do this for five days in a row, then rest for two and repeat for several weeks, or even months, if needed.

Helpful Supplements: Working from the Inside

Antioxidants, including beta-carotene, selenium, and vitamins E and C, are crucial since they help to get excess estrogen out of the body. A good, quality multivitamin/mineral is important to provide extra nutrients for healing. B vitamins are also important as they help to get rid of cysts.

If under-active thyroid is a factor, try thyroid-supporting nutrients such as L-tyrosine, kelp, and selenium.

If under-active adrenals are a problem, try using adrenal-supporting nutrients such as B vitamins, ginseng, vitamin C, calcium, magnesium, rhodiola, and ashwagandha (see Stress section).

If melatonin is low—another causative factor— try regulating with exercise, exposure to natural sunlight, and regular sleep hours. And try sleep herbs and nutrients such as valerian, 5-HTP, or melatonin.

For pain, try using a mixture of any of the following: turmeric, quercetin, cramp bark, white willow bark, ginger root, California poppy, and acupuncture.

Regular exercise also helps to reduce cysts and stops new ones from forming.

With a little time and effort, most cysts can be eliminated safely and without surgery.

*If a cyst ruptures, medical attention may be needed.

PREMENSTRUAL SYNDROME (PMS)

It is estimated that as many as 40 per cent of all women suffer from PMS. And this statistic is probably low, since many women who suffer from PMS do not seek help. At least, not at the doctor's office. PMS especially strikes women in their thirties and forties, although younger and older women suffer from it as well.

PMS was clinically defined over sixty years ago, but many doctors still do not take it seriously. As a result, doctors often do not give women the help they need for this illness, or they just give them antidepressant or anti-anxiety drugs or hormones, though the side effects of these drugs are far greater than any benefits they may offer.

The Symptoms and Causes of PMS

PMS occurs a few days to a couple of weeks before menstruation, at the time of ovulation. Symptoms of PMS include depression, fatigue, irritability, anxiety, tension, mood swings, altered sex drive, cravings for salt, sugar, and fat, acne, breast pain and tenderness, backache, headaches, bloating, water retention, weight gain, diarrhoea and/or constipation, dizziness, uterine cramping, and abdominal pain.

The main cause of PMS is elevated estrogen and lowered progesterone. Other important causes are hypothyroidism, elevated prolactin levels, elevated levels of the adrenal hormone aldosterone, which leads to water retention, and stress induced elevated levels of cortisol, another adrenal hormone. Failure of the corpus luteum to produce enough progesterone, depression, and nutritional deficiencies can all cause PMS[1].

How Does Too Much Estrogen Lead to the Symptoms of PMS?

To understand how to treat PMS, it is important to know what is happening in the body. The most common cause of PMS is an elevated estrogen-

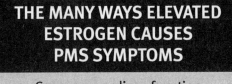

THE MANY WAYS ELEVATED ESTROGEN CAUSES PMS SYMPTOMS

Causes poor liver function
Reduces endorphins
Inhibits serotonin
Reduces the action of B6
Increases aldosterone
Increases prolactin

to-progesterone ratio.

If your liver is not working optimally, it can lead to a build-up of estrogen, since it is not being properly detoxified, causing PMS. Ironically, the build-up in estrogen now causes the liver to function more badly, leading to a further build-up of estrogen. Traditional Chinese medicine also attributes many of the symptoms of PMS to what they call blocked liver *qi* (liver *qi* stagnation), but it can also be caused by liver heat, phlegm fire, liver blood deficiency, liver and kidney *yin* deficiency, and spleen and kidney *yang* deficiency.

One of the ways that the liver detoxifies estrogen is by binding glucuronic acid to the estrogen and escorting it out of the body. But bad intestinal bacteria make an enzyme that breaks the bond between the glucuronic acid and the estrogen, setting the estrogen free to be reabsorbed by the body, leading to an increased amount of estrogen and PMS. Good bacteria help to get rid of those unfriendly bacteria, allowing the liver to detoxify excess estrogen. So if you suffer from PMS, it is a good idea to take probiotics.

Increased estrogen levels also reduce the body's endorphins, which leads to mood problems and an increase in pain. Women who suffer from PMS have low endorphin levels[2]. Stress also lowers endorphins, but exercise elevates them, so exercise regularly.

Increased estrogen also inhibits the body's sero-

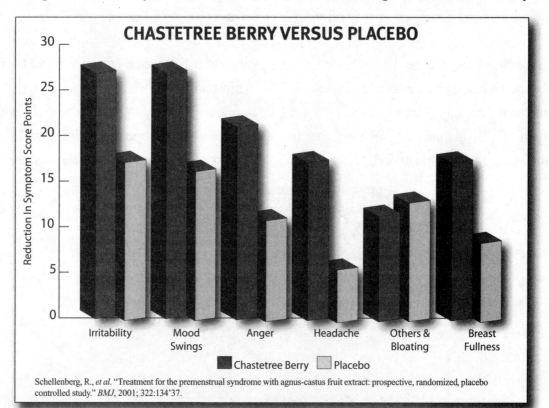

CHASTETREE BERRY VERSUS PLACEBO

Schellenberg, R., *et al.* "Treatment for the premenstrual syndrome with agnus-castus fruit extract: prospective, randomized, placebo controlled study." *BMJ*, 2001; 322:134'37.

onin, the brain's built-in antidepressant, leading to the depression that often accompanies PMS. Women with PMS have lower levels of serotonin, and PMS symptoms are typically more severe in depressed women[3]. As with endorphins, stress also decreases serotonin. To effectively treat PMS, stress must also be addressed, so it is important to support the adrenal glands (see section on Stress).

Increased estrogen also means reduced action of B6. But this vitamin is crucial to proper hormone balance and to the manufacture of serotonin. Taking B6 helps with PMS by reducing estrogen levels and increasing progesterone levels.

Increased estrogen also increases aldosterone levels, which leads to water retention, and in-creased prolactin, which leads to breast pain—two more common symptoms of PMS.

Estrogen levels can also be increased by plastics and chemicals.

Low Thyroid; Hi PMS

It is very important if you suffer from PMS to get your thyroid checked. *The New England Journal of Medicine* published a study that showed that over 94 per cent of women with PMS suffered from low thyroid function, compared to none in the control group. When they were treated for hypothyroidism, all of their PMS symptoms disappeared. As many as 20 per cent of all women suffer from hypothyroidism. Clinically, Linda sees

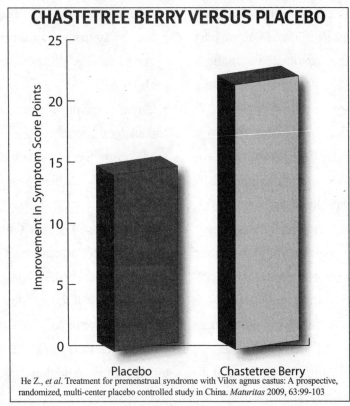

CHASTETREE BERRY VERSUS PLACEBO

He Z., *et al.* Treatment for premenstrual syndrome with Vilox agnus castus: A prospective, randomized, multi-center placebo controlled study in China. *Maturitas* 2009, 63:99-103

this again and again. It is often subclinical hypothyroidism.

Treating PMS

When a woman goes to a doctor and complains of PMS, she is usually given one or more of the following drugs: birth control pill, Prozac or other antidepressant drugs, Valium, a drug used for anxiety and insomnia or Naproxen, an aspirin-like pain killer. Yet these same drugs can actually contribute to PMS. For example, the birth control pill depletes magnesium, folic acid, B6, B1, B2, B3, B12, vitamin C, zinc, and manganese[5]. Levels of any of these same nutrients are already low in women with PMS, compared to healthy women, and they are the same nutrients used to effectively treat PMS. Drugs such as Prozac and Valium have a whole host of side effects associated with them, as does Naproxin.

Treating PMS with Diet

Women with PMS are often consuming the wrong foods. Compared to women without PMS, they eat more refined carbohydrates, sugar, dairy, and salt, and less iron, zinc, and manganese[6]. Christiane Northrup, M.D., reports that women with PMS also consume more animal fat and coffee, chocolate and soft drinks, and less whole grains and vegetables. All of these factors can worsen the symptoms of PMS. Low levels of magnesium and selenium, vitamin C, E and B vitamins are also found in women with PMS.

So what dietary changes can you make to help you avoid PMS? In fact, the same changes everyone who wants to be healthy should make.

- Follow a vegetarian diet, increasing your consumption of fibre from whole grains, fruits vegetables, legumes, seeds, and nuts, while reducing your consumption of saturated fats.
- Add essential fatty acids to your diet: they help to regulate the system. Use flaxseed and hempseed oil.
- Eliminate simple sugars and simple carbohydrates from your diet and avoid food allergies.
- Get all sources of caffeine out of your diet.
- Eliminate excess salt from the diet.
- Stay away from environmental sources of estrogen, such as plastics, pesticides, and other chemicals.
- Buy organic produce and avoid chemical-laden packaged foods.
- Make soy foods and sulphur-rich foods a regular part of your diet.

How Do these Dietary Changes Help?

The reason for a vegetarian diet is simple: it prevents and treats PMS. Vegetarian women eat more fibre and less of the bad fats and, as a result, they suffer less from PMS. Vegetarian women excrete two to three times more estrogen than non-vegetarian women. And they have 50 per cent less free estrogen in their blood.

Studies consistently show that decreasing the amount of saturated fat in the diet seriously reduces estrogen[7].

In addition to saturated fats, it is equally important to avoid trans-fatty acids, hydrogenated and partially hydrogenated fats, like those found in most margarines.

The reason for eliminating sugar is that it raises estrogen levels[8]. It also increases water retention, as does salt. Women who eat a lot of sugar have more frequent PMS symptoms, and one study found a high sugar diet to be the most important factor in the possibility of suffering from PMS[9]. Avoid alcohol for the same reason: it is a simple sugar.

To make the sugar problem even worse, many women crave chocolate prior to their periods, probably because chocolate has magnesium, and women with PMS are often low in magnesium. But chocolate is the most likely food to cause PMS symptoms[9]. Chocolate causes problems because it has sugar and caffeine-two especially bad things for women who suffer from PMS. Even one cup of coffee a day can lead to PMS. Caffeine makes the psychological symptoms of PMS worse and it contributes to breast pain and tenderness.

Why eat soy? Soy contains phtyoestrogens. Phytoestrogens balance estrogen levels. They accomplish this balancing act because they have very weak estrogen activity; they are only 2 per cent as strong as your own estrogen. If the body's estrogen is too low, as in menopause, then phytoestrogens can supply estrogen to receptor sites, increasing estrogen in the body; if estrogen is too high, as it is in PMS, then phytoestrogens steal receptors' sites, preventing your body's own estrogen from binding to them, lowering the body's estrogen.

Avoid chemicals as they can lead to an increase in estrogen-related conditions such as PMS. These chemicals include toxic pesticides that, once ingested, are stored in fat cells in the body and are believed to be one of the leading causes of growing estrogen-related health concerns[10].

Sunlight

It has also been found that women with PMS don't get enough natural sunlight. When these women were treated with two hours of bright light in the mornings, according to Christiane Northrup, M.D., their symptoms were reversed. Try a day lamp; it simulates sunlight without its harmful effects during the winter months to keep brain chemistry more balanced and prevent PMS.

If you still need a little help, there are a number of herbs and nutrients you can try.

Chastetree Berry

Chastetree berry is the most important herb for normalizing the menstrual cycle, and it is simply the best thing out there for PMS.

Two massive studies of over fifteen hundred women, found chastetree berry to partially or totally eliminate PMS symptoms in 90 per cent or more of women[11].

One study set out to determine just how good chastetree berry is by comparing it to vitamin B6, another amazing PMS remedy. In the study, 77.1 per cent of women reported improvements while taking the chastetree berry, compared to 60.6 per cent of the women using B6. Chastetree berry was better over the whole gamut of symptoms, including breast tenderness, edema, tension, headache, constipation, and depression[12].

And now, chastetree berry has been tested in two placebo-controlled studies and has stood up to the standard of modern medical research. In the first one hundred and seventy women with PMS were given chastetree berry extract or a placebo for three menstrual cycles. The chastetree berry group had significantly greater reduction in symptoms, including breast tenderness, bloating, headache, mood swing, and irritability. Fifty-two per cent of the women reduced their symptoms by 50 per cent or more, compared to only 24 per cent of the placebo group[13].

In the second, 202 women took either 40mg of chastetree berry extract or a placebo for three menstural cycles. PMS scores dropped significantly more in the chastetree berry group: 22.82 points versus 15.5 points. Women also self-rated their improvement on the herb as significantly better. There was no statistical difference in the number of adverse effects and none that did occur were serious, proving, once again, that chastetree berry is both safe and effective[14].

Why does chastetree berry work so well? Chastetree berry balances estrogen and progesterone. It balances out PMS by increasing progesterone and decreasing estrogen. It also decreases prolactin and is, therefore, especially useful for prolactin excess.

According to herbalist Michael Tierra, chastetree berry is the single most important herb for balancing mood before and during menstruation. In her clinic, Linda has seen scores of women, whose main PMS symptoms were emotional, use a combination of chastetree berry, liver herbs, vitamins, and minerals to regain their emotional health after three months of following their programs.

Why three months? Chastetree berry contains no hormones and does not do its work in a hurry; it takes time to normalize the cycle. Although chastetree berry may start working in only ten days, it really needs to be used for three months, and preferably longer. Herbalist Christopher Hobbs says that after one year, permanent relief from PMS is actually possible. If the imbalance has existed for a really long time, he says that it may be necessary to take chastetree berry for up to two years to correct the underlying problem. Chastetree berry has been shown in research not only to balance the female hormones, but also to actually cure PMS caused by abnormal levels of estrogen.

And if you have acne problems with your period, this amazing herb has a bonus for you. Linda has seen women who regularly suffered very bad outbreaks prior to their periods have their skin clear up after only three months of using chastetree berry and following a healthy, cleansing diet.

Licorice Root

Traditionally, licorice has been used for thousands of years for PMS. Licorice lowers estrogen levels and raises progesterone levels by preventing an enzyme from breaking down progesterone and by working as a phytoestrogen.

Licorice is extremely helpful for women who suffer from water retention. High levels of the hormone aldosterone cause sodium retention, and, therefore, water retention. Licorice binds to aldosterone receptors and, since its activity is only one-quarter as strong as the body's own aldosterone, it lowers the high levels of aldosterone found in women with PMS.

Licorice can also be used to support weak adrenal glands, as it contains substances that are similar to cortisol. The adrenal glands are in charge of dealing with stress, so licorice is particularly useful for women who suffer from stress-related PMS symptoms.

Black Cohosh

One of the great traditional women's herbs, black cohosh is a nervine with relaxing properties that make it useful for women who suffer from stress induced by PMS.

A standardized extract of black cohosh has shown significant benefits in treating PMS. Black cohosh significantly reduces feelings of depression, anxiety, tension, and mood swings[15].

Donq Quai

If you suffer from cramping along with your PMS, then donq quai is a good herb to try.

Donq quai is usually taken fourteen days after menstruation has begun and is taken until bleeding begins. It is taken throughout the period if pain is present. It should not be used by women who experience heavy bleeding during their periods, although they can usually take it up until the time that their periods begin.

B6

B6 benefits most women with PMS, according to studies. One double-blind study found that 84 per cent of women saw their symptoms decrease when they used B6[16]. And an analysis of the best studies on B6 concluded that the vitamin is more than twice as likely to help with PMS than a placebo[17].

B6 is a diuretic, so it helps with the water retention that so many women with PMS experience.

Another great choice for water retention is dandelion leaf, an amazing diuretic that also provides essential minerals to the body, including the potassium that is lost with most diuretics.

B6 has also been reported to alleviate the nervousness, irritability, depression, bloating, breast tenderness, weight gain, skin, and digestive problems of PMS.

B6 also helps PMS because magnesium helps PMS, and without B6, magnesium cannot get into the cells. Several studies have shown that B6 and magnesium taken together in a multi-vitamin/mineral supplement dramatically reduce PMS symptoms.

Magnesium

And, speaking of magnesium, most women don't eat enough foods rich in magnesium. And a low level of magnesium is a significant cause of PMS. Several studies have shown that red-blood-cell magnesium levels are lower in women with PMS[17]. This is why women often crave magnesium-laden chocolate before their periods.

A deficiency of magnesium may contribute to a lot of the symptoms of PMS, including headaches, fatigue, irritability, heart palpitations, stress, mood swings, nervous sensitivity, and aches and pains. And when women are given magnesium, their PMS symptoms improve. One study showed a reduction in nervousness in 89 per cent of the women, reduction in breast tenderness in 96 per cent, and a reduction in weight gain in 95 per cent[19].

Other studies have shown an extremely significant reduction in mood changes when magnesium is given.

Calcium

It is a myth that dairy is a good choice for calcium for anyone, but especially for women with PMS. Drinking a lot of milk is linked to PMS[18]. But PMS symptoms can improve with calcium supplementation. One study found a 48 per cent reduction in PMS symptoms with calcium supplements[20]. You can also increase calcium beneficially by eating more whole grains, deep green leafy vegetables, seaweed, nuts, seeds and legumes. Calcium doesn't only help you once you have PMS; new research shows that it can also help you not to get it in the first place[21]. Also, women with PMS have reduced bone density and are at a greater risk for osteoporosis, another reason to increase, not only the good sources of calcium, but magnesium and many other vitamins and minerals that healthy bones require as well (see section on Osteoporosis).

Vitamin E

It is a good idea to take vitamin E for PMS. Several studies have shown that vitamin E helps women with PMS[22]. Vitamin E helps reduce breast tenderness, nervous tension, headache, faigue, depression, anxiety, food cravings, weight gain, and insomnia.

Zinc

Women with PMS have lower levels of zinc than healthy women[23]. Low levels of zinc raise prolactin levels, and when levels of prolactin go up, PMS is worse. So women with elevated prolactin levels absolutely must take zinc to treat PMS.

For women who suffer from bad acne during their periods, zinc can be particularly helpful, since it is a crucial nutrient for acne control.

Chromium

Many women suffer from an imbalance of the body's regulation of insulin and cortisol when they have PMS. So it is a good idea to take chromium, which helps to balance blood-sugar levels and correct the problem. Like zinc, chromium is another crucial acne-control nutrient. Other useful aids for regulating insulin include herbs such as devil's club and dandelion root.

Essential Fatty Acids

Ninety per cent of all Americans are essential-fatty-acid deficient.

Women with PMS have deficiencies or abnormalities of essential fatty acids[24]. Gamma-inolenic acid (GLA) is the most common deficiency in women with PMS. To make GLA, the body requires zinc, B6, and magnesium-nu-

trients that women with PMS are already low in.

While not all the research on treating PMS with sources of GLA, such as evening primrose oil (omega-6), has been positive; the research on treating women with PMS with omega-3 essential fatty acids, such as flaxseed oil, has been better. So it is a good idea to supplement the diet of PMS sufferers with flaxseed oil, or with a mixture of omega-3 and 6, rather than just GLA.

5-HTP

In women with PMS, serotonin levels go down in the second half of the menstrual cycle. Serotonin helps you to sleep, prevents migraines and depression, and helps to stabilize both weight and mood-all problems experienced by women with PMS.

One of the best ways to increase serotonin naturally and safely is 5-HTP, and it can be a huge help to women whose PMS symptoms are due to low serotonin levels.

As a bonus, 5-HTP also raises endorphin levels[25]. Low levels of endorphins contribute to the mood problems and pain of PMS. SAMe is another great choice for increasing serotonin levels.

The Psychological Toll of PMS

Women with PMS who suffer from depression can try St. John's wort, which is simply the best antidepressant there is. If you suffer from anxiety from PMS, try kava kava—if you can get it. Kava is the very best treatment for anxiety. If you can't get kava, try passionflower, a herb that performs as well as anti-anxiety drugs, without the side effects. For women who are having difficulty sleeping, try valerian root. This herb will help you fall asleep faster, while encouraging a deep and natural sleep without a morning hangover. It is also great for anxiety. Or try hops, skullcap, lemon balm, oats, linden flower, vervain, or chamomile, all herbs that help to relax the nerves and encourage calmness and sleep. While it won't help you fall asleep, St. John's wort will help you to have a better, deeper sleep.

Liver-Supporting Herbs

Liver herbs are extremely important in treating PMS since they support the liver's jobs of detoxifying the body and breaking estrogen down into a safer form.

Milk thistle, dandelion root, yellow dock, black radish, artichoke, boldo, Oregon grape root, and curcumin are some of the many herbs that help the liver. These herbs detoxify a wide range of substances from the body, including chemicals, excess estrogen, and pesticides. Milk thistle and artichoke even rebuild damaged liver cells.

Herbs to Support Your Adrenals

Use herbs such as suma, rhodiola, eltheuro, and ashwagandha to help support the adrenal glands in order to help deal with the adrenal exhaustion that is involved in women with PMS. Also use vitamin C and a B-complex to support the adrenal glands. Licorice, as we have already seen, is a great PMS and adrenal support herb (not to mention liver herb).

Thyroid Support

Try using sea vegetables, such as kelp, nori, and dulse, and L-tyrosine and selenium, if an underactive thyroid is contributing to your PMS.

Wide Spectrum Multivitamin/Mineral

Women with PMS should take a wide-spectrum multivitamin/mineral. A double-blind study found that women who take a multivitamin feel better during their cycle[26]. A multivitamin can also help to correct underlying nutritional deficiencies.

Acupuncture

Also consider acupuncture. It is a great way of rebalancing the body to help get rid of PMS. One study showed a 78 per cent improvement in PMS sufferers who opted for acupuncture.

Women don't have to live with PMS anymore. PMS can be eliminated using a natural, comprehensive program that accounts for all of the factors involved.

Chapter Endnotes

1. Murray, M. T. *Premenstrual Syndrome*. Rocklin CA: Prima Publishing, 1997.

2. Chuong, C.J., et al. "Periovulatory betaendorphin levels in premenstrual syndrome." *Obstet Gynecol*, 1995; 83:755'60.

3. Barnhart, K. T., *et al.* "A clinician's guide to the premenstrual syndrome." *Med Clin North Am*, 1995; 79:1457'72.

4. Brayshaw, N. D., D.D. Brayshaw. "Thyroid hypofunction in premenstrual syndrome." *N Engl J Med*, 1986; 315:1486'87.

5. Brown, D., *et al. Healthnotes Clinical Essentials*, Vol.1. Portland OR: Healthnotes Inc., 2000; Hudson, T. *Women's Encyclopedia of Natural Medicine*. Los Angeles CA: Keats Publishing, 1999.

6. Abraham, G. E. "Nutritional factors in the etiology of the premenstrual tension syndromes." *J Reprod Med*, 1983; 28:446'64.

7. Longcope, C., *et al.* "The effects of a low fat diet on estrogen metabolism." *J Clin Endocinol Metab*, 1987; 64:1246'50.

8. Yudkin, J., O. Eisa. "Dietary sucrose and oestradiol concentration in young men." *Ann Nutr Metab*, 1988; 32:53'55.

9. Rossignol, A. M., H. Bonnlander. "Prevalence and severity of the premenstrual syndrome. Effects of foods and beverages that are sweet or high in sugar content." *J Reprod Med*, 1991; 36:132'36.

10. Falck, F., *et al.* "Pesticides and polychlorinated biphenyl residues in human breast lipids and their relation to breast cancer." *Archives of Environ Health*, 1992; 47:143'46.

11. Dittmar, F. W., *et al.* "Premenstrual syndrome: Treatment with a phytopharmaceutical." *TW Gynakologie*, 1992; 5:60'68; Loch, E-G., H. Selle, Nitz Bobl. "Treatment of premenstrual syndrome with a phytopharmaceutical formulation containing Vitex agnus castus." *Journal of Women's Health & Gender-Based Medicine*, 2000; 9:315'20.

12. Lauritzen, C., *et al.* "Treatment of premenstrual tension syndrome with Vitex agnus-castus. Controlled, double-blind study versus pyridoxine." *Phytomed*, 1997; 4:183'89.

13. Schellenberg, R., *et al.* "Treatment for the premenstrual syndrome with agnus-castus fruit extract: prospective, randomized, placebo controlled study." *BMJ*, 2001; 322:134'37.

14. He Z., *et al.* Treatment for premenstrual Syndrome with Vilox agnus castus: A prospective, randomized, multi-center placebo controlled study in China. *Maturitas* 2009, 63:99-103

15. Schildge, E. "Essay on the treatment of premenstrual and menopausal mood swings and depressive states." *Rigelh Biol Umsch*, 1964; 19:18'22.

16. Barr, W. "Pyridoxine supplements in the premenstrual syndrome." *Practitioner*, 1984; 228:425'27.

17. Wyatt, K. M., *et al.* "Efficacy of vitamin B-6 in the treatment of premenstrual syndrome: systematic review." *BMJ*, 1999; 318:1375-81.

18. Abraham, G. E. "Nutritional factors in the etiology of the premenstrual tension syndromes." *J Reprod Med*, 1983; 28:446'64; Piesse, J. W. "Nutritional factors in the premenstrual syndrome." *Int Clin Nutr Rev*, 1984; 4:54'81.

19. Abraham, G. E. "Nutritional factors in the etiology of the premenstrual tension syndromes." *J Reprod Med*, 1983; 28:446'64.

20. Thys-Jacobs, *et al.* "Calcium carbonate and the premenstrual syndrome: effects on premenstrual and menstrual symptoms." *Am J Obstet Gynecol*, 1998; 179:444'52.

21. Bertone-Johnson, E. R., *et al.* "Calcium and Vitamin D Intake and Risk of Incident Premenstrual Syndrome." *Arch Intern Med*, 2005; 165:1246'52.

22. London, R. S., *et al.* "The effect of alpha-tocopherol on premenstrual symptomatology: a double-blind study. II: endocrine correlates." *J Am Coll Nutr*, 1984; 3:351'56; London, R.S., *et al.* "The effect of alpha-tocopherol on premenstrual symptomatology: a double-blind study." *J Am Coll Nutr*, 1983; 2:115'22.

23. Chuong, C. J., E. B. Dawson. "Zinc and copper levels in premenstrual syndrome." *Fertility Sterility*, 1994; 62:313'20.

24. Erasmus, U. *Fats That Heal, Fats That Kill*. Burnaby, BC: Alive Books, 1995.

25. Murray, M. T. *5-HTP*. New York, NY: Bantam Books, 1998.

26. Chakmakjian, Z., *et al.* "The effects of a nutritional supplement, Optivate for Women, on premenstrual tension syndrome: effect of symptomatology, using a double-blind crossover design." *J Appl Nutr*, 1985; 37:12.

UTERINE FIBROIDS

Some estimate that as many as 70 per cent to 80 per cent or more of women over thirty-five or forty will get uterine fibroids. Seventy per cent of white women will get them and 80 per cent of black women will.

What is a uterine fibroid? It is a benign tumour that is usually solid and grows in or on the uterus. Some are tiny and cause no symptoms; some grow large or are numerous and can cause a whole host of symptoms such as pain, bleeding between periods, excessive bleeding during periods, and often anemia and fatigue, abdominal bloating, pressure or heaviness, enlarged abdomen, excessive vaginal discharge, irritation to the bladder, increased urination, blockage to the ureter, which results in enlarged kidneys, obstruction to the bowel, back pain, and pain during intercourse. They can even cause miscarriages and prevent pregnancy, cause a premature delivery, or increased blood loss during childbirth if they are very large, but this is rare.

Causes of Fibroids

While no on knows exactly what causes fibroids, they are known to grow in the presence of estrogen. Estrogen treatments, oral contraceptives, and pregnancy stimulate their growth. Menopause, when estrogen naturally drops, can allow them to shrink or even disappear altogether, unless they are malignant. Stress and a poor diet high in animal protein, dairy and fat, and low in fibre, also seem to be factors. Pesticides and heavy metals may be factors. Low thyroid, low progesterone, low physical activity, obesity, blood and *qi* stagnation in the pelvis, high amounts of growth hormone found in the liver, and low melatonin may also be causes. Some think that a fibroid represents an unfulfilled desire or stifled creativity or a need for children.

Treating Fibroids

While conventional medicine treats fibroids with drugs and surgery, it does not change the underlying problem, and fibroids can come back again. And, of course, the drugs are not without their side effects and risks. And the surgery that is performed often removes the uterus, which can cause a whole host of problems, such as bone problems and the prolapsing of organs.

The natural treatment aims to shrink the growths, rebalance the hormones, and cleanse the system, especially the liver and bowels, helping to prevent fibroids from coming back. It usually takes at least three to six full menstrual cycles for growths to begin to shrink or to disappear. Larger ones take longer.

Diet

Eat a diet rich in deep leafy greens, whole grains, fresh fruit and vegetables, and legumes, and low in dairy, eggs, meat, and bad fat. A vegan diet is best. Avoid peanuts. Avoid pesticides, heavy metals and chemicals, chocolate, coffee, and alcohol. Use 2 tsps of turmeric and 2 tbsps of flax seeds daily.

Herbal Help: Detoxification

Herbs that cleanse and detoxify the body, especially the bowels and the liver—which helps to break down and excrete excess estrogen-are used. So are cleansing herbs such as yellow dock root, Oregon grape root, wild yam root, dandelion root, tumeric (which also reduces inflammation), and milk thistle. Rosemary and ginger are also useful as they cleanse the body and increase circulation to the area.

Herbal Help: Shrinking Growth

Growth-shrinking and cleansing herbs such as burdock root, chaparral, and pau d'arco are used. The supplement indole-3-carbinol is effective. You can also consider using the mushrooms, such as shiitake, maitake, and reishi, to shrink growths and support the immune system.

Herbal Help: Balancing Hormones

Herbs that help to balance the hormones, such as chastetree berry and wild ya[...] Chastetree berry favours prog[...] can help to lower estrogen, helping to [...] growths. Women with fibroids may have a progesterone deficiency. In these cases, low doses of progesterone cream may be used as well.

Herbal Help: Toning the Lymphnatic System

Red root, cleavers, and echinacea are good herbs to help move lymph and stagnation, helping to shrink the growths.

Use a combination of herbs from each group—detoxifiers, growth shrinkers, hormone balancers, and lymph toners—for months at a time. For example, use dandelion root, wild yam root, tumeric, chastetree berry, pau d'arco, burdock, red root, and nettle.

More Natural Help

Castor oil packs, green-clay packs, and acupuncture are used very successfully to help remove stagnation and to break up and shrink growths. They are also cleansing and detoxifying to the body and can help to balance hormones. Acupuncture combined with herbs has proven to be very effective. Castor oil packs should be done three or more times per week. Sitz baths are also helpful. Alternate sitting in very hot and very cold water, back and forth, finishing with cold water, three times every day. Sitz baths also break up stagnation and shrink growths.

Herbalist Rosemary Gladstar uses vaginal boluses as part of her program. She uses 1 part each of yellow dock root powder, chaparral leaf powder, goldenseal root powder, witch hazel bark powder, 3 parts of slippery elm powder, 1/2 part black walnut powder, and 1 to 2 drops of essential oil of myrrh or tea tree oil. The bolus is inserted vaginally and used for five nights in a row, rest for two, and repeat for several weeks.

Another helpful herbal formula is 20 per cent each of wild yam root, lady's mantle, chastetree berry, 10 per cent each of calendula, burdock, red root, and cleavers. Use fifty drops of this tincture three times per day[1].

Lack of proper bowel function is another cause of uterine fibroids. Less than two to three bowel movements a day, an imbalance in proper bowel flora, and chemical and toxic overload in the body are all causes. So take probiotics (10 to 20 billion a day). Use extra fibre, such as flax or psyllium, to keep the bowels moving. And, if needed, use herbs such as senna (short-term), buckthorn, cascara sagrada (short term), aloe, or triphala as needed to relieve stubborn constipation. Remember, a castor oil pack is also wonderful for moving the bowels.

Low thyroid and melatonin deficiency can also be causes of fibroids. Determine if these are factors and address them if they are. If your thyroid levels are low, eat more sea vegetables, such as kelp, nori, hijiki, and dulse.

IGF-1, a growth hormone produced by the liver is found in higher amounts in uterine fibroid cells than in healthy uterine tissue and works with estrogen to stimulate fibroid growth. Avoiding sugar, refined carbohydrates, and moving toward a vegan diet can help control IGF-1.

Other factors linked to fibroids include low physical activity, excess weight, blood and energy stagnation in the pelvis, and toxins entering the lymph and blood circulation from an infected root canal. If weight is a factor, address this cause. Exercise forty minutes or more a day to break up stagnation. New research shows just how important exercise can be. Women who do vigorous exercise for at least four hours a week are less likely to develop fibroids, with the most active women being 39 per cent less likely to develop uterine fibroids than the least active women[2].

If your periods are heavy, use iron (see Anemia section) and vitamin C to help prevent anemia. Vitamin C will help with the absorption of iron and it will also help to detoxify the liver, helping to get rid of excess estrogen. Take up to 3 to 10 g a day. You can also use shepherd's purse, yarrow, or nettle to stop heavy bleeding.

Since stress is a causal factor, address adrenal function. Use herbs such as ashwagandha, ginseng and rhodiola, and vitamin C, a B-complex, calcium, and magnesium to correct adrenal problems and stress (see Stress section).

A high-potency multivitamin/mineral is also a good idea to help correct underlying deficiencies.

Nutrients that help to detoxify the liver such as inositol, choline, and L-methionine may also be useful.

Chapter Endnotes

1. Kaur, S. D., M. Danylak-Archanci, C. Dean. *The Complete Natural Medicine Guide to Women's Health.* Toronto, ON: Robert Rose, 2005.

2. Baird, D. D., *et al.* "Association of Physical Activity with Development of Uterine Leiomyoma." *Am J Epidemiol*, 2007; 165:157'63.

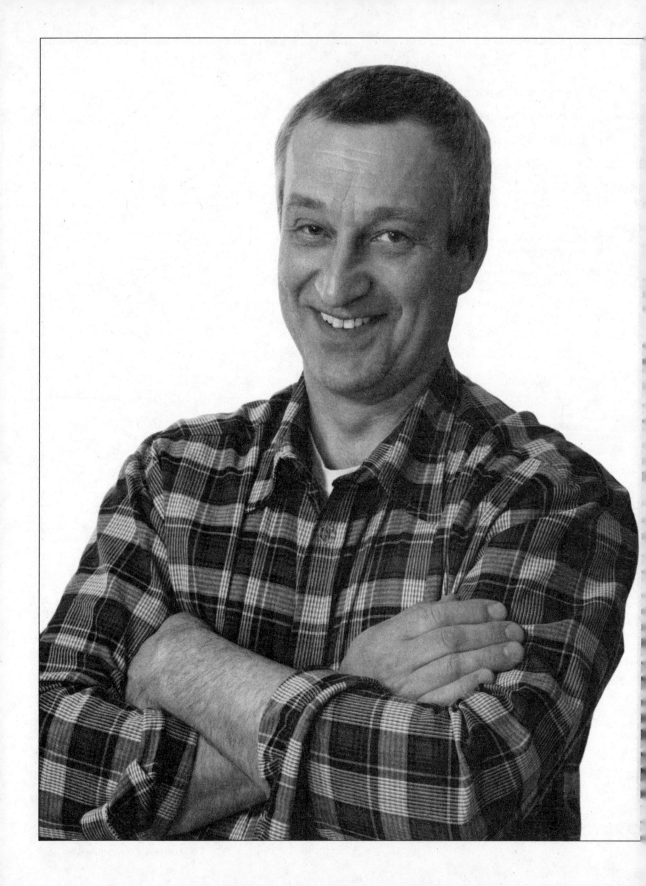

MEN'S HEALTH

Men have had a traditional role to play in our society that has changed drastically over the years, and the traditional health concerns for men have also changed. Men still have to worry about the same health concerns they always did have to worry about, but now there are other growing health concerns, issues that reflect the changes in our rapidly changing lives. Men suffer more from fertility issues and erectile dysfunction than they ever did before. And, although men figure prominently in our society, they have not necessarily had a lot of attention focused on their unique health issues: and certainly not a lot of attention focused in on their health from a natural health perspective. Well, this is what this section of the book is designed to do: give men a section that focuses on their unique health concerns, a section all for them.

And, of course, men still have all the regular health issues that are not unique just to them, but are some of the health concerns that can affect them the most. These health issues that men and women both face, like heart disease, are found in the whole family section of the book.

The male reproductive system is not as complex as the female system, but the problems are no less real. This section of the encyclopedia will look at male infertility, impotence, benign prostatic hyperplasia, prostate cancer and hair loss: very real, growing concerns for men.

BENIGN PROSTATIC HYPERPLASIA

Compared to the female system, the male system seems pretty simple. The prostate gland is one of the few things that can go wrong—but, boy, does it go wrong! Prostate cancer is the number-one cancer among men, and benign prostatic hyperplasia, enlargement of the prostate, affects more than half of all men in their lifetime, and over 90 per cent of men over eighty-five. But there is a lot you can do naturally to change these numbers.

Symptoms And Causes

Benign prostatic hyperplasia (BPH) is the guilty party responsible for those nighttime visits to the washroom, the frequent need to urinate, and the increased urgency but decreased force. It can also lead to urinary tract infections and kidney infection and damage. BPH results from the increased conversion of testosterone into the more powerful dihydrotestosterone (DHT).

Several lifestyle factors can help prevent BPH avoid pesticides, beer, stress, and high cholesterol Though beer is the worst, don't drink too much of any alcohol[1]. Get lots of exercise. Physical activity leads to less BPH, fewer symptoms of BPH and less surgery for BPH. Just walking for two to three hours a week leads to a 25 per cent lower risk of BPH[2].

Saw Palmetto Berry

By far the most important treatment for BPH is the herb saw palmetto berry. Tons of studies show that it is not only more effective than drugs for BPH, but also that it is faster acting and safer. Saw palmetto berry first went head to head with finasteride, a leading BPH drug, in 1996. It worked just as well, while causing fewer side effects, including erectile dysfunction[3]. A year later, the two met again. This time the herb was more effective than the drug, while

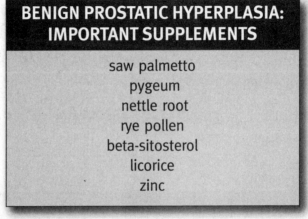

BENIGN PROSTATIC HYPERPLASIA: IMPORTANT SUPPLEMENTS

saw palmetto
pygeum
nettle root
rye pollen
beta-sitosterol
licorice
zinc

still being safer[4]. In 1998, the prestigious *Journal of the American Medical Association* reviewed the research on saw palmetto berry and ruled that it was just as effective as finasteride, while causing an unbelievable 90 per cent fewer adverse side effects[5]!

Since then, the drug world has offered nothing to dethrone saw palmetto berry. The new alpha-blockers have replaced finasteride as the most common BPH drugs, but the story is the same. Saw palmetto is just as effective as Flomax (tamsulosin) and is still safer to use[6].

Two new reviews of studies have found saw palmetto berry to have efficacy similar to drugs, and superior safety[7].

Take 320 mg a day of saw palmetto berry extract standardized for 85 to 95 per cent fatty acids and sterols.

Pygeum

Africa offers the next great herb for BPH. Years of research have shown the bark of the pygeum tree to be safe and effective for mild to moderate BPH[8]. A review of eighteen studies found that pygeum brought about significant improvement in men with BPH. Men on pygeum were twice as likely to have their symptoms improve[9]. Take 100 to 200 mg a day of pygeum extract standardized for 14 per cent triterpenes, including beta-sitosterol, and 0.5 per cent n-docosanol.

Nettle Root

Though it is often the leaf of the nettle plant that is used in natural medicine, it is the root that has shown great promise for BPH. Several studies have shown that it beats a placebo. Nettle root can reduce nighttime visits to the washroom by half[10] and improve urinary frequency and flow in over 90 per cent of men[11].

In the most recent double-blind study, 558 men were given either 120 mg of stinging nettle root extract or a placebo three times a day for six months; 81 per cent of the men improved with the nettle, compared to only 16 per cent with the placebo. Prostate symptoms went down by a significant 40 per cent in the nettle group, while dropping only 9 per cent in the placebo group. The nettle produced an 8-point drop on the symptom scale, compared to only a 1.5-point drop in the placebo group. The nettle root not only improved urinary flow and residual urine significantly better than the placebo, but what's really exciting is that this study showed for the first time that nettle root significantly shrank the enlarged prostate[12].

Take 120 mg of nettle root extract twice a day. Though, as we have seen, the most recent study used 120 mg three times a day.

Saw Palmetto Berry and Nettle: Powerful Combo

Since saw palmetto berry and stinging-nettle root both work so well, researchers have tried combining them and comparing the combination to Flomax. The herbs worked just as well as the drug, while producing fewer side effects[13]. This study is at least the sixth to prove the effectiveness of this combination. Two studies have found it to be safer than, and as effective as, finasteride[14].

Rye Pollen

Another exciting herb to add to the list is the little-discussed rye pollen. Double-blind studies confirm that this herb works[15]. Rye pollen was shown in one study to benefit 85 per cent of men. It improved urgency by 76.9 per cent, nighttime urination by 56.8 per cent, and incomplete emptying by 66.2 per cent[16]. Try taking 63 to 126 mg two to three times a day.

More Help for BPH

Beta-sitosterol has also been shown in double-blind studies to help[17]. Pumpkin seed oil also helps[18], as do essential fatty acids.

Another herb to consider, according to James Duke, Ph.D., is licorice, which possesses compounds that prevent testosterone from converting to DHT. And an exciting preliminary study of aged garlic extract produced a 32 per cent reduction in the size of the prostate, and significantly improved symptoms after one month[19].

The mineral, zinc, also helps prevent the conversion of testosterone to the prostate-dangerous DHT. One small study found that 150 mg of zinc shrank the prostate in 74 per cent of men[20].

Also, if force or retention of urine are particular problems, or even infection, try diuretics. Linda was once treating a man, who came to see her after not improving on a narual health plan, so she added corn silk and bucchu, and he normalized. Traditionally, diuretic herbs are often used.

Lycopenes as a supplement, or from tomato, pink grapefruit, and guava may also prove useful.

Chapter Endnotes

1. Chyou, P. H., *et al.* "A prospective study of alcohol, diet, and other lifestyle factors in relation to obstructive uropathy." *Prostate*, 1993; 22:253'64.

2. Platz, E. A., I. Kawachi, E. B. Rimm, *et al.* "Physical activity and benign prostatic hyperplasia." *Arch Intern Med*, 1998; 158:2349-56.

3. Carraro, J. C., J. P. Raynaud, G. Koch, *et al.* "Comparison of phytotherapy (Permixon®) with finasteride in the treatment of benign prostate hyperplasia: a randomized international study of 1,098 patients." *Prostate*, 1996; 29:231-40.

4. Bach, D., M. Schmitt, L. Ebeling. "Phytopharmaceutical and synthetic agents in the treatment of benign prostatic hyperplasia (BPH)." *Phytomedicine*, 1991; 3:309'13.

5. Wilt, T. J., A. Ishani, G. Stark, *et al.* "Saw palmetto extracts for treatment of benign prostatic hyperplasia. A systematic review." *JAMA*, 1998; 280:1604-09.

6. Debruyne, F., G. Koch, P. Boyle, *et al.* "Comparison of phytotherapeutic agent (Permixon®) with an alpha-blocker (Tamsulosin) in the treatment of benign prostatic hyperplasia: A 1-year randomized international study." *European Urology*, 2002; 41:497'506.

7. Boyle, P., *et.al.* "Updated meta-analysis of clinical trials of Serenoa repens extract in the treatment of symptomatic benign prostatic hyperplasia." *BJU International*, 2004; 93:751; Wilt T, Ishani A, MacDonald R. Serenoa repens for benign prostatic hyperplasia (Review). *Cochrane Database Syst Rev.* 2009; (Issue 1):CD001423. DOI: 10.1002/14651858.CD001423.

8. Duvia, R., G. P. Radice, R. Galdini. "Advances in the phytotherapy of prostatic hypertrophy." Med Praxis, 1983; 4:143'48; Andro, M. C., J.P. Riffaud. "Pygeum africanum extract for the treatment of patients with benign prostatic hyperplasia: a review of 25 years of published experience." *Curr Ther Res*, 1995; 56:796-817.

9. Ishani, A., *et al.* "Pygeum africanum for the treatment of patients with benign prostatic hyperplasia: A systematic review and quantitative meta-analysis." *Am J Med*, 2000; 109:654'64.

10. Stahl, H.P. "The treatment of prostatic nycturia with standardized extract of Radix Urticae (ERU)." *Allg Med*, 1984;.60:128'32.

11. Friesen, A. "Statistische analyse einer multizenter-langzeitstudie mit ERU." Cited in Mills, S., K. Bone. *Principles and Practice of Phytotherapy.* Toronto: Churchill Livingstone, 2000, pp. 494; Koch, E., A. Biber. "Pharmacological effects of sabal and urtica extracts as a basis for a rational medication of benign prostatic hyperplasia." *Urologue*, 1994; 334:90'95.

12. Safarineiead, M. R. "Urtica dioica for treatment of benign prostatic hyperplasia: a prospective, randomized, double-blind, placebo-controlled, crossover study." *J Herb Pharmacother*, 2005; 5:1'11.

13. Englemann, U., *et al.* "Efficacy and safety of a combination of sabal and urtica extract in lower urinary tract symptoms." *Arzneim Forsch/Drug Res*, 2006; 56:222'29.

14. Sökeland, J., J. Albrecht. "A combination of Sabal and Urtica extracts vs. Finasteride in BPH (Stage I and II acc. to Alken): a comparison of therapeutic efficacy in a one-year double-blind study." *Urologe*, 1997; 36;327'33; Sökeland, J. "Combined sabal and urtica extract compared with finasteride in men with benign prostatic hyperplasia: analysis of prostate volume and therapeutic outcome." *Br J Urol*, 2000; 86:439-42.

15. Buck, A. C., R. Cox, R.W. Rees, *et al.* "Treatment of outflow tract obstruction due to benign prostatic hyperplasia with the pollen extract, cernilton. A double-blind, placebo-controlled study." *Br J Urol*, 1990; 66:398-404; Becker, H., L. Ebeling. "Conservative therapy of benign prostatic hyperplasia (BPH) with Cernilton." *Urologe (B)*, 1988; 28:301-06.

16. Yasumoto, R., *et al.* "Clinical evaluation of long-term treatment using Cerniltin pollen extract in patients with benign prostatic hyperplasia." *Clinical Therapeutics*, 1995; 17:82'86.

17. Berges, R. R., J. Windeler, H. J. Trampisch, *et al.* "Randomized, placebo-controlled, double-blind clinical trial of beta-sitosterol in patients with benign prostatic hyperplasia." *Lancet*, 1995; 345:1529-32; Klippel, K.F., D.M. Hiltl, B. Schipp. "A multicentric, placebo-controlled, double-blind clinical trial of ß-sitosterol (phytosterol) for the treatment of benign prostatic hyperplasia." *Br J Urol*, 1997; 80:427-32.

18. Schiebel-Schlosser, G., M. Friederich. "Phytotherapy pf BPH with pumpkin seeds-a multicenter clinical trial." *Zeits Phytother*, 1998; 19:71-76; Friederich, M., C. Theurer, G. Schiebel-Schlosser. "Prosta Fink Forte capsules in the treatment of benign prostatic hyperplasia. Multicentric surveillance study in 2245 patients." *Forsch Komplementarmed Klass Naturheilkd*, 2000; 7:200-04.

19. Durak, I., E. Yilmaz, E. Devrim, *et al.* "Consumption of aqueous garlic extract leads to significant improvement in patients with benign prostatic hyperplasia and prostate cancer." *Nutr Res*, 2003; 23:199'204.

20. Bush, I. M., E. Berman, S. Nourkayhan, *et al.* "Zinc and the prostate." *Presented at the annual meeting of the American Medical Association Chicago*, 1974.

HAIR LOSS

Between the ages of fifteen and thirty, hair grows about half an inch each month. Many of us, though, are less interested in how fast hair grows than we are in how fast it is falling out. Most men have lost some hair by thirty-five, and 80 per cent of North American men are affected by hair loss.

Male-pattern baldness is a normal part of aging. Though it is less common or obvious, women are affected, too.

Historically, many exciting remedies have been tried. The ancient Egyptians, placed chopped romaine lettuce on their scalps. Not to be outdone, Hippocrates applied pigeon dung to his! You may prefer the following suggestions.

There can be many causes of hair loss. It is well known that chemotherapy drugs cause hair loss, but less well known that tons of other drugs can, too. Nonsteroidal anti-inflammatory drugs such as aspirin, antibiotics, blood thinners, antidepressants, heart, cholesterol, ulcer, and arthritis drugs can all cause hair loss.

Many nutrients are needed for full, healthy hair. Deficiency in several different nutrients could cause hair loss. The most important ones seem to be zinc, vitamin A, iron and essential fatty acids like those found in flaxseed oil. Other important nutrients include the full complex of B vitamins, and especially biotin, PABA, and folic acid, as well as silica, iodine, selenium, copper, and calcium. Foods rich in sulphur, such as Brussels sprouts, cabbage, beans, and garlic, can also help.

Since free radicals also contribute to baldness[1], Michael Murray, N.D., also recommends supplementing 1,000 to 1,500 mg of vitamin C and 400 IU of vitamin E every day.

A very powerful group of flavonoids known as proanthocyanidins has been shown to stimulate hair growth in people with male-pattern baldness[2]. Proanthocyanidins are found in many herbal supplements, including grape seed extract and pycnogenol.

Strangely, gluten intolerance can cause hair loss even in the absence of any obvious signs of celiac disease[3]. Another important cause of hair loss that needs to be treated if present is hypothyroidism. Stress can also be a factor.

One common cause of the normal hair loss that comes with aging is the conversion of testosterone into dihydrotestosterone (DHT), the same problematic conversion that is behind enlarged prostate. It is, however, a very common cause of female hair loss, too. Here, as for prostate problems, the most promising solution is saw palmetto berry. One study found a combination of saw palmetto and beta-sitosterol to be effective[4].

Dong quai has been shown to slow down male-pattern baldness, according to herbalist Terry Willard.

A good herb for keeping and returning both your hair and its colour is fo ti, also known as ho shou wu.

Applying extracts of rosemary, sage, chamomile, ginkgo, and hydrolized wheat protein can thicken and strengthen hair and revitalize the scalp. Rosemary, sage, and nettle tea can be taken internally. These herbs improve circulation to the scalp and improve hair growth. The essential oils of lavender, rosemary, thyme, sage, and cedar wood also help healthy hair by stimulating the scalp. An essential-oil combination of thyme, rosemary, lavender, and cedar wood in a carrier of jojoba and grape seed oil, applied topically, has been shown to stimulate hair growth in people suffering hair loss[5].

Finally, Japanese research has suggested that an important cause of balding is the large consumption of saturated animal fat so common in our culture[6]. The link may be the testosterone-increasing effect of saturated fat. Paul Pitchford, author of *Healing with Whole Foods*, also says that a high-fat, high-protein diet is a cause of hair loss, and he attributes this to the damaging effect this diet has on the kidneys and the role of the kidneys in influencing hair, according to traditional Chinese medicine.

Acupuncture also has a technique to offer, called tapping, in which the head is lightly tapped with a seven-star needle to increase circulation to the area.

Chapter Endnotes

1. Giralt M, *et al*. "Glutathione, glutathione S-transferase and reactive oxygen species of human scalp sebaceous glands in male pattern baldness." *J Invest Dermatol* 1996;107:154-8.

2. Takahashi, T., A. Kamimura, Y. Yokoo, *et al*. "The first clinical trial of topical application of procyanidin B-2 to investigate its potential as a hair-growing agent." *Phytother Res*, 2001; 15:331'36.

3. Corazza, G.R., *et al*. "Celiac disease and alopecia areata: Report of a new association." *Gastroenterology*, 1995; 109:1333'37.

4. Prager, N., *et al*. "A Randomized, Double-Blind, Placebo-Controlled Trial to Determine the Effectiveness of Botanically Derived Inhibitors of 5-'-Reductase in the Treatment of Androgenetic Alopecia." *The Journal of Alternative and Complementary Medicine*, 2002; 8:143-52.

5. Hay, J. C., M. Jamieson, A. D. Ormerod. 'Randomized trial of aromatherapy: successful treatment for alopecia areata.' *Archives of Dermatology*,1998; 134:1349'52.

6 Janowiak J. J., H. A., Carson "Practitioner's Guide to Hair Loss: Part 2—Diet, Supplements, Vitamins, Minerals, Aromatherapy, and Psychosocial Aspects." *Altern Comp Ther* 2004; 10:200-5.

MALE IMPOTENCE
(ERECTILE DYSFUNCTION)

It is estimated that ten to twenty million men suffer from erectile dysfunction. And, although 25 per cent of men over the age of fifty are affected, it is not aging that directly causes this problem. Men are capable of retaining their sexual virility well into their eighties. The causes of male impotence are many: depression, stress, anxiety, fatigue, diabetes, hypothyroidism, prostate disorders, low testosterone, or high estrogen can all be causes of impotence.

Cigarettes and Alcohol: Maybe this Will Make You Quit

Other causes include cigarette smoke and alcohol. Smoking just two cigarettes a day has been shown to inhibit erections produced by administration of a drug that dilates arteries and causes blood to flow to the penis[1]. Another study found that men who smoked a pack of cigarettes a day for five years were 15 per cent more likely to suffer clogging of the arteries supplying the penis, leading to erectile dysfunction. Alcohol, too, can cause erectile dysfunction since it can cause shrinking of the testes and decreased testosterone production. Another factor that can be responsible for causing erectile dysfunction is prescription drugs: the most common drugs that cause this problem are blood pressure lowering drugs.

Atherosclerosis: More than Just Heart Attacks and Strokes

One of the major causes of erectile dysfunction in men is hardening of the artery walls that lead to the penis, the same atherosclerosis that can cause a block in the blood flowing to the heart, causing a heart attack, and a block to the brain, causing a stroke. And like heart attacks and strokes, erectile dysfunction is on the rise in men. But although atherosclerosis is the cause of erectile dysfunction in 50 per cent of the men who suffer from it, it is not the only cause of erectile dysfunction.

As Dr. Dean Ornish has shown, lifestyle changes alone can help to reverse atherosclerosis. In Ornish's study, people were placed on a vegetarian diet, used stress-reduction methods, and exercised. At the end of one year, there was significant reduction in atherosclerosis. Interestingly, the control group who followed the American Heart Association diet and regular medical care got worse.

The Natural Approach

Drugs such as Viagra tend to give instant results. So why use the herbal approach? It's simple: The herbal approach goes deeper, helping to correct the underlying problem by improving the glandular system, the blood supply to erectile tissue, and by enhancing nerve signals.

All nutrients are needed to provide the overall energy and stamina required for sexual desire and performance. Some particularly helpful supplements for erectile dysfunction include antioxidants and inositol hexaniacinate. Antioxidants protect against atherosclerosis and, according to Michael Murray, N.D., inositol hexaniacinate not only reduces bad cholesterol but also increases the blood flow to the penis, aiding in cases of erectile dysfunction. The B-complex family of vitamins is especially important for energy, to help fight stress, and to calm the nervous system. Vitamin E is crucial to reproductive health and zinc is vital to prostate health.

Three of the best herbs for treating erectile dysfunction are ginkgo biloba, muira puama and ginseng.

Ginkgo biloba

Ginkgo biloba is known for its ability to increase circulation to the extremities, including the penis. For those who are suffering from erectile dysfunction caused by decreased blood flow, ginkgo biloba can be of aid. One study found that 50 per cent of men who had not responded to conventional drug therapy regained potency after six months of ginkgo biloba[2]. A second study has also proven ginkgo's effectiveness[3]. Research shows that ginkgo can resolve the difficulty by improving blood flow to the penis. It is recommended to take 120 to 240 mg of standardized ginkgo. Results usually take at least twelve weeks. But that is not all ginkgo can do. It can also help people on antidepressant drugs who suffer from loss of sexual desire or response, a common side effect of these drugs. In one study, 84 per cent of men and women using ginkgo resolved the sexual dysfunction they were experiencing because of antidepressant drugs[4].

Muira Puama

A herb from Brazil that can be very helpful for treating erectile dysfunction is muira puama. Herbalist Michael Tierra mentions the root of this herb for impotency. Muira puama seems to be able to help with both the physical and psychological problems associated with impotency. A study done by Dr. Jacques Waynberg of the Institute of Sexology in Paris found that of 262 men suffering from erectile dysfunction or from lack of sexual desire, 62 per cent of those with loss of desire were helped by muira puama, and 51 per cent of those with erectile dysfunction were benefitted by this herb[5]. Muira puama works because it is a nerve stimulant and aphrodisiac. Many traditional herbalists combine muira puama with other herbs, such as ho shou wu, ginseng, damiana, astragalus, spirulina, saw palmetto, and raspberry, that increase energy, glandular function, and sexual function.

Ginseng

Asian ginseng can also help erectile dysfunction. Ginseng was traditionally used as a treatment for impotence, but for a long time modern science was skeptical of this use. Not any more. In 1995, 1,800 mg of Korean red ginseng was discovered to significantly improve erectile dysfunction compared to both a placebo and a drug[6]. A year later, when thirty-five elderly men with erectile dysfunction were given either Korean red ginseng or a placebo, the herb once again defeated the placebo; ginseng helped a full 67 per cent of the men, while only 28 per cent of the placebo group improved[7]. In the most recent study, forty-five men with erectile dysfunction were given either 900 mg of powdered Korean red ginseng or a placebo three times a day for eight weeks. Sixty per cent of the men on the ginseng had improved erections. Erection scores increased by 42 per cent in the ginseng group, compared to only 16 per cent in the placebo group. Sexual function in the ginseng group improved by 36 per cent versus 10.4 per cent in the placebo group. Ginseng also improved their desire[8].

Another useful herb for male sexual vitality is eleuthero (formerly Siberian ginseng). According to *The Encyclopedia of Natural Healing*, eleuthero is helpful for aiding in cases of underdeveloped sex glands, impotence, and frigidity.

One placeobo-controlled study found that pycnogenol helps[9].

Other helpful herbs for increasing male sexual function are astragalus, damiana, sarsaparilla, saw palmetto, and yohimbe.

Chapter Endnotes

1. Morley, J. E. "Management of impotence." *Postgrad Med*, 1993; 93:65'72.

2. Sikora, R., *et al.* "Ginkgo biloba extract in the therapy of erectile dysfunction." *J Urol*, 1989; 141:188A.

3. Sohn, M., R. Sikora. "Ginkgo biloba extract in the therapy of erectile dysfunction." *J Sec Educ Ther*, 1991; 17:53-61.

4. Cohen, A. J., Bartlik, B. "Ginkgo biloba for antidepressant-induced sexual dysfunction." *J Sed Marital Ther*, 1998; 24:139'43.

5. Waynberg, J. "Contributions to the clinical validation of the traditional use of *Ptychopetalum guyanna*." Presented at the First International Congress on Ethnopharmacology, Strasbourg, France, June 5'9, 1990.

6. Choi, H. K., D. H. Seong, K. H. Rha. "Clinical efficacy of Korean red ginseng for erectile dysfunction " *Int J Impot Res*, 1995; 7:181'86.

7. *Korean J Ginseng Sci*, 1996.

8. Hong, B., *et al.* "A double-blind crossover study evaluating the efficacy of Korean red ginseng in patients with erectile dysfunction: A preliminary report." *The Journal of Urology*, 2002; 168:2070'73.

9. Durackova, Z., et al. "Lipid metabolism and erectile function improvement by Pycnogenol®, extract from the bark of Pinus pinaster in patients suffering from erectile dysfunction-a pilot study." Nutr Res, 2003; 23:1189-98.

MALE INFERTILITY

Not only are problems with erectile dysfunction occurring, but also problems with infertility. It is estimated that 15 to 20 per cent of all couples are having difficulty conceiving a child, and about 40 per cent of these cases of infertility are caused by problems in the male, and another 20 per cent are caused by problems in both the male and female. Six per cent of men between the ages of fifteen and fifty are infertile. Sperm count and sperm quality are plummeting; sperm counts are only 40 per cent of what they were in 1940[1].

Causes

The causes of this decreased sperm count are many. Obesity, hot tubs, saunas, excessively vigorous exercise, and tight-fitting clothes all cause the scrotum to be kept too warm, preventing sperm production. Infections can be a cause, as can candida, glandular diseases, heavy metals, and poor diets, too high in saturated fat and too low in fibre that increase the estrogen in the body. Chemicals found in pesticides and other materials and industrial chemicals have been found to mimic estrogen and to cause decreased sperm counts, infertility, undescended testes, and other developmental disorders of the male sexual system. Following a gluten-free diet has also enabled some men to produce viable sperm when they previously could not.

Other causes of male infertility include smoking, alcohol, caffeine, recreational and pharmaceutical drugs, stress, and not getting enough exercise.

Treating Infertility Naturally

Two of the most important supplements for treating male infertility are vitamin C and zinc.

Vitamin C

Vitamin C prevents sperm from clumping or sticking together (agglutination), improving the chances of fertilization. Sperm is also extremely sensitive to free-radical damage. Since vitamin C is an antioxidant, it is useful in preventing free-radical damage. In one study, when healthy men dropped their dietary vitamin C from 250 mg a day to 5 mg a day, there was a 91 per cent increase in the number of sperm with damaged DNA[2]. In another study, infertile men were given 1,000 mg of vitamin C, and after only one week their sperm counts went up by 140 per cent. After three weeks, their sperm count was still going up. Prior to the study, many of the men had agglutinated sperm (25 per cent of their sperm was agglutinated, enough to cause infertility), but after three weeks, only 11 per cent of their sperm was agglutinated. After sixty days, all of the men had conceived children with their wives; none of the men in the placebo group had[3].

Zinc

Zinc is among the most important factors in preventing infertility. Zinc helps in testosterone production, sperm formation, and motility[4]. In a study of thirty-seven men who had been infertile for at least five years, those who had low testosterone levels experienced a significant increase in both testosterone levels and sperm count when given 60 mg of zinc for forty-five to fifty days[5].

Selenium and Vitamin E

Supplementing with selenium can also be of aid, since deficiencies have been linked to reduced sperm counts and to sterility in both sexes. Selenium can increase sperm motility[6]. Vitamin E can also be of importance, since it is needed to balance hormone production. Vitamin E has been known as the sex vitamin or the antisterility vitamin. Vitamin E is called tocopherol: *Tokos* is Greek for childbirth or offspring, and *phero* means to bear. Vitamin A and the B-complex vitamins are also important in reproductive gland function.

Amino Acids

The amino acid L-arginine can also be of aid, since it improves both sperm count and motility[7]. It also improves sexual desire and ejaculation. Since sperm takes about three months to form, it will take at least this amount of time before results from nutritional supplements are achieved.

Another amino acid, L-carnitine, is also very important since it provides energy for the production and motility of sperm cells. Carnitine increases both sperm count[8] and motility[9].

Herbal Help

Herbally, ginseng has been shown to produce a rise in sperm count, motility, and testosterone, suggesting a role in infertility in addition to its role in impotence[10]. Ashwagandha root, a herb long used in India as an aphrodisiac, has also now been shown to improve sperm count, motility and testosterone[11].

Dietary Help

Helpful foods for treating the male sexual system include nuts and seeds, since they are high in zinc, essential fatty acids (essential for normal glandular functioning and activity in the reproductive system), fibre, and other nutrients. If estrogen is high or testosterone is low, soy foods can be of help since they are rich in phytoestrogens, which can lower estrogen when it is too high, and in phytosterols, which are similar to testosterone, and may be used by the body to produce hormones. For those who do not have candida, yeast is also a good food to use.

Acupuncture can also be of aid for both erectile dysfunction and lack of desire and infertility.

Chapter Endnotes

1. Carleson, E., *et al.* "Evidence for decreasing quality of semen during past 50 years." *Br Med J*, 1992; 305:609'13; Carlsen, E., *et al.* "Decline in semen quality from 1930 to 1991." *Ugeskr Laeger*, 1993; 155:2530'35.

2. Fraga, C., *et al.* "Ascorbic acid protects against endogenous oxidative DNA damage in human sperm." *Proc Natl Acad Sci*, 1991; 88:11003'06.

3. Dawson, E., *et al.* "Effect of ascorbic acid on male fertility." *Ann NY Acad Sci*, 1987; 498:312'23.

4. Prassad, A. S. "Zinc in growth and development and spectrum of human zinc deficiency." *J Am Coll Nutr*, 1988; 7:377'84.

5. Netter, A., *et al.* "Effect of zinc administration on plasma testosterone, dihydrotestosterone and sperm count." *Arch Androl*, 1982; 7:69'73.

6. Scott, R., *et al.* "The effect of oral selenium supplementation on human sperm motility." *Br J Urol*, 1998; 82:76-80.

7. Schacter, A., J. A. Goldman, Z. Zukerman. "Treatment of oligospermia with the amino acid arginine." *J Urol*, 1973; 110:311'13.

8. Costa, M., *et al.* "L-carnitine in idiopathic asthenozoospermia: a multicenter study." *Andologia*, 1994; 26:155'59; Vitali, G., R. Parente, C. Melotti. "Carnitine supplementation in human idiopathic asthenospermia: clinical results." *Drugs Exptl Clin* Res, 1995; 21:157'59.

9. Campaniello, E., *et al.* "Carnitine administration in asthenospermia." *IV International Congress of Andrology, Firenze*, May 14'18; Costa, M., *et al.* "L-carnitine in idiopathic asthenozoospermia: a multicenter study." *Andologia*, 1994; 26:155'59.

10. Salvati, G., *et al.* "Effects of Panax ginseng C.A. Meyer saponins on male fertility." *Panminerva Med*, 1996; 38:249-54.

11. Ahmad MK, *et al.* "*Withania somnifera* improves semen quality by regulating reproductive hormone levels and oxidative stress in seminal plasma of infertile males." *Fertil Steril*. Jun 5, 2009. [Epub ahead of print].

PROSTATE CANCER

Prostate cancer is the number-one cancer among men. The words "prostate" and "cancer" go together so often, that it is often the only way we think about the prostate gland. But it doesn't have to be that way.

The Importance of Diet: Overall Diet

As always, start with diet. The greatest risk factor of all for prostate cancer is a diet high in animal fat. Fat not only increases your chances of getting prostate cancer, a huge Harvard study of 48,000 men found that those who ate the most animal fat also have a greater risk of developing a more advanced form of prostate cancer[1]. And now Canadian researchers, in the very first study to look at nutrition and the progression of prostate cancer in men who already have it, have found that the men who eat the most saturated fat have more than triple the risk of dying of prostate cancer than men who eat the least[2]. Commenting on the study, Steve Austin, N.D., said that it is hard to imagine why anyone with prostate cancer would eat any red meat, dairy fat, egg yolks, or poultry.

Watching another kind of fat is crucial, too—yours! As your weight goes up, so does your risk of prostate cancer[3].

Recently, studies have shifted the focus away from what diets are risky for prostate cancer to a focus on what diets are good for preventing and fighting prostate cancer. The first compared men with early prostate cancer who made no lifestyle changes to men who switched to a vegan diet (no animal products) with lots of fruit, vegetables, legumes, whole grains, and little sugar and fat. They also had one serving of tofu and one soy protein drink each day and took 400 IU of vitamin E, 200 mcg of selenium, and 2g of vitamin C. In addition, they walked half an hour six days a week and did yoga and other relaxation techniques one hour each day. The healthy-lifestyle group dropped their PSA levels (a marker for prostate cancer) by 4 per cent, while PSA levels continued to climb another 6 per cent in the other group[4].

A second study looked simply at diet. Ten men with recurrent prostate cancer increased the amount of whole grains, fruits, vegetables, and legumes that they ate, while decreasing the amount of meat, dairy, and refined carbohydrates. At the end of the six-month study, PSA levels were rising significantly more slowly. Nine of the ten men had their PSA levels rising more slowly, and four of them actually had dropped their PSA levels to below where they were at the beginning of the study. Compared to the beginning of the study, PSA levels overall now doubled nearly ten times more slowly[5].

Special Foods: Garlic

There are also certain foods that are especially good at preventing prostate cancer. Recent research reveals that men who eat more foods in the garlic family—especially garlic and scallions—reduce their risk of developing prostate cancer by almost 50 per cent[6]. That's huge! That garlic is good for prostate cancer is not entirely surprising. In a 1997 interview for *Better Nutrition*, John Pinto, Ph.D., of Memorial Sloan-Kettering, told Linda that he has found that derivatives of garlic extract decrease the rate of proliferation of prostate cancer cells grown in culture.

Eat lots of soy, too. In countries where men eat a lot of soy, fewer men die of prostate cancer[7]. Interestingly, in Japan, where soy consumption is high, mortality from prostate cancer is the lowest in the world, even though Japanese men develop prostate cancer just as often as everyone else—they just don't die of it because the cancer grows so much slower.

Soy

Genistein, an isoflavone found in soy, seems to get much of the credit for soy's effect on prostate cancer. Genistein has been shown to inhibit the growth of prostate cancer cells in laboratories[8]. When men with prostate cancer were given either whole wheat bread or bread with 50 g of soy grits in it (containing 117 mg of soy isoflavones), the group who ate the soy bread had a significant drop in their PSA levels, compared to the regular bread group, suggesting that it shrank the tumour[9].

You can drink your soy, too. Preliminary research shows that men who drink soy milk more than once a day have a significantly lower risk of prostate cancer[10].

Tomatoes and Lycopene

The other spectacular anti-prostate cancer food is tomato. Tomatoes are loaded with lycopene, the most powerful carotene against human cancer cells[11]. Men who have the most lycopene in their diet are at lower risk of getting prostate cancer[12]. And men who eat more than ten servings a week of tomato-based foods decrease their risk of prostate cancer by a full 35 per cent, compared to men who eat less than one and a half servings[13]. Tomato juice, however, does not seem to offer the same benefits, perhaps due to the high salt content.

In a really exciting lycopene study, men with prostate cancer were given either 30 mg of lycopene or nothing for three weeks leading up to their prostatectomies. The lycopene group had smaller tumours and less spread of the cancer beyond the prostate (73 per cent confined versus only 18 per cent). The lycopene group also had lower PSA levels[14]. This is the second study to find that lycopene prevents the spread of prostate cancer while lowering PSA levels[15].

PSA levels also fell by 20 per cent in a group of men who ate 200 g of tomato sauce, containing 30 mg of lycopene, each day for three weeks. They also had less DNA damage in their prostate glands than those who did not eat the tomato sauce[16].

Though tomato is the main source of lycopene in our diet, lycopene is also found in watermelon, guava, papaya, apricot, and pink grapefruit.

Cruciferous Vegetables

Also, try eating a lot of cruciferous vegetables, such as broccoli, cauliflower, and cabbage, because preliminary research is pointing to them as yet another anti-prostate cancer food. If you eat three or more servings of cruciferous vegetables a week, your risk of prostate cancer is 41 per cent lower than if you eat less than one[17].

Herbal Help for Prostate Cancer

There are a number of less-discussed herbs and nutrients that are showing promise for prostate cancer. Since the isoflavones in soy are generating so much excitement, researchers decided to look at red clover, another source of isoflavones. They gave either 160 mg of isoflavones from red clover or nothing to a small group of men with prostate cancer. Apoptosis was significantly higher in the isoflavone group[18]. Apoptosis is a way in which the body kills cancer cells without harming the non-cancerous cells around them, unlike chemotherapy.

Another promising herb is maitake mushroom. Test-tube studies show that a component of the mushroom known as D-fraction causes almost complete cell death against aggressive prostate cancer cells[19]. Combining the D-fraction with vitamin C made it work even better. Like the isoflavones, maitake kills cancer cells without damaging the non-cancerous ones. Does it work in people as well as in laboratories? One study found that the clinical status of men with prostate cancer improved significantly with maitake D-fraction.

Another new treatment is curcumin. When prostate cancer becomes independent of hormones, it is very difficult to treat. But curcumin, a component of the herb turmeric, has now been shown to be a powerful inducer of apoptosis in both androgen-dependent and independent prostate cancer cells, making it an exciting candidate for preventing and treating advanced prostate cancer[20].

Milk thistle, the excellent liver herb, may also help the prostate. A component of milk thistle called silibinin, has been shown to be a strong fighter of prostate cancer cells in test tubes. And when prostate cancer cells were treated with either a chemotherapy drug, silibinin, or both, the silibinin boosted the chemo's ability to inhibit the growth of the cancer cells and powerfully increased apoptosis[21].

Perhaps the newest and most delicious ways

to combat prostate cancer are pomegranate juice and green tea. Forty-six men who had been treated for prostate cancer still had rising PSA levels, suggesting that their cancer was continuing to spread. But when they were given eight ozs of pomegranate juice daily for 33 months, the climbing PSA levels slowed significantly in 83 per cent of them. It actually went down in 15 per cent of them. When the study started, their PSA levels were doubling every 15 to 16 months; by the end of the study, it took 54.7 months for the level to double[22].

In a double-blind study, men with precancerous changes in their prostates were given either a green tea extract containing 600 mg of catechins or a placebo. After one year, 30 per cent of the men taking the placebo had developed prostate cancer, compared to only 3.3 per cent of the men taking the green tea. So, green tea may help prevent prostate cancer in men at high risk[23].

Vitamins, Minerals, and Other Nutrients

One of the best nutrients for fighting prostate cancer is selenium. A six-year study of 1,733 men found that the risk of developing prostate cancer was 31 per cent lower in men with high levels of selenium than it was in men with low levels[24]. And an interesting thirteen-year study found that among men with high levels of PSA, the ones with the highest blood levels of selenium had significantly less chance of developing prostate cancer than the ones with the lowest[25].

One amazing study found that when 974 men were given either 200 mcg of selenium or a placebo for four and a half years, the selenium reduced the risk of prostate cancer by an incredible 63 per cent, compared to the placebo[26].

Research also supports the use of vitamin D, antioxidants, and modified citrus pectin[27]. Shamsuddin and Yang (1995) found IP6 to be effective against prostate cancer cells in the laboratory. And the great prostate herb, saw palmetto berry, may also be helpful[28].

Other possible good fighters are pau d'arco, reishi, Essiac, CoQ10, indole-3-carbinol, and grape seed extract.

Chapter Endnotes

1. Giovannucci, E., *et al.* "A prospective study of dietary fat and risk of prostate cancer." *J Natl Cancer Inst*, 1993; 85(19):11571'79.

2. Fradet, Y., F. Meyer, I. Bairati, *et al.* "Dietary fat and prostate cancer progression and survival." *Eur Urol*, 1999; 35:388'91.

3. Talamini, R., C. La Vecchia, A. Decarli, *et al.* "Nutrition. Social factors and prostatic cancer in a Northern Italian poplualtion." *Br J Cancer*, 1986; 53:817'21; Andersson, S-O., A. Wolk, R. Bergstrom, et. al. "Body size and prostate cancer: a 20-year follow-up study among 135,006 Swedish construction workers." *J Natl Cancer Inst*, 1997; 89:385'89.

4. Ornish, D., *et al.* "Intensive lifestyle changes may affect the progression of prostate cancer." *Journal of Urolog*, 2005; 174:1065'70.

5. Saxe, Gordon A., *et al.* "Potential attenuation of disease progression in recurrent prostate cancer with plant-based diet and stress reduction." *Integr Cancer Ther*, 2006; 5: 206'13.

6. Hsing, Ann W., *et al.*, "Allium vegetables and risk of prostate cancer: a population-based study." *Journal of the National Cancer Institute*, 2002; 94:1648'51.

7. *Journal of Nutrition*, 1995.

8. Onozawa, Mizuki, *et al.* "Effects of soybean isoflavones on cell growth and apoptosis of the human prostatic cancer cell line LNCaP." *Japanese Journal of Clinical Oncology*, 1998; 28:360'63.

9. Dalais, F. S., *et al.* "Effects of a diet rich in phytoestrogens on prostate-specific antigen and sex hormones in men diagnosed with prostate cancer." *Urology*, 2004; 64:510'15.

10. Jacobsen, B. K., S. F. Knutsen, G. E. Fraser. "Does high soy milk intake reduce prostate cancer incidence? The Adventist Health Study." *Cancer Causes Control*, 1998; 9:553'57.

11. Levy, J., *et al.* "Lycopene is a more potent inhibitor of human cancer cell proliferation than either alpha-carotene or beta-carotene." *Nutr Cancer*, 1995; 24(3):257'66.

12. Gann, P. H., J. Ma, E. Giovannucci, W. Willett, *et al.* "Lower prostate cancer risk in men with elevated plasma lycopene levels: results of a prospective analysis." *Cancer Res*, 1999; 59:1225'30.

13. Giovannucci, E., A. Ascherio, E. Rimm, *et al.* "Intake of carotenoids and retinol in relation to risk of prostate cancer." *J Natl Cancer Inst*, 1995; 87:1767'76.

14. Kucuk, O., F. H. Sarkar, Z. Djuric, *et al.* "Effects of lycopene supplementation in patients with localized prostate cancer." *Exp Biol Med*, 2002; 227:881'85.

15. Kucuk, O., F. H. Sarkar, W. Sakr, *et al.* "Phase II randomized clinical trial of lycopene supplementation before radical prostatectomy." *Cancer Epidemiol Biomarkers Prev*, 2001; 10:861'68.

16. Chen, L., M. Stacewicz-Sapuntzakis, C. Duncan, *et al.* "Oxidative DNA damage in prostate cancer patients consuming tomato sauce-based entrees as a whole-food intervention." *J Natl Cancer Inst*, 2001; 93:1872-79.

17. Cohen, J. H., A. R. Kristal, J.L. Stanford. "Fruit and vegetable intakes and prostate cancer risk." *J Natl Cancer Inst*, 2000; 92:61'68.

18. Jarred, R.A., M. Keikha, C. Dowling, *et al.* "Induction of apoptosis in low to moderate-grade human prostate carcinoma by red clover-derived dietary isoflavones." *Cancer Epidemiol Biomarkers Prev*, 2002; 11:1689'96.

19. Fullerton SA, *et al.* "Induction of apoptosis in human prostatic cancer cells with beta-glucan (Maitake mushroom polysaccharide)." *Mol Urol* 2000;4:7-13.

20. Dorai, T., N. Gehani, A. Katz. "Therapeutic potential of curcumin in human prostate cancer-I. Curcumin induces apoptosis in both androgen-dependent and androgen-independent prostate cancer cells." *Prostate Cancer Prostatic Dis*, 2000; 3:84'93.

21. Tyagi, Anil K., *et al.* "Silibinin Strongly Synergizes Human Prostate Carcinoma DU145 Cells to Doxorubicin-induced Growth Inhibition, G2-M Arrest, and Apoptosis." *Clinical Cancer Research*, 2002; 8:3512'19.

22. Pantuck, A. J., *et al.* "Phase II study of pomegranate juice for men with rising prostate-specific antigen following surgery or radiation for prostate cancer." *Clinical Cancer Research*, 2006; 12:4018'26.

23. Bettuzzi, S., M. Brausi, F. Rizzi, *et al.* "Chemoprevention of human prostate cancer by oral administration of green tea catechins in volunteers with high-grade prostate intraepithelial neoplasia: a preliminary report from a one year proof-of-principle study." *Cancer Res*, 2006; 66:1234'40.

24. Van den Brandt, Piet A., P. Maurice, A. Zeegers, Peter Bode, R. Alexandra Goldbohm. "Toenail Selenium Levels and the Subsequent Risk of Prostate Cancer: A Prospective Cohort Study." *Cancer Epidemiology, Biomarkers and Prevention*, 2003; 12:866'71.

25. Li, Haojie, *et al.* "A Prospective Study of Plasma Selenium Levels and Prostate Cancer Risk." *Journal of the National Cancer Institute*, 2004; 96:696'703.

26. Clark, L. C., B. Dalkin, A. Krongrad, *et al.* "Decreased incidence of prostate cancer with selenium supplementation: results of a double-blind cancer prevention trial." *Br J Urol*, 1998; 81:730'34.

27. Strum, S., M. Scholz, J. McDermed, *et al.* "Modified citrus pectin slows PSA doubling time: a pilot clinical trial." *Presentation: International conference on Diet and Prevention of Cancer*, Finland. May 28, 1999"June 2, 1999.

28. Vacherot, F., *et al.* "Induction of apoptosis and inhibition of cell proliferation by the lipido-sterolic extract of Serenoa repens (LSESr, Permixon) in benign proatatic hyperplasia." *Prostate*, 2000; 45:259'66; Iguchi, K., *et al.* "Myristoleic acid, a cytotoxic component in the extract form of Serenoa repens, induces apoptosis and necrosis in human prostatic LNCaP cells." *Prostate*, 2001; 47:59'65.

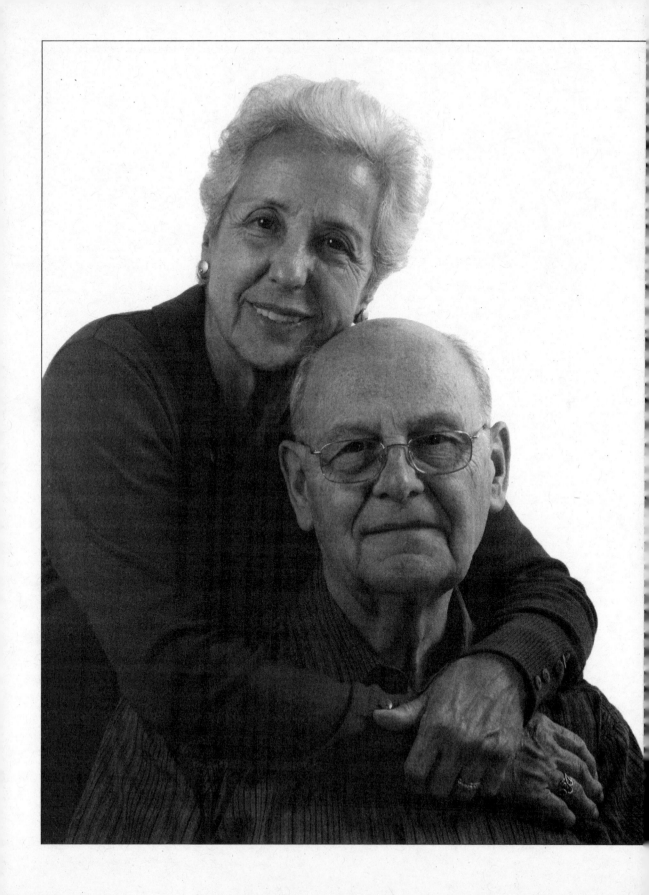

SENIORS' HEALTH

As well as having the same needs as everybody else, seniors also have a whole variety of special health needs that are best addressed in this section of the book. Seniors face aging and all the issues that aging brings to their lives. And this section of the book will take a comprehensive look at seniors' health needs in a healthy, holistic way.

To feel healthy and fit, both mentally and physically, can be a challenge as you get older. Nutritional needs may change, as does the need for supplements that help to promote longevity, sound mind and healthy body. As you get older, issues that affect the bones, joints, brain function, blood sugar, heart, eyes, ears and every other part of the body can become a problem.

This section will look at Alzheimer's disease, diabetes and hypoglycemia, osteoporosis, hearing loss, cataracts, glaucoma, macular degeneration, cholesterol, high blood pressure, congestive heart failure, Parkinson's disease, osteoarthritis, rheumatoid arthritis and gout.

ALZHEIMER'S DISEASE

In a culture that already fears old age, what could be more terrifying than an old age that robs you of your memory, concentration, and ability to reason, learn, and speak? Alzheimer's is old age's nightmare, and it is becoming a more and more common nightmare. Alzheimer's numbers are unbelievable, affecting about 10 per cent of all people over sixty-five and a seemingly impossible 50 per cent of all people over eighty-five. Clearly, we need to find more effective ways of preventing and treating Alzheimer's. And, fortunately, nature has much to offer.

Ginkgo Biloba: The Most Promising Alzheimer's Treatment of Them All

The most important supplement for Alzheimer's is the herb ginkgo biloba. Ginkgo has demonstrated its amazing ability to help memory, cognition, and daily living skills in people with Alzheimer's in study after study[1]. When researchers reduced the pile of ginkgo studies to just four very well-designed ones, they found strong evidence that ginkgo helps people with Alzheimer's[2]. In all of these studies, the herb's safety has stood out as much as its effectiveness.

So, given ginkgo's safety and effectiveness, the obvious question is: How does it stack up against the best drugs medicine has to offer? The answer might surprise you. When a comparison was done between studies that used ginkgo and studies that used two conventional cognitive drugs, all three treatments were found to help significantly, but the side effects were lowest with ginkgo[3]. A second study found that more people respond, and respond better, to ginkgo than to the drug tacrine[4]. Tacrine is a cholinesterase inhibitor, which is the dominant class of drugs for Alzheimer's. Another study comparing ginkgo to the cholinesterase inhibitors also found it to be better and safer than tacrine. This study also found ginkgo to be comparable to the latest drug the pharmacy has to offer, donepezil[5]. More recent research has again found that ginkgo is as good as donepezil and, in fact, better because it is better tolerated[6]. The conclusion then is not that ginkgo is the best herbal treatment for Alzheimer's, but that it is the best treatment for Alzheimer's.

Anti-Alzheimer's Antioxidants

Free-radical damage plays an important role in the development of Alzheimer's. People who have Alzheimer's have significantly lower antioxidant activity than people who don't. So it is not surprising to find that, as in so many other diseases, antioxidants can help protect against and treat Alzheimer's disease. The antioxidant vitamins C and E appear to stand out.

There is a lot of evidence from several large studies that the combination of vitamins C and E prevents Alzheimer's[7]. Higher blood levels of vitamin E in middle-aged and older people also correlate with better brain function[8], and elderly people who get the most vitamin E have a lot less cognitive decline than people who get the least[9].

What if someone already has Azheimer's? There is evidence for vitamin E here, too. In an important study published in the *New England Journal of Medicine*, people with Alzheimer's given vitamin E lived longer. Those who were given an Alzheimer's drug outlived a placebo group by 215 days, while those given vitamin E outlived them by 230 days. Vitamin E also helped them take care of themselves longer. While 39 per cent of the placebo group and 33 per cent of the drug group had to be institutionalized, only 26 per cent of the vitamin E group did[10].

Thinking with Your Heart

Have you ever been told not to think with your heart? Well, think again! A number of factors usually thought of for heart health are turning out to be important factors for brain health, too. If you have high blood pressure or cholesterol in midlife,

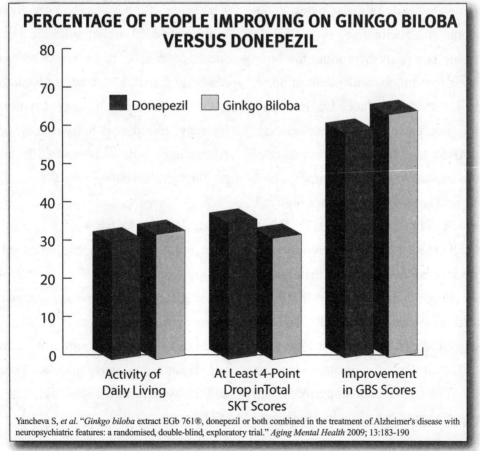

PERCENTAGE OF PEOPLE IMPROVING ON GINKGO BILOBA VERSUS DONEPEZIL

Yancheva S, *et al.* "*Ginkgo biloba* extract EGb 761®, donepezil or both combined in the treatment of Alzheimer's disease with neuropsychiatric features: a randomised, double-blind, exploratory trial." *Aging Mental Health* 2009; 13:183-190

for example, you have a significantly higher risk of developing Alzheimer's. If you have both high blood pressure and elevated cholesterol, you have 3.5 times the risk of those with neither[11]. The increased risk of Alzheimer's may be because these factors increase the risk of atherosclerosis, and atherosclerosis is another heart factor that increases the risk of Alzheimer's.

Homocysteine is an important risk factor for heart disease that is much less known, but that is starting to get more attention. Maybe it should be getting more attention for Alzheimer's as well, because we now know that people with high levels of homcysteine are nearly twice as likely to develop symptoms of Alzheimer's[12].

Homocysteine is a nasty byproduct the body produces from the amino acid methionine. A group of B vitamins that includes B6, B12, and, especially, folic acid prevents homocysteine levels from rising. And it now seems that this power of the B vitamins can help prevent Alzheimer's. Low levels of folic acid seem to be linked to a high risk of Alzheimer's[13], as do low levels of B12[14]. When over 10,000 people took a thinking and memory test, it was discovered that the higher their homocysteine, the poorer their recall, and the lower their folic acid, the poorer their recall[15]. And, excitingly, research has also found that folic acid, B6, and B12 seem to protect against Alzheimer's[16]. The most recent study found that seniors who got the most folic acid had the lowest incidence of Alzheimer's[17].

In an interesting study, 370 people over the age of seventy-five who had no Alzheimer's or other dementias had their folate and B12 levels measured and then were followed for three years. People who had normal levels of both B vitamins were the least likely to develop Alzheimer's. Those who were low in both had a geater chance of getting Alzheimer's than those who were only low in one[18].

Phosphatidylserine: Amazing Results

Another exciting nutrient in the fight against Alzheimer's is phosphatidylserine. Three hundred milligrams of phosphatidylserine a day has been shown to significantly improve memory in double-blind research[19]. A large double-blind study also found significant improvement in memory, learning, mood, and behaviour in people with Alzheimer's who were given 300 mg of phosphatidylserine a day[20].

Other Helpful Nutrients

Coenzyme Q10 and melatonin might also help. Giving coenzyme Q10 to people with Alzheimer's has been shown in preliminary research to slow down the progress of the disease, and one study has found melatonin to improve memory significantly in elderly people whose cognitive abilities were mildly impaired[21].

The mineral, silica, might also help. When silica

was given to elderly women who were followed for seven years, it was found to decrease their risk of Alzheimer's[22].

And most studies of acetyl L-carnitine have found that 1 gram taken three times a day delays the progress of Alzheimer's and improves memory[23].

Helpful Herbs: Beyond Ginkgo

Though ginkgo is the star here, several other herbs can contribute. Though new to the science of memory, many of them are not new in their use for memory. As its name suggests, sage has long been associated with improving memory. And now science has started to confirm that use. Sixty drops a day of sage extract for four months led to significant improvement in people with mild to moderate Alzheimer's. While Alzheimer's scores climbed by 22 per cent in a group given a placebo, they went down by 26 per cent in the group given sage[24]. Herb expert James Duke, Ph.D., says that research reveals that sage can prevent the breakdown of the neurotransmitter acetylcholine, deficiency of acetylcholine is linked to Alzheimer's.

In *Hamlet*, Ophelia says, "There's rosemary, that's for remembrance." And it seems she was right. Rosemary is loaded in antioxidants and it has several compounds that prevent the breakdown of acetylcholine.

Lemon balm is another herb that frequently gets mentioned for Alzheimer's. When a lemon balm extract was put to the test in people with Alzheimer's, cognitive function improved significantly and agitation was reduced[25].

Muira puama and ginseng are other herbs that might help. Though better known as a herb for impotence, muira puama has also been used traditionally in South America for memory problems. Research has now found that it does enhance cognitive and physical performance[26]. It may also help in the case of Alzheimer's.

Lifestyle Changes

One thing you can do is eat and drink more fruits and vegetables. Eating more fruits, vegetables and, especially, fibre has been shown to improve brain function in the elderly[27]. And drinking more fruits and veggies helps, too. People who drink at least three glasses of fruit or vegetable juice a week have an incredible 76 per cent lower chance of developing Alzheimer's[28].

The Mediterranean diet has also been shown to prevent Alzheimer's. This diet is high in fruits, vegetables, grains, nuts, seeds, beans, olive oil, and may include fish. It is low in meat and dairy. People who follow the Mediterranean diet have an incredible 40 to 48 per cent reduced risk of Alzheimer's[29].

One thing you might want to avoid is aluminum, since it may contribute to Alzheimer's. A preliminary study has found that people with Alzheimer's are more likely to have eaten foods that are high in aluminum additives[30]. Avoiding aluminum foil, aluminum pots, aluminum additives, drinks in aluminum cans, antacids, cake and pancake mixes, processed cheese, frozen dough, pickles, tap water, and many antiperspirants may be a good idea.

And, finally, staying physically and mentally active can help prevent Alzheimer's. People who play musical instruments, garden, exercise, or play board games are less likely to develop the disease[31]. And when people with Alzheimer's were given one hour of exercise twice a week and had their progress compared to those who received standard medicalcare after one year, the ability to perform daily living activities had decreased by 29 per cent in the medical care group, but by only 19 per cent in the exercise group, indicating that exercise slowed down the progress of the disease by a third[32].

Chapter Endnotes

1. Hofferberth, B. "The efficacy of EGb 761 in patients with senile dementia of the Alzheimer type, a double-blind, placebo-controlled study on different levels of investigation." *Hum Psychopharmacol*, 1994; 9:215-22; Kanowski, S., et al. "Proof of efficacy of the Ginkgo biloba special extract EGb 761 in outpatients suffering from mild to moderate primary degenerative dementia of the Alzheimer type or multi-infarct dementia." *Pharmacopsychiatry*, 1996; 29:47-56; Maurer, K., et al. "Clinical efficacy of Ginkgo biloba special extract EGb 761 in dementia of the Alzheimer's type." *J Psychiatr Res*, 1997; 31:645-55; Le Bars, P.L., et al. "A placebo-controlled, double-blind, randomized trial of an extract of Ginkgo biloba for dementia. North American EGb Study Group." *JAMA*, 1997; 278:1327'32.

2. Oken, Barry S., et al. "The Efficacy of Ginkgo biloba on Cognitive Function in Alzheimer Disease." *Arch Neurol*, 1998; 55:1409'15.

3. Letzel, H, J., Haan, W.B. Feil Nootropics: "Efficacy and tolerability of products from three active substance classes." *J Drug Dev Clin Pract*, 1996;8:7794.

4. Itil, T.M., et al. "The pharmacological effects of Ginkgo biloba, a plant extract, on the brain of dementia patients in comparison with tacrine." *Psychopharmacol Bull*, 1998; 34:391'97.

5. Wettstein, A. "Cholinesterase inhibitors and Ginkgo extracts—are they comparable in the treatment of dementia? Comparison of published placebo-controlled efficacy studies of at least six months' duration." *Phytomed*, 2000; 6:393'401.

6. Mazza, M., et al. "Ginkgo biloba and donepezil: a comparison in the treatment of Alzheimer's dementia in a randomized placebo-controlled double-blind study." Euro J Neurol, 2006; 13:981'85. Yancheva S, et al. "Ginkgo biloba extract EG 761®, donepezil or both combined in the treatment of Alzheimer's disease with neuropsychiatric features: a randomised, double-blind, exploratory trial." *Aging Mental Health* 2009; 13:183-190.

7. Morris, M.C., et al. "Vitamin E and vitamin C supplement use and risk of inciden Alzheimer disease." *Alzheimer Dis Assoc Disord*, 1998; 12:121-26; Engelhart M.J., et al. "Dietary Intake of Antioxidants and Risk of Alzheimer Disease." *JAMA*, 2002; 287:3223'29; Zandi, P.P., et al. "Reduced Risk of Alzheimer Disease in Users of Antioxidant Vitamin Supplements. The Cache County Study." *Arch Neurol*, 2004; 61:82'88.

8. Schmidt, R., et al. "Plasma antioxidants and cognitive performance in middle-age and older adults: results of the Austrian Stroke Prevention Study." *J Am Geriat. Soc*, 1998; 46:1407-10.

9. Morris, M.C., et al. "Vitamin E and Cognitive Decline in Older Persons." *Arch Neurol*, 2002; 59:1125'32.

10. Sano, M., et al. "A controlled trial of selegiline, alpha-tocopherol, or both as treat ment for Alzheimer's disease." *N Engl J Med*, 1997; 336:1216-22.

11. Kivipelto, M., et al. "Midlife vascular risk factors and Alzheimer's disease in later life: longitudinal, population based study." *BMJ*, 2001; 322:1447'51.

12. Seshadri, S., et al. "Plasma Homocysteine as a Risk Factor for Dementia and Alzheimer's Disease." *N Engl J Med*, 2002; 346:476'83.

13. Ebly, E.M., et al. "Folate status, vascular disease and cognition in elderly Canadians." *Age Ageing*, 1998; 27:485-91; Snowdon, D.A., et al. "Serum folate and the severity of atrophy of the neocortex in Alzheimer disease: findings from the Nun study." *Am J Clin Nutr*, 2000; 71:993-98. Clarke R., et al. "Folate, vitamin B12, and serum total homocysteine levels in confirmed Alzheimer disease." *Arch Neurol* 1998;55:1449-55; Wang H. X., et al. "Vitamin B(12) and folate in relation to the development of Alzheimer's disease." *Neurology* 2001;56:1188-94.

14. McCaddon A., et al. "Familial Alzheimer's Disease and Vitamin B12 Deficiency." *Age Ageing* 1994; 23:334-7; M. A., Bernard, P. A., T. M., Nakonezny Kashne "The effect of vitamin B12 deficiency on older veterans and its relationship to health." *J Am Geriatr Soc*. 1998;46:1199-1206; Clarke R., et al. "Folate, vitamin B12, and serum total homocysteine levels in confirmed Alzheimer disease." *Arch Neurol* 1998;55:1449-55; H. X., Wang, et al. "Vitamin B(12) and folate in relation to the development of Alzheimer's disease." *Neurology* 2001;56:1188-94; Joosten E., et al. "Is metabolic evidence for vitamin B-12 and folate deficiency more frequent in elderly patients with Alzheimer's disease?" *J Gerontol A Biol Sci Med Sci*, 1997;52:M76-M79.

15. Morris, M. S., et al. "Hyperhomocysteinemia associated with poor recall in the third National Health and Nutrition Examination Survey." *Am J Clin Nutr* 2001;73:927-33.

16. Riggs, K. M., "Relations of vitamin B-12, vitamin B-6, folate , and homocystein to cognitive performance in the Normative Aging Study." *Am J Clin Nutr* 1996;63:306-14.

17. Luchsinger, J.A., et al. "Relation of Higher Folate Intake to Lower Risk of Alzheimer Disease in the Elderly." *Arch Neurol*, 2007; 64:86'92.

18. Wang, H.X., et al. "Vitamin B12 and folate in relation to the development of Alzheimer's disease." *Neurology*, 2001; 56:188'94.

19. Crook, T., et al. "Effects of phosphatidylserine in Alzheimer's disease." *Psychopharmacol Bull*, 1992; 28:61-66.

20. Cenacchi, T., *et al*. "Cognitive decline in the elderly: A double-blind, placebo-controlled multicenter study on efficacy of phosphatidylserine administration." *Aging: Clinical and Experimetal Research*, 1993; 5:123'33.

21. Jean-Louis G., von H., Gizycki, F., Zizi, "Melatonin effects on sleep, mood, and cognition in elderly with mild cognitive impairment." *J Pineal Res* 1998;25:177-83; see also L. I., Brusco, M., Marquez, D. P., Cardinali, "Monozygotic twins with Alzheimer's disease treated with melatonin: Case report." *J Pineal Res* 1998;25:260-3.

22. Gillette-Guyonnet, S., *et al*. "Cognitive impairment and composition of drinking water in women: findings of the EPIDOS Study." *Am J Clin Nutr*, 2005;.81:897'902.

23. Pettegrew, J.W., *et al*. "Clinical and neurochemical effects of acetyl-L-carnitine in Alzheimer's disease." *Neurobiol Aging*, 1995; 16:1-4; Salvioli, G., M. Neri. "L-acetylcarnitine treatment of mental decline in the elderly." *Drugs Exp Clin Res*, 1994; 20:169-76; Rai, G., *et al*. "Double-blind, placebo controlled study of acetyl-L-carnitine in patients with Alzheimer's dementia." *Curr Med Res Opin*, 1990; 11:638-47; Sano, M., *et al*. "Double-blind parallel design pilot study of acetyl levocarnitine in patients with Alzheimer's disease." *Arch Neurol*, 1992; 49:1137-41; Cucinotta, D., *et al*. "Multicenter clinical placebo-controlled study with acetyl-L-carnitine (LAC) in the treatment of mildly demented elderly patients." *Drug Development Res*, 1988; 14:213-16; Bonavita, E. "Study of the efficacy and tolerability of L-acetylcarnitine therapy in the senile brain." *Int J Clin Pharmacol Ther Toxicol*, 1986; 24:511-16; Calvani, M., *et al*. "Action of acetyl-L-carnitine in neurodegeneration and Alzheimer's disease." *Ann NY Acad Sci*, 1992; 663:483-86.

24. Akhondzadeh, S., *et al*. "Salvia officinalis extract in the treatment of patients with mild to moderate Alzheimer's disease: a double-blind, randomized and placebo-controlled trial." *J Clin Pharm Ther*, 2003; 28:53-59.

25. Akhondzadeh, S., *et al*. "Melissa officinalis extract in the treatment of patients with mild to moderate Alzheimer's disease: a double-blind, randomised, placebo controlled trial." *J Neurol Neurosurg Psychiatry*, 2003; 74:863-66.

26. Elisabetsky, E., *et al*. "Antioxidant and Memory Enhancing Properties of *Ptychopetalum olacoides*." Poster Presentation, 48th Annual Meeting of the International Congress of the Society of Medicinal Plant Research, P2A/28, Sept. 5, 2000.

27. Eur J Clin Nutr, 2001. "Scarmeas N, et al. Mediterranean Diet and Mild Cognitive Impairment." *Arch Neurol* 2009;66:216-25; Féart C., *et al*. Mediterranean diet and cognitive function in older adults." *Curr Opin Clin Metab Care* 2010; 13:14-18.

28. Dai, Q., *et al*. "Fruit and vegetable juices and Alzheimer's disease: the Kame Project." *Am J Med*, 2006; 119:751'59.

29. Liu R. H., Eur J Clin Nutr 2001; "Health benefits of fruit and vegetables are from additive and synergistic combinations of phytochemicals." *Am J Clin Nutr 2003*; 78:517S

30. Rogers, M.A., D.G Simon,. "A preliminary study of dietary aluminium intake and risk of Alzheimer's disease." *Age Ageing*, 1999; 28:205-09.

31. Friedland, R. American Academy of Neurology's 52nd Annual Meeting in San Diego, CA, April 29-May 6, 2000.

32. Rolland, Y., *et al*. "Program for nursing home residents with Alzheimer's disease: a 1-year randomized, controlled trial." *J Am Geriatr Soc*, 2007; 55:158'65.

BALANCING BLOOD-SUGAR: DIABETES AND HYPOGLYCEMIA

It can be too high or it can be too low—one way it is diabetes and the other it is hypoglycaemia. Both are diet-related and can benefit from herbs and other supplements as well as dietary changes. Over two million Canadians have diabetes, and the numbers are getting worse. What's even more worrisome is that more young people are getting what used to be considered adult-onset diabetes[1].

So what can you do to help control blood-sugar levels? Switch to whole grains and avoid simple sugar, processed foods, and refined carbs, and, so that you keep your sugar levels well balanced, don't skip meals. Eat a diet that is high in complex carbohydrates and high-fibre foods. Saturated and hydrogenated fats should be kept to a minimum. It is also a good idea to consume legumes, as they can help to stabilize blood-sugar levels. A very important recent study has now shown that a vegan diet improves blood-sugar control in diabetics better than the standard American Diabetic Association diet[2].

Get a copy of the glycemic index of foods and try to eat the ones that are best for diabetes. And exercise. Proper exercise is known to help regulate blood-sugar levels.

Diabetics are two to three times more likely than non-diabetics to die prematurely of heart disease or stroke, so a supplement that can help control blood-sugar and can also reduce risk factors for heart disease and stroke in diabetics is literally a lifesaver. There are a number of supplements that can address both factors, including fenugreek, cinnamon, psyllium, zinc, and vitamin C.

There are several herbs and nutrients that help with blood-sugar control issues. Some, like cinnamon and fenugreek, are common spices.

HERBS THAT BALANCE BLOOD-SUGAR

As Simple as Cinnamon?

We became intrigued when we met someone who said they knew of a family in which every member had developed diabetes, except one son. When they looked into the reason for this anomaly, they found that although this son ate the exact same diet as every other member of the family, there was one difference: The son added a generous portion of cinnamon to his cereal each day. The cinnamon was believed to be the reason for his not developing diabetes. Studies are currently ongoing to ascertain whether cinnamon might contain a powerful component for preventing diabetes. It is thought that adding cinnamon every day to the diet may reduce the risk of diabetes. Cinnamon is one of those herbs that addresses both diabetes and cardiovascular disease because in addition to significantly lowering glucose levels, it also lowers LDL and total cholesterol, and triglycerides[3].

Fenugreek: Ancient Remedy, Modern Science

Fenugreek is one of the oldest recorded spices used medicinally. It has been used to treat diabetes for many years, and now the seeds of fenugreek have been shown in studies to have significant antidiabetic effects. The active ingredient in fenugreek is in the defatted portion of the seed. Results from studies indicate that both diabetics and hypoglycaemics could benefit from including fenugreek seeds in their diet. In those with insulin-dependent diabetes (type I), 50 g of defatted fenugreek seed powder, two times per day for ten days resulted in significant improvement in their diabetes. Compared to a placebo, there was a significant reduction in blood-sugar and improvement in glucose tolerance[4].

When non-insulin-dependent (type II) diabetics were given 15g of powdered fenugreek seed soaked in water, there was a significant drop in after-meal glucose levels[6]. A later study gave 25g of fenugreek to sixty type II diabetics for twenty-four weeks and produced a significant 25 per cent drop in blood-sugar levels. And when type II diabetics not successfully managed by the drug sulfonylureas added either fenugreek total saponins or a placebo, there was a significantly greater drop in blood-sugar levels, symptom scores and other important markers of diabetes in the fenugreek group[7].

Bilberry and Ginkgo: Diabetic Retinopathy and Other Problems

Another useful herb for treating diabetes is bilberry, best known for improving eyesight. This herb grows well in Europe, where it has a long history of use in treating diabetes. Bilberry is especially useful in cases of diabetic retinopathy, the leading cause of blindness among diabetics[8].

Although the herb ginkgo biloba is best known for its ability to improve memory, it is also very useful for diabetes and hypoglycaemia. Ginkgo biloba has been shown in studies to increase blood flow to the brain, resulting in increase in oxygen and glucose utilization. Both diabetics and hypoglycaemics can suffer from reduced blood flow to the extremeties, and ginkgo can help to correct this problem. Research suggests that ginkgo is another herb that holds promise against diabetic retinopathy[9].

Human See, Human Do

Noticing the reactions of people and animals to what they eat has led to the discovery that certain plants are helpful for certain conditions. An uncommon herb known as saltbush was found to be useful for type II diabetics after it was noticed that when the sand rats stopped eating the herb, they developed severe diabetes. When the sandrats resumed eating saltbush, the diabetes disappeared. This observation led researchers to test saltbush on people, and they found that it is helpful for type II diabetes.

Onions and Garlic: Fighting Diabetes Deliciously

Onions and garlic are wonderful for balancing sugar levels. The active compounds in these foods, the sulphur and flavonoids , have been shown to be effective in reducing blood-sugar levels. They seem to work by competing with insulin for insulin-activating sites in the liver, resulting in an increase in free insulin. Eating raw garlic and onions is recommended for both diabetics and hypoglycaemics.

Diabetes Superstars: Bitter Melon and Gymnema Sylvestre

Bitter melon, which is popular for getting rid of pinworms, is also very useful for treating blood-sugar problems. Bitter melon has been used for years to treat diabetes, and research has confirmed the blood-sugar-lowering effects of this fruit. Charantin, one of this fruit's several compounds effective against blood-sugar problems, fights hypoglycaemia better thatn chemical drugs. And one of its other compounds, a

polypeptide, has been found to lower blood-sugar levels in a similar way to insulin without insulin's side effects.

Research suggests that the fresh juice of the melon is probably the best form to use. When 100 ml of fresh bitter melon juice was given to type II diabetics, 73 per cent of them improved significantly[10]. And when type II diabetics were given either 5 g of dried bitter melon powder three times a day or 100 ml of aqueous extract once a day for three weeks, the dry powder lowered blood-sugar levels by 25 per cent and the extract by 54 per cent[11]. Michael Murray, N.D., recommends two ozs of the juice a day.

The herb Gymnema sylvestre can help both type I and type II diabetes. In type I diabetes, the beta cells of the pancreas, which are responsible for insulin production, have been destroyed. Nonetheless, when *Gymnema sylvestre* was given to twenty-seven type I diabetics who were on insulin, the insulin requirements were reduced by almost 50 per cent. Blood-sugar decreased and blood-sugar control improved. The herb seems to have enhanced the action of insulin and also to have regenerated the beta cells[12].

When twenty-two type II diabetics on oral diabetes drugs were given the herb, every one of them had a significant improvement in blood-sugar control. All but one of them were able to reduce their drug dosage, and five of them were able to stop the drug altogether[13].

Rising Star: Berberine

Berberine is the active ingredient in the herb goldenseal. And it may be very active against diabetes. In the first of a two-part study, diabetics were given either 500 mg of berberine or 500 mg of the drug metformin three times a day. The two treatments had the identical effect on blood glucose and insulin, but the berberine had the advantage of lowering triglycerides and cholesterol while the drug did not. In the second part, type II diabetics whose diabetes was not being adequately controlled by drugs and diet added 500 mg of berberine three times a day. Adding the berberine significantly lowered blood glucose, a long-term marker of blood sugar control, triglycerides, total cholesterol and harmful LDL cholesterol. The study's authors called berberine a potent hypoglycemic agent[14].

These results have now been confirmed by a second study, which also had two parts. The first found that treating cells with berberine in a laboratory increases the number and responsiveness of insulin receptor cells. The second gave 97 type II diabetics either 1 g of berberine, 1.5 g of the drug metformin, or 4 mg of the drug rosiglitazone for two months. The effectiveness of the berberine was similar to that of the drugs. The berberine significantly lowered fasting blood glucose levels, insulin, triglyc-erides and a marker of long-term blood-sugar control. The researchers said that "berberine increases insulin receptors in humans and that this is associated with its glucose-lowering effect. We believe that berberine . . . is an ideal medicine for type 2 diabetes"[15].

More Herbal Help

Other valuable herbs for treating blood-sugar problems include blueberry, devil's club, and jambolan seed. All three have been used traditionally to treat both diabetes and hypoglycaemia. Some herbalists believe that devil's club may be one of the most effective herbs for treating blood-sugar problems. Herbalist Terry Willard says that devil's club reduces cravings for sweets and helps control sugar metabolism.

Another useful supplement is pycnogenol. When 100 mg of pycnogenol was added to standard diabetes treatment, it significantly lowered glucose levels[16].

Green tea can also be helpful for diabetics and hypoglycaemics since it is a source of the flavonoid, epicatechin, which has been shown to improve both diabetes and hypoglycaemia.

VITAMINS AND MINERALS THAT BALANCE BLOOD-SUGAR

There are numerous supplements—zinc, vitamin C, magnesium, fibre, lipoie acid, CoQ10, essential fatty acids, and vitamin D—that can aid in the treatment of diabetes and hypoglycaemia but probably the most important is the mineral, chromium.

Chromium: The Key to Controlling Blood-Sugar

Chromium is vital to blood-sugar control. Studies have confirmed chromium's ability to help both diabetics and hypoglycaemics. Many believe that an underlying chromium deficiency may be the root cause of diabetes. Chromium is essential for insulin to do its work. Without chromium, insulin can't transport sugar from the blood into the cells, and blood-sugar rises. Several controlled studies show that chromium improves impaired glucose tolerance[17]. It helps both insulin-dependent diabetes (type I) and non-insulin-dependent diabetes (type II). A 1991 study found that only 200 mcg of chromium a day for three months improved glucose tolerance in diabetics[18]. When a later double-blind, placebo-controlled study compared 200 mcg of chromium to 1,000 mcg in 180 type II diabetics for four months, the 1,000 mcg dose dropped glucose levels significantly more effectively. This higher dose had no toxicity[19].

In probably the most important study on chromium to date, type II diabetics who were already on the diabetes drug, glipizide, were also put on either 500 mcg of chromium or a placebo twice a day for ten months. The chromium significantly improved insulin sensitivity compared to the placebo and also led to less weight gain and less diabetes-caused tissue damage[20]. If medical science is truly science-based, then this double-blind, placebo-controlled study should end any doubt about this natural treatment for diabetes.

Unlike type II diabetics, type I diabetics will require insulin. But chromium can help even here. When type I diabetics were given 200 mcg of chromium a day, 71 per cent of them were able to decrease their insulin by 30 per cent[21].

Chromium also helps pregnant women who are suffering from gestational diabetes[22].

It is also useful in the treatment of hypoglycemia[23].

Crucial Zinc

Zinc is crucial for diabetics for two reasons. The first is that zinc deficiency contributes to the development of diabetes[24], and, in a vicious circle, diabetes contributes to deficiencies of zinc. Diabetics lose too much zinc in their urine, so they need to supplement it.

According to Murray, zinc is necessary for the production and use of insulin. It also protects the beta cells from destruction. Even in type I diabetics, zinc lowers blood-sugar levels[25].

Diabetic men who took zinc were able to lower their total cholesterol and triglycerides while raising their levels of beneficial HDL cholesterol[26], making it one of those supplements that helps with both diabetes and heart-disease risk.

Vitamin C: Getting Enough

Insulin is necessary not only for the transport of sugar into the cells, but also of vitamin C. For that reason, many diabetics don't get enough vitamin C into their cells and, therefore, need more of the nutrient than non-diabetics. Research shows that 1 to 2 g of vitamin C per day can help prevent many of the complications of diabetes[27]. Vitamin C may also improve glucose tolerance. Vitamin C is one of the nutrients that also helps address the cardiovascular risk of diabetics: 500 mg of vitamin C lowers blood pressure in type II diabetics nearly as well as medications, and it reduces the stiffness of the arteries[27].

Magnesium

Diabetics are also commonly low in magnesium[29]. Supplementing magnesium corrects the deficiency[30] and may prevent some of the complications of diabetes. It has been shown in some studies to reduce insulin requirements in type I diabetics[31] and to improve insulin production in elderly type II diabetics[32].

The Amazing Power of Fibre

The New England Journal of Medicine reports a very significant study for diabetics[33]. It compared the American Diabetic Association Diet (24 g of fibre) to a high fibre diet (50 g of fibre) in type II diabetics. The high fibre diet led to significantly lower glucose levels. In fact, it reduced glucose similarly to oral diabetes drugs. That means that simply eating more fibre could reduce or eliminate the need for drugs.

A 1983 study had already also concluded that high fibre diets decrease the need for insulin or oral diabetes drugs[34].

Other fibre studies have looked at psyllium in type II diabetics. One gave only 5.1 g or a placebo twice a day. Glucose levels went down in the psyllium group and up in the placebo group. The difference after lunch was 19.2 per cent and, all day, 11 per cent[35]. A larger dose of 15 g per day dose produced a significant 80 per cent drop in glucose[36].

Psyllium is also able to address complications of diabetes. It significantly lowers blood-sugar levels while elevating the good HDL cholesterol[37]. Psyllium also significantly lowers glucose absorption, the harmful LDL cholesterol, and total cholesterol[38]. LDL is the cholesterol that causes heart disease and stroke, and HDL cholesterol is the one that prevents it. So psyllium not only improves blood-sugar control in diabetics but also reduces the risk of heart disease.

Other fibre supplements shown to help include guar gum[39], pectin[40], and oat bran[41].

A related study showed that eating whole rather than refined grains reduced the risk for diabetes[42].

Lipoic Acid

Lipoic acid, a powerful antioxidant, may help diabetics convert sugar into energy. Clinically, it has been shown to aid in diabetic neuropathy, a common complication of diabetes in which nerve function is lost in the peripheries. Diabetic neuropathy leads to tingling, numbness, pain, and loss of function of that part of the body. It can become very serious. Studies show that lipoic acid leads to an improvement in blood-sugar metabolism, reduces glycosylation of proteins, improves blood flow and, incredibly, helps regenerate nerve fibres, making it extremely valuable for diabetics. In fact, lipoic acid is so valuable to diabetics that many lipoic acid-using diabetics are able to reduce their insulin intake.

Richard Podell, M.D., reports that at least a dozen studies have shown lipoic acid to help diabetic neuropathy. One study giving 600 mg 3 times a day found a significant improvement compared to a placebo[43]. Several other double-blind studies, usually using lower doses, have also proven the remarkable value of lipoic acid for diabetic neuropathy[44].

A dose of 600 mg was also found to significantly improve insulin sensitivity[45].

Essential Fatty Acids

Bad fats, such as saturated fat[46] and trans-fatty acids[47] are bad for diabetics, and good fats, such as vegetable fats and omega-3 fatty acids, like those found in flaxseed oil, are good for them[48]. Studies show that diets that are high in saturated fats and low in essential fatty acids reduce the fluidity of cell membranes, reducing insulin sensitivity and action. Omega-3s work in exactly the opposite way, so increasing essential fatty acids improves the symptoms of diabetes and decreases the risk of getting it.

Coenzyme Q10

Recently, disturbances in the mitochondria have been blamed as another culprit in diabetes[49]. CoQ10 increases mitochondrial function. In one study, 60 mg of CoQ10 improved blood glucose and insulin synthesis and secretion[50].

Vitamin D Helps Diabetes

Simply getting enough vitamin D could help reduce your chances of getting diabetes. A recent study of healthy young people has found that lower levels of vitamin D are associated with a greater degree of insulin resistance and a reduced capacity of the pancreas to secrete insulin. Thus it is thought that optimal amounts of vitamin D may positively affect blood-sugar levels and possibly help to prevent insulin resistance and diabetes[51].

This study was not the first to suggest that vitamin D may help prevent diabetes[52]. A thirty-year follow-up study that looked at over ten thousand children found that the ones who took vitamin D regularly had an 80 per cent reduced risk of getting type I diabetes. The ones with deficiencies of vitamin D had a 300 per cent increased risk of having type I diabetes[53].

Other Herbal Nutrients

Other particularly good nutrients for blood-sugar stability and its related factors include B12, L-glutamine, vitamin E, the B vitamins, manganese, potassium, grape seed, and other flavonoids.

Be sure to monitor your blood-sugar levels carefully when taking any supplement, as they could alter your levels and your requirements for insulin and oral medications. It is a good idea to work with a professional health-care worker when trying to monitor sugar levels.

Chapter Endnotes

1. Duncan, G. E. "Prevalence of Diabetes and Impaired Fasting Glucose Levels Among US Adolescents." *Arch Pediatr Adolesc Med*, 2006; 160:523'28.

2. Barnard, N. D., *et al*. "A Low-Fat Vegan Diet Improves Glycemic Control and Cardiovascular Risk Factors in a Randomized Clinical Trial in Individuals With Type 2 Diabetes." *Diabetes Care*, 2006; 29:1777'83.

3. Khan, A., *et al*. "Cinnamon improves glucose and lipids of people with type 2 diabetes." *Diabetes Care*, 2003;2 6:3215'18.

4. Sharma, R. D., T. C., Raghuram, N.S. Rao. "Effect of fenugreek seeds on blood glucose and serum lipids in type I diabetes." *Eur J Clin Nutr*, 1990; 44:301-06.

5. Madar, Z., *et al*. "Glucose-lowering effect of fenugreek in non-insulin dependent diabetics." *Eur J Clin Nutr*, 1988; 42:51-54.

6. Sharma, R.D., *et al*. "Use of fenugreek seed powder in the management of non-insulin dependent diabetes mellitus." *Nutr Res*, 1996; 16:1131-39. Lu F. R., *et al*. "Clinical observation on trigonella foenum-graecum L. total saponins in combination with sulfonylureas in the treatment of type 2 diabetes mellitus." *Chin J Integr Med*. 2008; 14:56-60.

7. Lu F.R., *et al*. Clinical observation on trigonella fuenum-graecum L. total saponins in combination with sulfonylureas in the treatment of type 2 diabetes mellito. *Chin L Integr Med* 2008;14:36-60

8. Perossini, M., *et al*. "Diabetic and hypertensive retinopathy therapy with *Vaccinium myrtillus anthocyanosides* (Tegens): double-blind placebo controlled clinical trial." *Ann Ottalmol Clin Ocul*, 1987; 113:1173'88.

9. Lanthony, P., J. P. Cosson. "The course of color vision in early diabetic retinopathy treated with *Ginkgo biloba* extract. A preliminary double-blind versus placebo study." *J Fr Ophtalmol*, 1988; 11:671-74; Huang, S. Y., *et al*. "Improved haemorrheological properties by *Ginkgo biloba* extract (Egb 761) in type 2 diabetes mellitus complicated with retinopathy." *Clin Nutr*, 2004; 23:615'21.

10. Welihinda, J., *et al*. "Effect of *Momordica charantia* on the glucose tolerance in maturity onset diabetes." *J Ethnopharmacol*, 1986; 17:277-82.

11. Srivastava, Y., *et al*. "Antidiabetic and adaptogenic properties of *Momordica charantia extract*: An experimental and clinical evaluation." *Phytother Res*, 1993; 7:285-89.

12. Shanmugasundaram, E.R.B., *et al*. "Use of *Gymnema sylvestre* leaf extract in the control of blood glucose insulin-dependent diabetes mellitus." *J Ethnopharmacol*, 1990; 30:281-94.

13. Baskaran, K., *et al*. "Antidiabetic effect of a leaf extract from Gymnema sylvestre in non-insulin dependent diabetes mellitus patients." *J Ethnopharmacol*, 1990; 30:295'305.

14. Yin, J., H., Xing, J., Ye "Efficacy of berberine in patients with type 2 diabetes mellitus." *Metab Clin Exper*. 2008; 57: 712-717.

15. Zhang H., *et al*. "Berberine lowers blood glucose in type 2 diabetes mellitus patients through increasing insulin receptor expression." *Metabolism*, 2010; 59:285-92.

16. Liu, X., *et al*. "Antidiabetic effect of Pycogenol French maritime pine bark extract in patients with diabetes type II." *Life Sci*, 2004; 75:2502'13.

17. Mertz, W. "Chromium in human nutrition: a review." *J Nutr*, 1993; 123:626'33.

18. Anderson, R.A., *et al*. "Supplemental-chromium effects on glucose, insulin, glucagons, and urinary chromium losses in subjects consuming controlled low-chromium diets." *Am J Clin Nutr*, 1991; 54:909'16.

19. Anderson, R.A., *et al*. "Elevated intakes of supplemental chromium improve glucose and insulin variables in individuals with type 2 diabetes." *Diabetes*, 1997; 46:1786'91'.

20. Martin, J., *et al*. "Chromium Picolinate Supplementation Attenuates Body Weight Gain and Increases Insulin Sensitivity in Subjects With Type 2 Diabetes." *Diabetes Care*, 2006; 29:1826-32.

21. Fox, G.N., Z. Sabovic. "Chromium picolinate supplementation for diabetes mellitus." *J Fam Pract*, 1998; 46:83'86.

22. Jovanovic, L., M. Gtierres, C.M. Peterson. "Chromium supplementation for women with gestational diabetes mellitus." *J Trace Elem Exp Med*, 1999; 12:91'97.

23. Anderson, R.A. *et al*. "Chromium supplementation of humans with hypoglycemia." *Fed Proc*, 1984; 43:471; Anderson, R.A., *et al*. "Effects of supplemental chromium on patients with symptoms of reactive hypoglycemia." *Metab*, 1987; 36:351'55; Clausen, J. "Chromium induced clinical improvement in symptomatic hypoglycemia." *Biol Trace Elem Res*, 1988; 17:229'36.

24. Mooradian, A.D., J.E. Morley. "Micronutrient status in diabetes mellitus." *Am J Clin Nutr*, 1987; 45:877'95.

25. Rao, K.V.R., V. Seshiah, T.V. Kumar. "Effect of zinc sulfate therapy on control and lipids in type I diabetes." *J Assoc Physicians India*, 1987; 35:52.

26. Partida-Hernandez, G., *et al*. "Effect of zinc replacement on lipids and lipoproteins in type 2-diabetic patients." *Biomed Pharmacother*, 2006; 60:161'68.

27. Davie, S.J., B.J. Gould, J.S. Yudkin. "Effect of vitamin C on glycosylation of proteins." *Diabetes*, 1992; 41:167'73; Will, J.C., T. Tyers. "Does diabetes mellitus increase the requirement for vitamin C?" *Nutr Rev*, 1996; 54:193-202 [review].

28. Mullan, B.A., *et al.* "Ascorbic Acid Reduces Blood Pressure and Arterial Stiffness in Type 2 Diabetes." *Hypertension*, 2002; 40:804'09.

29. Paolisso, G., *et al.* "Magnesium and glucose homeostasis." *Diabetologia*, 1990; 33:511-14; De Leeuw, I., *et al.* "Effect of intensive magnesium supplementation on the in vitro oxidizability of LDL and VLDL in Mg-depleted type 1 diabetic patients." *Magnes Res*, 1998;.11:179-82.

30. Eibl, N.L., *et al.* "Hypomagnesemia in type II diabetes: effect of a 3-month replacement therapy." *Diabetes Care*, 1995; 18:188.

31. Sjorgren, A., C.H. Floren, A. Nilsson. "Oral administration of magnesium hydroxide to subjects with insulin dependent diabetes mellitus." *Magnesium*, 1988; 121:16-20.

32. Paolisso, G., *et al.* "Improved insulin response and action by chronic magnesium administration in aged NIDDM subjects." *Diabetes Care*, 1989; 12:265-69.

33. Chandalia, M., *et al.* "Beneficial effects of high dietary fibre intake in patients with type 2 diabetes mellitus." *New Engl J Med*, 2000; 342:1392-98.

34. Acta Med Scand, 1983.

35. Anderson, J.W., *et al.* "Effects of psyllium on glucose and serum lipid responses in men with type 2 diabetes and hypercholesterolemia." *Am J Clin Nutr*, 1999; 70:466-73.

36. Rodríguez-Morán, M., F. Guerrero-Romero, G. Lazcano-Burciaga. "Lipid- and glucose-lowering efficacy of *plantago psyllium* in type II diabetes." *J Diab Comp*, 1998; 12:273-78.

37. Seyed, A.Z., *et al.* "Psyllium decreased serum glucose and glycosylated hemoglobin significantly in diabetic outpatients." *Journal of Ethnopharmacology*, 2005; 102:202'07.

38. Sierra, M., *et al.* "Therapeutic effects of psyllium in type 2 diabetic patients." *European Journal of Clinical Nutrition*, 2002; 56:830'42.

39. Landin, K., *et al.* "Guar gum improves insulin sensitivity, blood lipids, blood pressure, and fibrinolysis in healthy men." *Am J Clin Nutr*, 1992; 56:1061-65.

40. Schwartz, S.E., *et al.* "Sustained pectin ingestion: effect on gastric emptying and glucose tolerance in non-insulin-dependent diabetic patients." *Am J Clin Nutr*, 1988; 48:1413-17.

41. Hallfrisch, J., D.J. Scholfield, K.M. Behall. "Diets containing soluble oat extracts improve glucose and insulin responses of moderately hypercholesterolemic men and women." *Am J Clin Nutr*, 1995; 61:379-84.

42. Liu, S., *et al.* "A prospective study of whole-grain intake and risk of type 2 diabetes mellitus in US women." *American Journal of Public Health*, 2000; 90:1409'15.

43. Ruhnau, K.J., *et al.* "Effects of 3-week oral treatment with the antioxidant thiotic acid (alpha-lipoic acid) in symptomatic diabetic polyneuropathy." *Diabet Med*, 1999; 16:1040-43.

44. Reljanovic M, *et al.* "Treatment of diabetic polyneuropathy with the antioxidant thiotic acid (alpha-lipoic acid): a two year multicenter randomized double-blind placebo-controlled trial (ALADIN II). Alpha Lipoic Acid in Diabetic Neuropathy." *Free Radic Res* 1999;31:171-9; Ziegler D, *et al.* "Effects of treatment with the antioxidant alpha-lipoic acid on cardiac autonomic neuropathy in NIDDM patients. A 4-month randomized controlled multicenter trial (DEKAN Study)." *Diabetes Care* 1997;20:369-73; Ziegler D, *et al.* "Treatment of symptomatic diabetic polyneuropathy with the antioxidant alpha-lipoic acid: a 7-month multicenter randomized controlled trial (ALADIN III Study). ALADIN III Study Group. Alpha-Lipoic Acid in Diabetic Neuropathy." *Diabetes Care* 1999;22:1296-301.

45. Jacob, S., *et al.* "Oral administration of RAC-alpha-lipoic acid modulates insulin sensitivity in patients with type-2 diabetes mellitus: a placebo-controlled pilot trial." *Free Radic Biol Med*, 1999; 27:309-14.

46. Feskens, E.J., *et al.* "Dietary factors determining diabetes and impaired glucose tolerance. A 20-year follow-up of the Finnish and Dutch cohorts of the Seven Countries Study." *Diabetes Care*, 1995; 18:1104-12; Feskens, E.J., D. Kromhout. "Habitual dietary intake and glucose tolerance in euglycaemic men: the Zutphen Study." *Int J Epidemiol*, 1990; 19:953-59; Marshall, J.A., *et al.* "Dietary fat predicts conversion from impaired glucose tolerance to NIDDM. The San Luis Valley Diabetes Study." *Diabetes Care*, 1994; 17:50-56; Marshall, J.A., R.F. Hamman, J. Baxter. "High-fat, low-carbohydrate diet and the etiology of non-insulin-dependent diabetes mellitus: the San Luis Valley Diabetes Study." *Am J Epidemiol*, 1991; 134:590-603.

47. Salmeron, J., *et al.* "Dietary fat intake and risk of type 2 diabetes in women." *Am J Clin Nutr*, 2001; 73:1019'26.

48. Salmeron, J., *et al.* "Dietary fat intake and risk of type 2 diabetes in women." *Am J Clin Nutr*, 2001; 73:1019'26; Rivellese, A.A., C. DeNatale, S. Lilli. "Type of dietary fat and insulin resistance." *Ann NY Acad Sci*, 2002; 967:329'35; Uusitupa, M., *et al.* "Effects of two high-fat diets with different fatty acid compositions on glucose and lipid metabolism in healthy young women." *Am J Clin Nutr*, 1994; 59:1310-16; Sarkkinen, E., *et al.* "The effects of monounsaturated-fat enriched diet and polyunsaturated-fat enriched diet on lipid and glucose metabolism in subjects with impaired glucose tolerance." *Eur J Clin Nutr*, 1996; 50:592-98; Garg, A., *et al.* "Comparison of a high-carbohydrate diet with a high-monounsaturated-fat diet in patients with non-insulin dependent diabetes mellitus." *N Engl J Med*, 1988; 319:829-34; Colditz, G.A., *et al.* "Diet and risk of clinical diabetes in women." *Am J Clin Nutr*, 1992; 55:1018'23.

49. Lamson, D.W., S. Plaza. "Mitochondrial factors in the pathogenesis if diabetes: a hypothesis for treatment." *Altern Med Rev*, 2002; 7:94'111.

50. McCarty, M.F. "Can correction of sub-optimal coenzyme Q status improve beta-cell function in type II diabetics?" *Med Hypotheses*, 1999; 52:397'400.

51. Chiu, K.C. "Hypovitaminosis D is associated with insulin resistance and beta cell dysfunction." *Am J Clin Nutr*, 2004; 79:820'25.

52. Hypponen, E., *et al.* "Intake of vitamin D and risk of type 1 diabetes: a birth-cohort study." *Lancet*, 2001; 358:1500'03; Littorin, B., *et al.* "Lower levels of plasma 25-hydroxyvitamin D among young adults at diagnosis of autoimmune type 1 diabetes compared with control subjects: results from the nationwide Diabetes Incidence Study in Sweden (DISS)." *Diabetologia*, 2006; 49:2847'52.

53. Hypponen, E., *et al.* "Intake of vitamin D and risk of type 1 diabetes: a birth-cohort study." *Lancet*, 2001; 358:1500'03.

CHOLESTEROL

Wouldn't it be great if there were a safe, natural way to raise cholesterol?

If you answered yes, you're right. If you answered no, you're also right. How can both answers be right, and how can it be great to raise cholesterol? Because, although everyone talks about cholesterol as if it is one thing, there are actually two kinds of cholesterol: one good and one bad.

Introducing the Cholesterols

When people talk about lowering cholesterol, they are talking about lowering low-density lipoprotein, or LDL, cholesterol. LDL cholesterol is harmful and elevated levels are a risk factor for heart disease. Less talked about are the other bad guys that we want to lower: very low-density, or VLDL, cholesterol and triglycerides. Even more dangerous is the worst cholesterol of them all, the almost never talked about lipoprotein (a), or Lp(a).

But what is even less talked about is that there is also a good cholesterol: high-density lipoprotein, or HDL, cholesterol. We need to stop neglecting this beneficial cholesterol because raising your HDL cholesterol is actually more important for preventing heart disease than lowering your LDL cholesterol is.

Because LDL and VLDL carry cholesterol from your liver to your cells, but HDL carries it from the cells to the liver, where it is broken down and eliminated, LDL contributes to heart disease while HDL prevents it. So the goal—and here's why the answer to our question was yes and no—is to lower your LDL cholesterol while raising your HDL cholesterol. Every single percentage point you can lower your LDL cholesterol reduces your risk of having a heart attack by 2 per cent; every single per cent you can raise your HDL cholesterol reduces your risk of having a heart attack by 3 to 4 per cent[1]. Controlling Lp(a) is even more important because an elevated Lp(a) level is ten times riskier than an elevated LDL cholesterol level for heart disease.

So the natural approach to cholesterol problems goes well beyond taking drugs to lower your LDL cholesterol. It is much more comprehensive, focusing on lowering all the bad guys and raising the good guy.

Nothing's More Important than Diet

By far the most important part of any serious plan for controlling cholesterol is diet. And the most important part of diet is shifting from an animal-based diet toward a plant-based, or vegetarian diet. Vegetarians have lower cholesterol than people who eat meat[2], and vegans have the lowest levels of all[3]. The reasons are simple.

Only foods that come from animals—meat, dairy, and eggs—contain cholesterol. So when you eliminate animal foods from your diet, you stop putting cholesterol into your body. Plant foods, on the other hand, contain no cholesterol and are rich in fibre. Fibre helps eliminate the cholesterol that is already in your body. Animal foods are also high in saturated fat, and eating saturated fat increases cholesterol[4]. Instead of saturated fats, plant foods are rich in heart-healthy unsaturated fats that help to reduce cholesterol.

The overall goal of the cholesterol diet is to heavily reduce or eliminate the saturated fat animal-based foods and to start eating a lot more whole grains, legumes, raw nuts, raw seeds, fruits, and vegetables. You should also eliminate trans fats because they raise your LDL cholesterol and lower your HDL cholesterol. Sugar is also bad because it lowers the beneficial HDL cholesterol[5]

What about eggs? Egg yolks are very high in cholesterol, and eating eggs increases your cholesterol[6], though eating foods high in saturated fat increases cholesterol even more. The real danger of eggs may be that the cholesterol in eggs oxidizes when it is exposed to air or heat, and it is when cholesterol is oxidized that it becomes really dangerous for your heart.

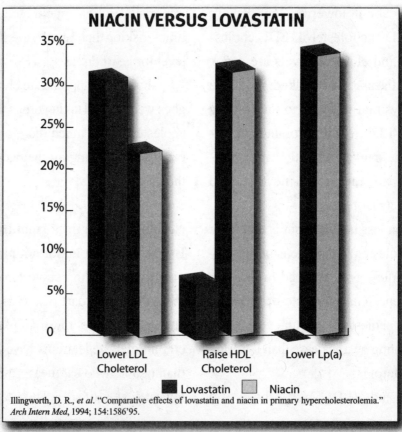

NIACIN VERSUS LOVASTATIN

Illingworth, D. R., *et al*. "Comparative effects of lovastatin and niacin in primary hypercholesterolemia." *Arch Intern Med*, 1994; 154:1586'95.

Soy: A Special Food

Though better known as a food for hormonal conditions such as menopause and breast and prostate cancer, one of the things soy does best is lower cholesterol. In 1995, a meta-analysis of thirty-eight placebo-controlled studies confirmed soy's ability to significantly lower total and LDL cholesterol[7]. Since then, several more double-blind studies have found the same positive result[8]. By replacing animal foods with soy foods, you will improve your cholesterol levels and actually lower your risk of coronary artery disease.

Nuts and Seeds

The often expressed warning that nuts are fattening has given nuts an undeservedly bad rap. Not only are they not fattening, but, along with seeds, they improve cholesterol and reduce the risk of heart disease[9]. Of all the nuts, almonds[10] and walnuts[11] may be the best. But hazelnuts[12], pistachio nuts[13], and pecans have all been shown to help, too. And now a meta-analysis of twenty-five controlled studies has proven once again that nuts are good for controlling cholesterol. The study found that eating nuts lowers total cholesterol by 5.1 per cent and the heart-harmful LDL cholesterol by 7.4 per cent compared to controls. Eating nuts also lowered triglycerides. The benefit was found for several kinds of nuts, including, again, walnuts, almonds, hazelnuts and pistachios[14]. Sesame seeds have also been shown to help[15]. And a meta-analysis of twenty-eight studies has found that adding flaxseed to the diet significantly lowers total cholesterol and LDL cholesterol[16].

Supplements: When You Need More than Diet

When dietary changes are not enough, there is a host of natural supplements that lower LDL cholesterol, and raise HDL cholesterol or both.

One of the simplest things to try is fibre. Of course, the best way to increase fibre is dietary, by moving toward a more vegetarian diet. Of the two basic kinds of fibre, it is the soluble fibre that so effectively lowers cholesterol[17]. One of the easiest and tastiest ways to increase your cholesterol-lowering soluble fibre is by eating oatmeal or oat bran. All kinds of studies show that this simple breakfast change significantly lowers cholesterol[18]. Michael Murray, N.D., says that one bowl of oat bran cereal or oatmeal can lower total cholesterol by 8 to 23 per cent in people with high cholesterol.

Several other sources of soluble fibre have also been shown to improve cholesterol levels, including legumes[19], flaxseeds[20], psyllium[21], pectin[22], and glucomannan[23].

Niacin: Powerful Cholesterol Fighter

Whether you are looking in the drugstore or the health food store, you won't find a more powerful cholesterol fighter than niacin. Niacin looks after all of the good and bad cholesterols that we talked about. It lowers LDL cholesterol, Lp(a), and triglycerides, while it raises the beneficial HDL cholesterol[24].

Just how good is niacin? It's better than the cholesterol-lowering drug lovastatin! When the two went head to head in a study, while lovastatin lowered the bad LDL cholesterol by 32 per cent, compared to niacin's 23 per cent, niacin raised the beneficial HDL cholesterol by a whopping 33 per cent, compared to a meager 7 per cent by lovastatin. Remember, raising HDL is more important than lowering LDL. And while lovastatin had no power over the most dangerous Lp(a), niacin lowered it by a remarkable 35 per cent[25].

A number of studies have duplicated this superiority of niacin over lovastatin and also over the drug gemfibrozil when it comes to raising the heart-healthy HDL cholesterol[26]. In one study, niacin raised the HDL cholesterol by 30 per cent, compared to only 10 per cent by gemfibrozil and 6 per cent by lovastatin.

Two hundred and eight people with, or at high risk of, coronary artery disease who were on statins, had either niacin or a second cholesterol drug added to their statin. The dose of niacin was 500 mg, increased to a maximum of 2,000 mg. There was a significant decrease in atherosclerosis in the niacin group, but no change in the double drug group. And while 5 per cent of the double drug group suffered a major cardiovascular event, only 1 per cent of the niacin group did. Niacin also significantly decreased triglycerides and the bad LDL cholesterol beyond the improvement achieved on statins, and significantly increased the good HDL cholesterol[27].

With numbers like these, it should come as no surprise that niacin has actually been shown to reduce mortality by 11 per cent, compared to a placebo[28].

There are some drawbacks to niacin. It can cause flushing and, more importantly, liver damage. Trying to solve these problems with a time-release formula improved the former, but only made the latter worse. Niacin can also affect glucose tolerance. Therefore, it should not be used by diabetics or people with liver disease. However, it has recently been suggested that the effect of niacin on blood-sugar is minor and that niacin is, in fact, safe for diabetics[29].

And as for niacin's potential liver toxicity, there is a simple solution. A special form of niacin called inositol hexaniacinate is safer, causing no toxicity, and actually works even a little better than ordinary niacin[30]. That makes inositol hexaniacinate the niacin of choice. The dose is 500 mg three times a day for the first two weeks, and then increase to 1,000 mg three times a day after that.

The next three natural cholesterol fighters are truly bizarre!

Sugar Cane Wax Extract

Sounds strange, but it's true. In sugar's only appearance as a healthy plant, an extract of the wax of the sugar cane—if all its claims are true—just may be the best cholesterol fighter of them all, including inositol hexaniacinate.

Sugar cane wax extract has beaten virtually every kind of cholesterol-lowering drug in existence. Sugar cane wax extract lowers LDL cholesterol every bit as well as lovastatin, but while lovastatin actually lowered the beneficial HDL cholesterol in this head-to-head study, sugar cane wax extract raised it by 17 per cent. And while lovastatin is toxic to the liver, sugar cane wax extract is not. The sugar cane wax also had fewer of the other side effects.

Sugar cane wax extract is also better and safer than pravastatin[31] and at least as good as, and safer than, simvastatin[32]. Sugar cane wax trumps not only the statins but also fibrate drugs, probucol[33] and acipimox. In the acipimox study, in addition to benefiting both LDL and HDL cholesterol, sugar cane wax also lowered the dangerous Lp(a) by 32.6 per cent[34].

Sugar cane wax extract should lower LDL cholesterol by 20 to 30 per cent and raise HDL cholesterol by 15 to 25 per cent.

Start by taking 10 mg with dinner. If after two months there is no effect, try taking 20 mg. Sugar cane wax extract is completely safe for diabetics with cholesterol problems[32] and is not toxic to the liver.

Here's the rub, though. Many of these extraordinary studies were done in Cuba—where the sugar cane comes from—or in Russia. Recent studies done outside of these countries have not been able to duplicate these results. Whether sugar cane extract's benefits are trumped-up or whether it is the victim of political assassination awaits determination. Linda has had excellent results in her clinic. But since the herb was always used in conjunction with dietary changes, it is hard to isolate the effectiveness of the sugar cane wax.

Stranger Sounding Still: Gugulipid

If you thought sugar cane wax sounded strange, meet gugulipid, India's ancient answer to cholesterol. Gugulipid is every bit as good as the drugs, without the side effects.

Gugulipid has the ability to lower total cholesterol by 14 to 27 per cent, LDL cholesterol by 25 to 35 per cent, triglycerides by 22 to 30 per cent, and to raise HDL cholesterol by 16 to 20 per cent. Several studies have shown how well it works[35].

The dose of gugulipid is 500 mg, standardized for 25 mg of guggulsterone, three times a day.

Red Yeast Rice: One More Strange Herb

First you ferment the rice with red yeast, then you kill off the yeast, and, presto, you have red yeast rice, an ancient traditional Chinese food and medicine.

The studies on this little known herb have been impressive. Together they show that red yeast rice can lower total cholesterol by 16 to 26 per cent, LDL cholesterol by 21 to 33 per cent, and triglycerides by 20 to 34 per cent, while raising HDL cholesterol by 14 to 20 per cent[37]. In one study, fifty-nine people who were forced to stop taking statins because the drug caused muscle pain and weakness were put on red yeast rice for twenty-four weeks. Both their total and LDL cholesterol went down significantly more than the placebo group's[38]. A recent meta-analysis of ninety-three controlled studies has confirmed red yeast rice's ability to significantly reduce total and LDL cholesterol as well as triglycerides, while raising HDL cholesterol[39].

Try taking 2.4 mg a day in divided doses.

Other Useful Nutrients

Strangely, though vitamin B5 (pantothenic acid) has no beneficial powers against cholesterol, its active form, pantethine, has significant powers[40]. Pantethine can lower total cholesterol by 19 per cent, LDL cholesterol by 21 per cent, and triglycerides by 32 per cent, while raising HDL cholesterol by 23 per cent. It has no toxicity and is safe for diabetics.

Vitamin C lowers LDL cholesterol[41] and protects it from the damage that makes it a danger to the heart[42]. High blood levels of vitamin C have also been shown to lower triglycerides and raise the heart-healthy HDL cholesterol[43]. Vitamin E also protects LDL cholesterol from the damage that makes it a threat.

Better known as the most valuable nutrient for diabetes, the mineral chromium may also be valuable for cholesterol problems. Though not all studies have been positive, several have found chromium to both lower LDL cholesterol[44] and raise HDL cholesterol[45]. Some, but not all, studies have also found that calcium helps[46].

In addition to the major cholesterol herbs discussed above, a number of other herbs can also help. Green tea has wide powers, lowering total, LDL, and VLDL cholesterol and triglycerides, while raising HDL cholesterol[47].

Green tea is not the only delicious way to improve cholesterol. Artichoke helps, too. In a double-blind study, artichoke extract lowered total cholesterol by 18.5 per cent, compared to only 8.6 per cent in the placebo group, and LDL cholesterol by 22.9 per cent, compared to only 6.5 per cent in the placebo group[48]. Artichoke is also able to lower triglycerides[49].

A less expected entry on the cholesterol list is berberine, the active ingredient in goldenseal. Berberine is much better known as a remarkable antimicrobial, but now research has shown berberine to lower cholesterol by an impressive 29 per cent[50]. Berberine has also been shown in at least two studies to lower cholesterol in diabetics[51].

Several other herbs help, as well. In fact, it seems like almost every herb can help with cholesterol. Check out this list: ho shou wu (fo ti), fenugreek, alalfa, ginseng, eleuthero (formerly known as Siberian ginseng), hawthorn, cayenne, cinnamon, devil's claw, licorice, reishi and maitake mushrooms, turmeric, and wild yam.

The Liver and Cholesterol

Since the liver is involved with cholesterol, it is often quite effective to work on defatting the liver to help correct cholesterol problems. Perhaps that is why herbs such as artichoke and goldenseal are effective. Other good liver supplements include the lipotrophic factors; choline, methionine, inositol, and liver herbs such as boldo, milk thistle, dandelion root, and yellow dock.

Lifestyle Changes

Finally, as always, there are some lifestyle changes that can help. While smoking[52] and weight gain[53] lower the healthy HDL cholesterol, exercise raises it[54]. Exercise also lowers total and LDL cholesterol[55]. And, although it sounds strange, eating several small meals a day instead of eating the same amount in three big meals lowers cholesterol.

Chapter Endnotes

1. Wilson, P. W. F. "High-density lipoprotein, low-density lipoprotein and coronary artery disease." *Am J Cardiol*, 1990; 66:7A'10A.

2. Thorogood, M., *et al.* "Plasma lipids and lipoprotein cholesterol concentrations in people with different diets in Britain." *Br Med J*, (Clin Res Ed) 1987; 295:351-53.

3. Resnicow, K., *et al.* "Diet and serum lipids in vegan vegetarians: a model for risk reduction." *J Am Dietet Assoc*, 1991; 91:447-53.

4. Kromhout, D., *et al.* "Dietary saturated and trans fatty acids and cholesterol and 25-year mortality from coronary heart disease: the Seven Countries Study." *Prev Med*, 1995; 24:308-15.

5. Yudkin, J., S. S. Kang, K. R. Bruckdorfer. "Effects of high dietary sugar." *Br Med J*, 1980; 281:1396.

6. Connor, S. L., W. E. Connor. "The importance of dietary cholesterol in coronary heart disease." *Prev Med*, 1983; 12:115-23 [review].

7. Anderson, J. W., B. M. Johnstone, M. E. Cook-Newell. "Meta-analysis of the effects of soy protein intake on serum lipids." *N Engl J Med*, 1995; 3333:276-82.

8. Baum, J. A., *et al.* "Long-term intake of soy protein improves blood lipid profiles and increases mononuclear cell low-density-lipoprotein receptor messenger RNA in hypercholesterolemic, postmenopausal women." *Am J Clin Nutr*, 1998; 68:545-51; Crouse, J. R., 3rd, *et al.* "A randomized trial comparing the effect of casein with that of soy protein containing varying amounts of isoflavones on plasma concentrations of lipids and lipoproteins." *Arch Intern Med*, 1999; 159:2070-76; Sirtori, C. R., *et al.* "Double-blind study of the addition of high-protein soya milk v. cows' milk to the diet of patients with severe hypercholesterolaemia and resistance to or intolerance of statins." *Br J Nutr*, 1999; 82:91-96; Teixeira, S. R., *et al.* "Effects of feeding 4 levels of soy protein for 3 and 6 wk on blood lipids and apolipoproteins in moderately hypercholesterolemic men." *Am J Clin Nutr*, 2000; 71:1077-84.

9. Abbey, M., *et al.* "Partial replacement of saturated fatty acids with almonds or walnuts lowers total plasma cholesterol and low-density-lipoprotein cholesterol." *Am J Clin Nutr*, 1994; 59:995-99; Hu, F. B., M. J. Stampfer. "Nut consumption and risk of coronary heart disease: a review of epidemiologic evidence." *Curr Atheroscler Rep*, 1999; 1:204-09.

10. Spiller, G.A., *et al.* "Effect of a diet high in monounsaturated fat from almonds on plasma cholesterol and lipoproteins." *J Am Coll Nutr*, 1992; 11:126-30; Spiller, G.A., *et al.* "Nuts and plasma lipids: an almond-based diet lowers LDL-C while preserving HDL-C." *J Am Coll Nutr*, 1998; 17:285-90; Jambazian, P.R., *et al.* "Almonds in the diet simultaneously improve plasma alpha-tocopherol concentrations and reduce plasma lipids." *J Am Dietetic Association*, 2005; 105:449'54.

11. Sabaté, J., *et al.* "Effects of walnuts on serum lipid levels and blood pressure in normal men." *N Engl J Med*, 1993; 328:603-07; Zambon, D., *et al.* "Effects of walnuts on the serum lipid profile of hypercholesterolemic subjects: the Barcelona Walnut Trial." *FASEB J*, 1998; 12:A506 [abstract]; Zambon, D., *et al.* "Substituting walnuts for monounsaturated fat improves the serum lipid profile of hypercholesterolemic men and women. A randomized crossover trial." *Ann Intern Med*, 2000; 132:538-46; Rogelio, U. A., *et al.* "Effects of walnut consumption on plasma fatty acids and lipoproteins in combined hyperlipidemia." *Am J Clin Nutr*, 2001; 74:72'79.

12. Durak, I., *et al.* "Hazelnut supplementation enhances plasma antioxidant potential and lowers plasma cholesterol levels." *Clin Chim Actia*, 1999; 284:113-15 [letter].

13. Edwards, K., *et al.* "Effect of pistachio nuts on serum lipid levels in patients with moderate hypercholesterolemia." *J Am Coll Nutr*, 1999; 18:229-32.

14. Sabaté J., *et al.* "Nut Consumption and Blood Lipid Levels: A Pooled Analysis of 25 Intervention Trials." *Arch Intern Med,* 2010; 170:821-27.

15. Chena P. R., *et al.* "Dietary sesame reduces serum cholesterol and enhances antioxidant capacity in hypercholesterolemia." *Nutrition Research* 2005; 25:559-67; Wu W. H., *et al.* "Sesame ingestion affects sex hormones, antioxidant status, and blood lipids in postmenopausal women." *J Nutr 2006,* 136:1270-75.

16. Pan A. *et al.* "Meta-analysis of the effects of flaxseed interventions on blood lipids." *Am J Clin Nutr,* 2009; 90:288-97.

17. Glore, S. R., *et al.* "Soluble fibre and serum lipids: a literature review." *J Am Dietet Assoc,* 1994; 94:425-36.

18. Ripsin, C. M., *et al.* "Oat products and lipid lowering-a meta-analysis." *JAMA,* 1992; 267:3317-25; Romero, A. L., *et al.* "Cookies enriched with psyllium or oat bran lower plasma LDL cholesterol in normal and hypercholesterolemic men from Northern Mexico." *J Am Coll Nutr,* 1998; 17:601-08; Uusitupa, M. I., *et al.* "A controlled study on the effect of beta-glucan-rich oat bran on serum lipids in hypercholesterolemic subjects: relation to apolipoprotein E phenotype." *J Am Coll Nutr,* 1992; 11:651-59; Braaten, J. T., *et al.* "Oat beta-glucan reduces blood cholesterol concentration in hypercholesterolemic subjects." *Eur J Clin Nutr,* 1994; 48:465-74; Davidson, M. H., *et al.* "The hypocholesterolemic effects of beta-glucan in oatmeal and oat bran. A dose-controlled study." *JAMA,* 1991; 265:1833-39.

19. Anderson, J.W., W.J.L. Chen. "Legumes and their soluble fibre: effect on cholesterol-rich lipoproteins." In: *Furda, I., ed. Unconventional Sources of Dietary Fibre. Washington, DC: American Chemical Society,* 1983.

20. Bierenbaum, M. L., R. Reichstein, T. R. Watkins. "Reducing atherogenic risk in hyperlipemic humans with flaxseed supplementation: a preliminary report." *J Am Coll Nutr,* 1993; 12:501-04; Cunnane, S. C., *et al.* "High alpha-linolenic acid flaxseed (Linum usitatissimum): some nutritional properties in humans." *Br J Nutr,* 1993; 69:443-53; Arjmandi, B. H., *et al.* "Whole flaxseed consumption lowers serum LDL-cholesterol and lipoprotein(a) concentrations in postmenopausal women." *Nutr Res,* 1998; 18:1203-14.

21. Romero, A. L., *et al.* "Cookies enriched with psyllium or oat bran lower plasma LDL cholesterol in normal and hypercholesterolemic men from Northern Mexico." *J Am Coll Nutr,* 1998;.17:601-08; Anderson, J. W., *et al.* "Cholesterol-lowering effects of psyllium intake adjunctive to diet therapy in men and women with hypercholesterolemia: meta-analysis of 8 controlled trials." *Am J Clin Nutr,* 2000; 71:472-79; Olson, B. H., *et al.* "Psyllium-enriched cereals lower blood total cholesterol and LDL cholesterol, but not HDL cholesterol, in hypercholesterolemic adults: results of a meta-analysis." *J Nutr,* 1997; 127:1973-80.

22. Miettinen, T. A., S. Tarpila. "Effect of pectin on serum cholesterol, fecal bile acids and biliary lipids in normolipidemic and hyperlipidemic individuals." *Clin Chim Acta,* 1977; 79:471-77.

23. Walsh, D. E., V. Yaghoubian, A. Behforooz. "Effect of glucomannan on obese patients: a clinical study." *Int J Obes,* 1984; 8:289-93; Zhang, M.Y., *et al.* "The effect of foods containing refined Konjac meal on human lipid metabolism." *Biomed Environ Sci,* 1990; 3:99-105; Arvill, A., L. Bodin. "Effect of short-term ingestion of konjac glucomannan on serum cholesterol in healthy men." *Am J Clin Nutr,* 1995; 61:585-89; Vuksan, V., *et al.* "Konjac-mannan (glucomannan) improves glycemia and other associated risk factors for coronary heart disease in type 2 diabetes. A randomized controlled metabolic trial." *Diabetes Care,* 1999; 22:913-19.

24. DiPalma, J. R., W. S. Thayer. "Use of niacin as a drug." *Annu Rev Nutr,* 1991; 11:169'87.

25. Illingworth, D. R., *et al.* "Comparative effects of lovastatin and niacin in primary hypercholesterolemia." *Arch Intern Med,* 1994; 154:1586'95.

26. Guyton, J. R., *et al.* "Extended-release niacin vs gemfibrozil for the treatment of low levels of high-density lipoprotein cholesterol. Niaspan-Gemfibrozil Study Group." *Arch Intern Med,* 2000; 160:1177-84; Vega, G. L., S. M. Grundy. "Lipoprotein responses to treatment with lovastatin, gemfibrozil, and nicotinic acid in normolipidemic patients with hypoalphalipoproteinemia." *Arch Intern Med,* 1994; 154:73'82.

27. Taylor A. J., *et al.* "Extended-release niacin or ezetimibe and carotid intima-media thickness." *N Engl J Med* 2009; 361:2113-22.

28. Canner, P. L., *et al.* "Fifteen year mortality in Coronary Drug Patients: Long-term benefits with niacin." *J Am Coll Cardiol,* 1986; 8:1245'55.

29. Guyton, J. R., H. E. Bays. "Safety considerations with niacin therapy." *Am J Cardiol,* 2007; 99:22C'31C.

30. Welsh, A. L., M. Ede. "Inositol hexaniocotinate for improved nicotinic acid therapy." *Int Record Med,* 1961; 174:9'15; El-Enein, A. M. A., *et al.* "The role of nicotinic acid and inositol hexaniacinate as anticholesterolemic and antilipemic agents." *Nutr Rep Intl,* 1983; 28:899'911; Sunderland, G. T., *et al.* "A double-blind randomized placebo controlled trial of hexopal in primary Raynaud's disease." *Clin Rheumatol,* 1988; 7:46'49.

31. Benitez, M., *et al.* "A comparative study of policosanol versus pravastatin in patients with type II hypercholesterolemia." *Curr Ther Res Clin Exp,* 1997; 58:859'67; Castano, G., *et al.* "Effects of policosanol and parvastatin on lipid profile, platelet aggregation and endothelemia in older hypercholesterolemic patients." *Int J Clin Pharmacol Res,* 1999; 29:105'16.

32. Illnait, J., *et al.* "A comparative study on the efficacy and tolerability of policosanol and simvastatin for treating type II hypercholesterolemia." *Can J Cardiol,* 1997; 13:342B.

33. Pons, P., *et al.* "A comparative study of policosanol versus probucol in patients with hypercholesterolemia." *Curr Ther Res Clin Exp,* 1997; 58:26'35.

34. Alcocer, L., *et al.* "A comparative study of policosanol versus acipimox in patients with type II hypercholesterolemia." *Int J Tissue React,* 1999; 21:85'92.

35. Torres, O., *et al.* "Treatment of hypercholesterolemia in NIDDIM with policosanol." *Diabetes Care,* 1995; 18:393'97; Crespo, N., *et al.* "Effects of policosanol on patients with non-insulin-dependent diabetes mellitus and hypercholesterolemia: a pilot study." *Curr Ther Res Clin Exp,* 1997; 58:44'51; Crespo, N., *et al.* "Comparative study of the efficacy and tolerability of policosanol and lovastatin in patients with hypercholesterolemia and noninsulin dependent diabetes mellitus." *Int J Clin Pharmacol Res,* 1999; 29:117'27.

36. Agarwal, R.C., *et al.* "Clinical trial of gugulipid new hypolipidemic agent of plant origin in primary hyperlipidemia." *Indian J Med Res,* 1986; 84:626-34; Nityanand, S., J. S. Srivastava, O. P. Asthana. "Clinical trials with Gugulipid-a new hypolipidemic agent." *J Assoc Phys India,* 1989; 37:323-28; Tripathi, S. N., B. N. Upadhyay. "A clinical trial of Commiphora mukul in the patients of ischaemic heart disease." *Journal of Molecular and Cellular Cardiology,* 1978; 10 (Supp 1):124.

37. Wang, J., *et al.* "Multicenter clinical trial of the serum lipid-lowering effects of a Monascus purpureus (red yeast) rice preparation from traditional Chinese medicine." *Curr Ther Res,* 1997; 58:964'78; Heber, D., *et al.* "Cholesterol-lowering effects of a proprietary Chinese red-yeast-rice dietary supplement." *Am J Clin Nutr,* 1999; 69:231'36; Rippe, J., K. Bonovich, H. Colfer. "A multi-center, self-controlled study of Cholestinin subjects with elevaqted cholesterol." 39th Annual Conference on Cardiovascular Disease Epidemiology and Prevention. Orlando, FL, 1999; March 24'27:1123.

38. Becker D. J., *et al.* "Red Yeast Rice for Dyslipidemia in Statin-Intolerant Patients: A Randomized Trial." *Ann Intern Med,* 2009; 150:830-39.

39. Liu, J., *et al.* "Chinese red yeast rice (Monascus purpureus) for primary hyper-

lipidemia: a meta-analysis of randomized controlled trials." *Chin Med*, 2006; 1:4.

40. Arsenio, L., *et al*. "Effectiveness of long-term treatment with pantethine in patients with dyslipidemia." *Clin Ther*, 1986; 8:537-45; Prisco, D., *et al*. "Effect of oral treatment with pantethine on platelet and plasma phospholipids in IIa hyperlipoproteinemia." *Angiology*, 1987; 38:241-47; Gaddi, A., *et al*. "Controlled evaluation of pantethine, a natural hypolipidemic compound, in patients with different forms of hyperlipoproteinemia." *Atherosclerosis*, 1984; 50:73-83.

41. Simon, J. A. "Vitamin C and cardiovascular disease: a review." *J Am Coll Nutr*, 1992; 11:107-27; Gatto, L.M., *et al*. "Ascorbic acid induces a favorable lipoprotein profile in women." *J Am Coll Nutr*, 1996; 15;154-58.

42. Frei, B. "Ascorbic acid protects lipids in human plasma and low-density lipoprotein against oxidative damage." *Am J Clin Nutr*, 1991; 54:1113-8S.[is this correct?]

43. Hallfrisch, J., *et al*. "High plasma vitamin C associated with high plasma HDL- and HDL2 cholesterol." *Am J Clin Nutr*, 1994; 60:100'05.

44. Press, R. I., J. Geller, G. W. Evans. "The effect of chromium picolinate on serum cholesterol and apolipoprotein fractions in human subjects." *West J Med*, 1990; 152:41-45; Hermann, J., *et al*. "Effects of chromium or copper supplementation on plasma lipids, plasma glucose and serum insulin in adults over age fifty." *J Nutr Elderly*, 1998; 18:27-45.

45. Riales, R., M. J. Albrink. "Effect of chromium chloride supplementation on glucose tolerance and serum lipids including high-density lipoprotein of adult men." *Am J Clin Nutr*, 1981; 34:2670-78; Roeback, J.R., *et al*. "Effects of chromium supplementation on serum high-density lipoprotein cholesterol levels in men taking beta-blockers." *Ann Intern Med*, 1991; 115:917-24.

46. Bell, L., *et al*. "Cholesterol-lowering effects of calcium carbonate in patients with mild to moderate hypercholesterolemia." *Arch Intern Med*, 1992; 152:2441-44; Karanja, N., C. D. Morris, D. R. Illingworth. "Plasma lipids and hypertension: response to calcium supplementation." *Am J Clin Nutr*, 1987; 45:60-65.

47. Kono, S., *et al*. "Green tea consumption and serum lipid profiles: a cross-sectional study in Northern Kyushu, Japan." *Prev Med*, 1992; 21:526-31; Sagesaka-Mitane, Y., M. Milwa, S. Okada. "Platelet aggregation inhibitors in hot water extract of green tea." *Chem Pharm Bull*, 1990; 38(3):790-93; Stensvold, I., *et al*. "Tea consumption. Relationship to cholesterol, blood pressure, and coronary and total mortality." *Prev Med*, 1992; 21:546-53; Imai, K., K. Nakachi. "Cross sectional study of effects of drinking green tea on cardiovascular and liver diseases." *BMJ*, 1995; 310:693'96; Kono, S., *et al*. "Green tea consumption and serum lipid profiles: a cross-sectional study in northern Kyushu, Japan." *Prev Med*, 1992; 21:526'31.

48. Englisch, W., *et al*. "Efficacy of artichoke dry extract in patients with hyperlipoproteinemia." *Arzneimittelforschung*, 2000; 50:260-65.

49. Fintelmann, V. "Antidyspeptic and lipid-lowering effect of artichoke leaf extract." *Zeitschirfit fur Allgemeinmed*, 1996; 72:1-19.

50. Kong, W., *et al*. "Berberine is a novel cholesterol-lowering drug working through a unique mechanism distinct from statins." *Nat Med*, 2004; 10:1344-51.

51. Zhang Y., *et al*. "Treatment of Type 2 Diabetes and Dyslipidemia with the Natural Plant Alkaloid Berberine." *J Clin Endocrinol Metab*, 2008;93:2559-65; Yin J., Xing J., J., Ye "Efficacy of berberine in patients with type 2 diabetes mellitus." *Metab Clin Exp*, 2008; 57:712-27.

52. Dwyer, J. H., *et al*. "Low-level cigarette smoking and longitudinal change in serum cholesterol among adolescents." *JAMA*, 1988; 2857-62.

53. Glueck, C. J., *et al*. "Plasma high-density lipoprotein cholesterol: association with measurements of body mass: the Lipid Research Clinics Program Prevalence Study." *Circulation*, 1980; 62(Suppl IV):IV62-69.

54. Reaven, P. D., *et al*. "Leisure time exercise and lipid and lipoprotein levels in an older population." *J Am Geriatr Soc*, 1990; 38:847-54; Duncan, J. J., N. F. Gordon, C. B. Scott. "Women walking for health and fitness-how much is enough?" *JAMA*, 1991; 266:3295-99.

55. Tran, Z. V., A. Weltman. "Differential effects of exercise on serum lipid and lipoprotein levels seen with changes in body weight: a meta-analysis." *JAMA*, 1985; 254:919-24.

56. Edelstein, S. L., *et al*. "Increased meal frequency associated with decreased cholesterol concentrations; Rancho Bernardo, CA, 1984-1987." *Am J Clin Nutr*, 1992; 55:664-69; Jenkins, D. J. A., *et al*. "Effect of nibbling versus gorging on cardiovascular risk factors: serum uric acid and blood lipids." *Metabolism*, 1995; 44:549-55.

CONGESTIVE HEART FAILURE

Congestive heart failure is a serious problem that occurs when the heart is no longer able to do its job of pumping blood effectively.

Since the three most important heart supplements are probably hawthorn, coenzyme Q10 and magnesium, it is no surprise to find that all of them are important for congestive heart failure.

Hawthorn

Hawthorn is the most amazing and versatile of all the heart herbs, and it may just be the most exciting of all the congestive-heart-failure remedies. Many double-blind studies show that hawthorn makes the heart pump more efficiently[1], and a meta-analysis confirms hawthorn's significant benefit[2]. Most excitingly, while these studies were done on stage II congestive heart failure, placebo-controlled research now shows that hawthorn even works on the more severe stage III congestive heart failure[3]. One study found that hawthorn works at least as well as the ACE inhibitor captopril[4]. Studies in stages I and II have used 900 mg of hawthorn extract. For the more severe stage III, the dose is 1800 mg.

Coenzyme Q10

Another powerful and versatile heart nutrient is coenzyme Q10. CoQ10 is important for virtually any kind of heart problem, including congestive heart failure. CoQ10 is often deficient in people with congestive heart failure. Though not every study has found a benefit for congestive heart failure, several double-blind studies have found it to be effective[5], including an analysis of eight controlled studies[6]. Many CoQ10 studies have used it in conjunction with conventional medications. Most studies have used 100 mg to 200 mg a day. A good way to dose CoQ10 is to take 2 mg for each kilogram of body weight.

Magnesium

Magnesium is another crucial heart nutrient that is often deficient in people with congestive heart failure. People with congestive heart failure who have normal magnesium levels have 71 per cent one-year survival rates, and 61 per cent two-year survival rates, compared to 45 per cent and 42 per cent for those with lower levels of magnesium[7]. As you can see, magnesium is very important. Even if you are on medication for congestive heart failure, you should consider adding magnesium for two reasons. The first is that magnesium boosts the postitive effects of the meds[8], and the second is that supplementing magnesium prevents the arrhythmias caused by the magnesium-depleting effect of congestive-heart-failure drugs.

Another nutrient that addresses deficiencies caused by congestive heart failure drugs is vitamin B1. Furosemide (lasix), a drug commonly used in congestive heart failure, causes B1 deficiencies. Adding 200 mg to 240 mg of B1 a day to congestive heart failure regimens has been shown to lead to improvements[9].

Amino Acids

People with congestive heart failure are low in L-carnitine[10], and several double-blind studies have shown that supplelmenting L-carnitine improves heart function in people with congestive heart failure. The amount of time people with congestive heart failure are able to exercise and the amount of blood the heart is able to pump with each beat increases when they are given a form of carnitine called propionyl-L-carnitine[11]. The dose of L-carnitine is 500 mg two to three times a day.

Two other amino acids, arginine and taurine, have also been shown to help. Because taurine increases the force of the heart muscle's contraction, it helps correct congestive heart failure[12]. The dose is 2 g, three times a day: 5.6 g to 12.6 g a day of arginine has also been shown in double-blind research to be of value in congestive heart failure[13].

Berberine

One surprising congestive-heart-failure remedy is the herb goldenseal. Way better known as a powerful antimicrobial herb. A double-blind study tried adding either berberine—an active ingredient in goldenseal—or a placebo to the conventional treatment for congestive heart failure. After eight weeks on 300 mg to 500 mg of berberine four times a day, there was significantly greater improvement in heart function, arrhythmias and exercise capacity than on the placebo. Even more importantly, there were significantly fewer deaths in the berberine group during the long-term follow-up[14].

More Heart Help

Other herbs that might help incude *coleus forskohlii* and ginseng. An extract from an obscure herb from India called arjuna bark has been shown in double-blind research to significantly help people with congestive heart failure[15], and herbalist David Hoffmann calls linden and garlic, along with hawthorn, essential.

Though too much exercise is dangerous for people with congestive heart failure, appropriate, supervised exercise is helpful[16]. And one last caution to be aware of: Though the study didn't look at low-dose aspirin (which has its own risks), nonsteroidal anti-inflammatory drugs seem to significantly increase the risk of congestive heart failure[17].

Chapter Endnotes

1. Schmidt, V., *et al*. "Efficacy of the Hawthorn (Crataegus) preparation LI 132 in 78 patients with chronic congestive heart failue defined as NYHA functional class II." *Phytomed*, 1994; 1:17'24; Weikl, A., *et al*. "Crataegus extract WS 1442. Evidence-based evaluation of its effect on patients with Stage II congestive heart failure (NYHA II)." *Fortschr Med*, 1996; 114:291'96; Degenring, F. H., *et al*. "A randomised double-blind placebo controlled clinical trial of a standardised extract of fresh Crataegus berries (Crataegisan®) in the treatment of patients with congestive heart failure NYHA II." *Phytomed*, 2003; 10:363'69.

2. Pittler, M. H., R., Guo, E.,Ernst, "Hawthorn extract for treating chronic heart failure." *Cochrane Database of Systematic Reviews*, 2008; 1: Art No.: CD005312.

3. Tauchert, M. "Efficacy and safety of *Crataegus* extract WS 1442 in comparison with placebo in patients with chronic state New York Heart Association class-III heart failure." *American Heart Journal*, 2002; 143:910'15.

4. Tauchert, M., M. Ploch, W. Hubner. "Efficacy of Hawthorn extract LI 132 in comparison with Captopril. Double-blind, multicentre study involving 1332 patients with stage II congestive heart failure (NYHA II)." *Munch Med Wschr*, 1994; 136(Suppl 1):S27'33.

5. Hofman-Bang, C., N. Renquist, K. Swedberg. "Coenzyme Q10 as an adjunctive treatment of congestive heart failure." *J Am Coll Cardiol*, 1992; 19:216A; Morisco, C., B. Trimarco, M. Condorelli. "Effect of coenzyme Q10 therapy in patients with congestive heart failure: a long-term multicenter randomized study." *Clin Investig*, 1993; 71(Suppl 8):S134'6; Baggio, E., *et al*. "Italian multicenter study of the safety and efficacy of coenzyme Q10 as adjunctive therapy in heart failure. CoQ10 Drug Surveillance Investigators." *Mol Aspects Med*, 1994; 15(Suppl):S287'94.

6. Soja, A. M., S. A. Mortensen. "Treatment of chronic cardiac insufficiency with coenzyme Q10, results of meta-analysis in controlled clinical trials." *Ugeskr Laeger*, 1997; 159:7302-08.

7. Gottlieb, S. S., *et al*. "Prognostic importance of serum magnesium concentrations in patients with congestive heart failure." *J Am Coll Cardiol*, 1990; 16:827'31.

8. Gottlieb, S. S. "Imporance of magnesium in congestive heart failure." *Am J Cardiol*, 1989; 63:39G'42G.

9. Leslie, D., M. Gheorghiade. "Is there a role for thiamine supplementation in the management of heart failure?" *Am Heart J*, 1996; 131:1248'50.

10. Suzuki, Y., *et al*. "Myocardial carnitine deficiency in chronic heart failure." *Lancet*, 1982; i:116 (letter).

11. Mancini, M., *et al*. "Controlled study on the therapeutic efficacy of propionyl-L-carnitine in patients with congestive heart failure." *Arzneimittelforschung*, 1992; 42:1101-04; Pucciarelli, G., *et al*. "The clinical and hemodynamic effects of propionyl-L-carnitine in the treatment of congestive heart failure." *Clin Ther*, 1992; 141:379-84.

12. Azuma, J., *et al*. "Taurine for treatment of congestive heart failure." *Int J Cardiol*, 1982; 2:303-04; Azuma, J., *et al*. "Double-blind randomized crossover trial of taurine in congestive heart failure." Curr Ther Res, 1983; 34(4):543-57; Azuma, J., *et al*. "Therapy of congestive heart failure with orally administered taurine." *Clin Ther*, 1983; 5(4):398-408; Azuma, J., *et al*. "Taurine and failing heart: experimental and clinical aspects." *Prog Clin Biol Res*, 1985; 179:195-213.

13. Rector, T. S., *et al*. "Randomized, double-blind, placebo-controlled study of supplemental oral L-arginine in patients with heart failure." *Circulation*, 1996; 93:2135'41.

14. Zeng, X. H., X. J. Zeng, Y. Y. Li. "Efficacy and safety of berberine for congestive heart failure secondary to ischemic or idiopathic dilated cardiomyopathy." *Am J Cardiol*, 2003; 92:173-76.

15. Bharani, A., A. Ganguly, K. Bhargava. "Salutory effect of Terminalia arjuna in patients with severe refractory heart failure." *Int J Cardiol*, 1995; 49:191'99.

16. Coats, A. J. S. "Effects of physical training in chronic heart failure." Lancet, 1990; 335:63-66; Belardinelli, R., *et al*. "Randomized, controlled trial of long-term moderate exercise training in chronic heart failure." *Circulation*, 1999; 99:1173-82; Oka, R. K., *et al*. "Impact of a home-based walking and resistance training program on quality of life in patients with heart failure." *Am J Cardiol*, 2000; 85:365-69.

17. Page, J., D. Henry. "Consumption of NSAIDs and the development of congestive heart failure in elderly patients." *Arch Intern Med*, 2000; 160:777-84.

EYE DISEASES

Sight is one of the most beautiful gifts that there is. And most people would do everything they could to prevent or slow down the progression or prevent visual impairment and blindness. Fortunately, nature has a lot to offer three of the most significant diseases of the eyes: cataracts, glaucoma, and macular degeneration.

CATARACTS

Free Radicals and Antioxidants

Cataracts cloud the normally transparent lenses of the eye and are the most common cause of impaired vision and blindness. Most people over the age of sixty have some degree of cataracts, so prevention becomes important for everyone.

The leading cause of cataracts is free-radical damage, and the leading preventers of cataracts are the antioxidants that fight free radicals. That is why people who eat a lot of foods rich in vitamins C and E, carotenes, and selenium have a much lower risk of developing cataracts. So, eating lots of fruits and vegetables is the first prescription for healthy eyes. Studies show that if you have low levels of antioxidants and if you eat few antioxidant-rich fruits and vegetables, then you have a high risk of developing cataracts[1].

You also increase your risk for cataracts if your diet is high in fat and salt[2]. Donald Brown, N.D., suggests avoiding fried foods and animal products, including milk

There are also nondietary risk factors for cataracts. Smokers are more likely to develop cataracts, as are people who have used steroids for a long time.

Just as a diet rich in antioxidants is important for fighting cataracts, the supplements that help the most are antioxidants. Supplements probably cannot reverse advanced cataracts, but it is possible for them to reverse cataracts in the early stages, and they can stop the progress.

Stopping Cataracts with Vitamin C

Vitamin C is one of the most important antioxi-

FOOD SOURCES OF LUTEIN, ZEAXANTHIN AND LYCOPENE

Lutein	Zeaxanthin	Lycopene
Spinach, kale, collard greens, also corn, potato, carrot, tomato, fruit	Spinach, kale, collard greens also paprika, corn, fruit	Tomato, watermelon, pink grapefruit also carrot, green pepper, apricot

dants, so it is no surprise that it can help fight cataracts. Several studies show that vitamin C can stop the progress of cataracts and sometimes can even significantly improve vision. A 1939 study found that vitamin C could significantly reduce the development of cataracts. During the long eleven-year study, most of the people on vitamin C had no progression of their cataracts and few needed surgery, though similar cases usually do[3].

Vitamin C can help if you already have cataracts, but what if you don't? Take it anyway. Several studies have shown that people who supplement vitamin C are at lower risk for developing cataracts[4]. Murray and Pizzorno suggest using 1g of vitamin C three times per day.

Selenium and Vitamin E

Other antioxidants are also important. One major risk factor for cataracts is low levels of selenium. Selenium levels in the lenses of the eyes of people with cataracts are only 15 per cent of normal[5], so taking selenium is a good idea. Vitamin E and selenium work closely together. So it is not surprising to find that supplementing vitamin E protects against cataracts[6].

Lutein and Zeaxanthin

Carotenes are also important. They protect the lens of the eye against damage from light. People who eat a lot of spinach and kale (a delicious and underused health food), which is rich in the carotenes zeaxanthin and lutein, have a lower risk for developing cataracts[7]. And when people who got the most lutein and zeaxanthin in their diet were compared with the people who got the least, they were found to have only half the risk of developing cataracts[8]. A small placebo-controlled study found that lutein could actually significantly improve vision in people with cataracts. Eighty per cent of the lutein group suffered no progress in their cataracts over two years, compared to only 20 per cent in the placebo group[9]. Try using mixed carotenes for optimal protection.

Making Superoxide Dismutase

Zinc, copper, and manganese are not usually at the top of the list of antioxidants. But they are important components of the antioxidant superoxide dismutase (SOD); which decreases in the eyes as cataracts increase. Taking SOD as a supplement does not help to raise SOD levels, but taking zinc, copper, and manganese does.

Bilberry: Eye Herb Supreme

Herbally, the most promising cataract fighter is the superstar eye herb, bilberry. In one study, bilberry and vitamin E stopped the progression of cataracts in an amazing 48 out of 50 people[10].

You can also try taking quercetin and B3 for cataracts. As a preventative for cataracts, herb authority James Duke, Ph.D., suggests infusing a herbal tea made from the antioxidant-rich herbs catnip and rosemary, and says that you might also add some lemon balm, ginger, and turmeric.

GLAUCOMA

Like cataracts, glaucoma is a leading cause of blindness. Glaucoma is a condition caused by increased pressure within the eyeball. The focus in treating glaucoma is on improving collagen, which keeps the tissue of the eye strong and intact, and on reducing pressure in the eye.

As in treating cataracts, vitamin C and bilberry are crucial.

Vitamin C and Bilberry Again

Vitamin C is perfectly suited to treating glaucoma because it addresses both of the goals of glaucoma treatment. It is crucial for the manufacture of collagen and it reduces pressure in the eyeball. Seven studies have looked at whether vitamin C can significantly reduce pressure in the eyeball in people with glaucoma, and six of them have confirmed that it does[11].

And don't forget bilberry. Bilberry is rich in flavonoids called anthocyanosides, which not only increase vitamin C levels, but strengthen collagen in their own right. Bilberry has actually been shown to improve vision in people with glaucoma[12].

Like bilberry, the herb Ginkgo Biloba is rich in proanthocyanidin flavonoids. At least two studies have shown ginkgo to help glaucoma[13].

Improving Vision with Minerals: Magnesium and Chromium

Other good choices for treating glaucoma include the minerals magnesium and chromium. One study found that when people with glaucoma were given 121.5 mg of magnesium twice a day for a month, their vision improved, though the improvement did not quite reach statistical significance[14]. And another study found that deficiencies of vitamin C or chromium were associated with increased pressure in the eyeball[15].

A 1979 study that found that people with glaucoma usually have lower blood levels of vitamin B1[16].

Avoid Allergens and Corticosteroids

There are also two notable things to avoid if you have glaucoma. One is any food you are allergic to. Every single person in a 1964 study suffered an immediate rise in pressure in the eyeball when exposed to an allergen[17]. So find out what you are allergic to and avoid it. The other thing to avoid is corticosteroids. Corticosteroids inhibit the synthesis of collagen, causing glaucoma to develop.

MACULAR DEGENERATION? MACULAR REGENERATION!

Sound too good to be true? Well, there is actually reason to believe that diet and supplements can prevent, stop, and perhaps even reverse macular degeneration.

While less well-known than cataracts or glaucoma, macular degeneration is one of the leading causes of blindness in people over fifty-five. The macula is the area of the retina responsible for fine vision. If it degenerates, central vision (but not peripheral) and fine details degenerate with it. There are many things that can contribute to macular degeneration, and each of them must be addressed if they are involved. Smoking, atherosclerosis, high blood pressure, and diabetes are all risk factors. Free-radical damage and reduced blood and oxygen supply lead to macular degeneration, and each of these factors can contribute to those causes.

Eat Lots of Fruits and Vegetables

In preventing and treating macular degeneration, diet is one of the most important factors to start with, and that diet has to be rich in fruits and vegetables. Studies have found that such diets, because of their wealth of antioxidants, reduce the risk of macular degeneration[18]. One group of antioxidants stands out—a group of carotenes that includes lutein, zeaxanthin, and lycopene and that has been found to be especially powerful.

Lutein, Zeaxanthin and Lycopene

One study reported in the *Journal of the American Medical Association* found that people who ate the most lutein and zeaxanthin had a remarkable 57 per cent lower risk of macular degeneration than people who ate the least[19]. Collard greens, spinach, and kale are all good sources of lutein and zeaxanthin. Lutein and zeaxanthin concentrate in the macula and, by protecting it from free-radical damage, protect it from macular degeneration. Another study found that lutein can not only prevent macular degeneration, but also significantly improve your vision if you have it[20].

And don't forget lycopene. Though better known for preventing prostate cancer, this carotene, found abundantly in tomato, watermelon, and pink grapefruit, also prevents macular degeneration. People with the least lycopene are twice as likely to develop macular degeneration[21].

Antioxidant Protection

The more well-known antioxidants also help prevent macular degeneration. One study found lower risk of macular degeneration in people with the highest levels of antioxidants in their blood[22]; another found a 70 per cent lower risk of macular degeneration in people with the highest levels of selenium and vitamins C and E[23]. When over four thousand people aged fifty-five or more who did not have macular degeneration were followed for fourteen years, the ones who got more vitamin C, vitamin E, beta-carotene, and zinc in their diet were 35 per cent less likely to develop macular degeneration[24].

Herbs for the Eyes

Another group of antioxidants that really stands out for the prevention and treatment of macular degeneration is the flavonoids, and the best choices here are three flavonoid-rich herbs: bilberry, grape seed, and ginkgo biloba.

These herbs address both causes of macular degeneration: free radical damage and reduced blood and oxygen supply. The flavonoids they supply are powerful antioxidants, and they help blood flow to the retina. Several studies have proven the ability of all of these herbs to stop the progression of the loss of sight due to macular degeneration and perhaps even to improve vision again. According to one study, ginkgo biloba may reverse damage in the retina[25].

Bilberry: The Vision Herb

Though all three of these herbs are great for the eyes, the best may be bilberry. The flavonoids in this herb have a particular affinity for the part of the retina affected by macular degeneration. Bilberry also strengthens the capillaries in the retina, which also helps slow macular degeneration. One herb expert recommends a tea that blends bilberry with butcher's broom, gotu kola, and ginger. Butcher's broom and gotu kola are both good herbs for increasing circulation and strengthening capillaries, and ginger is an effective herb for circulation.

Avoid fried and grilled foods in order to avoid additional free radicals. Eat plenty of legumes and fruits and vegetables, especially berries that are loaded in flavonoids, such as blueberries, blackberries, cranberries, and cherries.

The Latest Research

The latest research has added two more macular degeneration supplements: vitamin D and omega-3 essential fatty acids. Researchers have now found that people with the highest levels of vitamin D in the blood are 36 per cent less likely to have macular degeneration than people with the lowest levels[26]. And several studies are now linking omega-3 essential fatty acids to reduced risk of macular degeneration.

Chapter Endnotes

1. Jacques, P. F., L. T. Chylack, Jr. "Epidemiologic evidence of a role for the antioxidant vitamins and carotenoids in cataract prevention." *Am J Clin Nutr*, 1991; 53:352S-55S; Knekt, P., *et al*. "Serum antioxidant vitamins and risk of cataract." *BMJ*, 1992; 305:1392-94.

2. Tavani, A., *et al*. "Food and nutrient intake and risk of cataract." *Ann Epidem*, 1996; 6:41'46.

3. Bouton, S. "Vitamin C and the aging eye." *Arch Int Med*, 1939; 63:930'45.

4. Jacques, P. F., L. T. Chylack, Jr. "Epidemiologic evidence of a role for the antioxidant vitamins and carotenoids in cataract prevention." *Am J Clin Nutr*, 1991; 53:352S-55S; Jacques, P. F., *et al*. "Antioxidant status in persons with and without senile cataract." *Arch Ophthalmol*, 1988; 106:337-40; Robertson, J. McD., A. P. Donner, J. R. Trevithick. "A possible role for vitamins C and E in cataract prevention." *Am J Clin Nutr*, 1991; 53:346S-51S; Hankinson, S. E., *et al*. "Nutrient intake and cataract extraction in women: a prospective study." *BMJ*, 1992; 305:335-39; Jacques, P. F., *et al*. "Long-term vitamin C supplement use and prevalence of early age-related lens opacities." *Am J Clin Nutr*, 1997; 66:911-16.

5. Swanson, A., A. Truesdale. "Elemental analysis in normal and cataractous human lens tissue." *Biochem Biophys Res Comm*, 1971; 45:1488'96.

6. Robertson, J. McD., A.P. Donner, J.R. Trevithick. "A possible role for vitamins C and E in cataract prevention." *Am J Clin Nutr*, 1991; 53:346S-51S; Leske, M.C., *et al*. "Antioxidant vitamins and nuclear opacities. The Longitudinal Study of Cataract." *Ophthalmology*, 1998; 105:831-36.

7. Hankinson, S. E., *et al*. "Nutrient intake and cataract extraction in women: a prospective study." *BMJ*, 1992; 305:335-39; Chasan-Taber, L., *et al*. "A prospective study of carotenoid and vitamin A intakes and risk of cataract extraction in U.S. women." *Am J Clin Nutr*, 1999;.70:509-16.

8. Lyle, B.J., *et al*. "Antioxidant intake and risk of incident age-related nuclear cataracts in the Beaver Dam Eye Study." *Am J Epidemiol*, 1999; 149:801-09.

9. Olmedilla, B., *et al*. "Lutein, but not alpha-tocopherol, supplementation improves visual function in patients with age-related cataracts: a 2-y double-blind, placebo-controlled pilot study." *Nutrition*, 2003; 19:21-24.

10. Bravetti, G. "Preventive medical treatment of senile catarcts with vitamin E and anthocyanosides: clinical evaluation." *Ann Ottalmol Clin Ocul*, 1989; 115:109.

11. Ringsdorf, W. M. Jr., E. Cheraskin. "Ascorbic acid and glaucoma: a review." *J Holistic Med*, 1981; 3:167-72.

12. Caselli, L. "Clinical and electroretinographic study on activity of anthocyanosides." *Arch Med Int*, 1985; 37:29'35.

13. Merte, H. J., W. Merkle. "Long-term treatment with Ginkgo biloba extract of circulatory disturbances of the retina and optic nerve." *Klin Monatsbl Augenheilkd*, 1980; 177:577'83; Quaranta, L., *et al*. "Effect of Ginkgo biloba extract on preexisting visual field damage in normal tension glaucoma." *Ophthalmology*, 2003; 110:359-62.

14. Gaspar, A. Z., P. Gasser, J. Flammer. "The influence of magnesium on visual field and peripheral vasospasm in glaucoma." *Ophthalmologica*, 1995; 209:11-13.

15. Lane, B. C. "Diet and glaucomas." *J Am Coll Nutr*, 1991; 10:536.

16. Asregadoo, E. R. "Blood levels of thiamine and ascorbic acid in chronic open-angle glaucoma." *Ann Opthalmol*, 1979; 11:1095'1100.

17. Raymond, L.F. "Allergy and chronic simple glaucoma." *Ann Allergy*, 1964 22:146-50.

18. Eye Disease Case Control Study Group. "Antioxidant status and neovascular age-related macular degeneration." *Arch Opthalmol*, 1993; 111:104'09; Mares-Perlman, J.A., *et al*. "Serum antioxidants and age-related macular degeneration in a population-based case-control study." *Arch Opthalmol*, 1995; 113:1518'23; Snodderly, D.M. "Evidence for protection against age-related macular degeneration by carotenoids and antioxidant vitamins." *Am J Clin Nutr*, 1995; 62(6 suppl):1448S'61S.

19. Seddon, J.M., *et al*. "Dietary carotenoids, vitamins A, C, and E, and advanced age-related macular degeneration." *JAMA*, 1994; 272:1413-20.

20. Seddon, J.M., *et al*. "Dietary carotenoids, vitamins A, C, and E, and advanced age-related macular degeneration." *JAMA*, 1994; 272:1413-20.

21. Mares-Perlman, J.A., *et al*. "Serum antioxidants and age-related macular degeneration in a population-based case-control study." *Arch Opthalmol*, 1995 113:1518'27.

22. West, S., *et al*. "Are anti-oxidants or supplements protective of age-related macula degeneration?" *Arch Ophthalmol*, 1994; 112:222-27.

23. Eye Disease Case-Control Study Group. "Antioxidant status and neovascular age related macular degeneration." *Arch Ophthalmol*, 1993; 111:104-09.

24. Van Leeuwen, R., *et al*. "Dietary Intake of Antioxidants and Risk of Age-Related Macular Degeneration." *JAMA*, 2005; 294:3101'07.

25. Lebuisson, D.A., L. Leroy, G. Reigal. "Treatment of senile macular degeneration with Ginkgo biloba extract: a preliminary double-blind study versus placebo." *Presse Med*, 1986; 15:1556'58.

26. Parekh, N., *et al*. "Association Between Vitamin D and Age-Related Macular Degeneration in the Third National Health and Nutrition Examination Survey, 1988 Through 1994." *Arch Opthalmol*, 2007; 125:661'69.

GOUT

Gout is a type of arthritis that is caused by excessive uric acid. When the level of uric acid in the body is normal, it is believed to be beneficial for you, acting as an antioxidant. But when levels rise too high, the uric acid can form sharp crystals that cause inflammation and damage in the joints and other tissue, a painful arthritic condition known as gout. Aside from gout, high levels of uric acid may also be a risk factor for heart disease. So treating this condition may have additional health benefits.

Over 90 per cent of people with gout are men over thirty. Strangely, the big toe is often the site of the first attack, and the pain can be excruciating.

Diet: The Most Important Treatment for Gout

The cause of gout is fairly straightforward, and so, fortunately, so is the treatment. Uric acid is a breakdown product of purine, which is found in many foods. Since purine raises uric acid levels, and raised uric acid levels cause gout, the goal is to lower uric acid levels. For most people, this can be achieved by diet alone. In order to reduce uric acid by diet, you must eliminate the foods that are the richest sources of purine. These foods include meat, organ meats, goose, gravy, broth, bouillon, consommé, shellfish, shrimp, mussels, scallops, anchovies, sardines, mackerel, herring, fish roe, brewer's and baker's yeast, dried legumes, asparagus, peanuts, and mushrooms. Though common in meat-eaters, gout is rare in vegetarians.

In addition to eliminating foods that are high in purine, there are a number of other dietary factors that help either by decreasing uric acid production or by increasing uric acid excretion. Alcohol both increases uric acid production and decreases uric-acid excretion. Therefore, avoiding alcohol—and especially beer—can reduce the number of gout attacks[1]. For many sufferers of gout, eliminating alcohol is all they need to do to reduce their level

FOOD SOURCES OF PURINE

meat	consommé	sardines	dried legumes
organ meats	shellfish	mackerel	asparagus
goose	shrimp	herring	peanuts
gravy	mussels	fish roe	mushrooms
broth	scallops	brewer's and	
bouillon	anchovies	baker's yeast	

of uric acid and prevent gout[2].

Refined sugar should be eliminated since it increases uric acid[3]. In general, refined carbohydrates increase the production of uric acid. High protein also increases production of uric acid, and saturated fats decrease its excretion. Drinking lots of fluids helps to increase the excretion of uric acid.

Obesity and high blood pressure increase the risk of gout[4]. People with gout are often overweight, and losing that extra weight significantly reduces their levels of uric acid and decreases the number of attacks[5].

Pharmaceutical Drugs and Uric Acid

Certain drugs, including diuretics, aspirin, cyclosporine, and the Parkinson's drug levodopa, can also decrease the body's ability to excrete uric acid. High-dose niacin can also raise uric acid levels. Lead toxicity can also cause gout.

NATURAL SUPPLEMENTS FOR GOUT

Cherries

Though these dietary changes are usually enough to control gout, there are a number of natural supplements that offer additional help. One of the tastiest is cherries. In addition to the many people who swear by this remedy, one study found that eating half a pound of cherries or drinking the equivalent amount of cherry juice each day was very effective in lowering levels of uric acid and

in preventing attacks of gout[6]. Pomegranate and other berries may help.

Vitamin C

Another study found that people who were given 500 mg of vitamin C a day dropped their uric acid levels by 10 per cent, while those who were not given the vitamin C had theirs go up. The difference was statistically significant[7].

Folic Acid

Folic acid also might help. It has been shown to reduce the enzyme that makes uric-acid[8] and, in high enough doses, to reduce the uric acid itself[9]. The dose of folic acid needed seems to be high— 10 to 40 mg a day. This dose is safe but should be taken with B12 and under supervision. A dose this high could interfere with drugs prescribed for epilepsy.

Herbal Help

Herbally, the arthritis and painkilling herb devil's claw has been shown to reduce uric acid levels and relieve joint pain[10]. Other herbs that could be useful include nettle and celery seed and juice. Herb authority James Duke, Ph.D., highly recommends celery seed extract and says that he has personally managed to successfully replace his gout medication with it. He also reports that, though there is no scientific support for the claim, Amazonian healers use avocado for gout.

More Help

Quercetin is a powerfully anti-inflammatory bioflavonoid that also inhibits uric acid production[11], so it also may help. Omega-3 essential fatty acids, such as flaxseed oil, can also help because they reduce the inflammatory leukotrienes, which are the main cause of the inflammation and tissue damage in gout. The anti-inflammatory bromelain might also help.

Other possible choices that may help include herbs that detoxify the urinary tract system, helping to get rid of uric acid, such as corn silk, bucchu, uva ursi, juniper berries, cleavers, dandelion, and burdock.

Chapter Endnotes

1. Ralston, S. H., H. A. Capell, R. D. Sturrock. "Alcohol and response to treatment of gout." *BMJ*, 1988; 296:1641'42; Scott, J.T. "Alcohol and gout." *BMJ*, 1989; 298:1054.

2. Foller, J., I. H. Fox. "Ethanol-induced hyperuricemia." *N Engl J Med*, 1982; 307:1598'1692.

3. Emmerson, B. Y. "Effect of oral fructose on urate production." *Ann Rheum Dis*, 1974; 33:276'80.

4. Loenen, H., *et al.* "Serum uric acid correlates in elderly men and women with special reference to body composition and dietary intake (Dutch Nutrition Surveillance System)." *J Clin Epidemiol*, 1990; 43:1297'1303.

5. Lin, K. C., H. Y. Lin, P. Chou. "The interaction between uric acid level and other risk factors on the development of gout among asymptomatic hyperuricemic men in a prospective study." *J Rheumatol*, 2000; 27:1501'05; Dessein, P.H., *et al.* "Beneficial effect of weight loss associated with moderate calorie/carbohydrate restriction and increased proportional intake of protein and unsaturated fats on serum urate and lipoprotein levels in gout: a pilot study." *Ann Rheum Dis*, 2000; 59:539'43.

6. Blau, L. W. "Cherry diet control for gout and arthritis." *Tex Rep Biol Med*, 1950; 8:309'11.

7. Huang, H. Y., L. J. Appel, M. J. Choi, *et al.* "The effects of vitamin C supplementation on serum concentrations of uric acid: results of a randomized controlled trial." *Arthritis Rheum*, 2005; 52:1843'47.

8. Lewis, A. S., *et al.* "Inhibition of mammalian xanthine oxidase by folate compounds and amethopterin." *J Biol Chem*, 1984; 259:12'15.

9. Oster, K. A. "Xanthine oxidase and folic acid." *Ann Intern Med*, 1977; 87:252'53 [letter].

10. Brady, L. R., V. E. Tyler, J. E. Robbers. Pharmacognosy 8th ed. Philadelphia, *PA: Lea & Febiger*, 1981.

11. Bindoli, A., M. Valente, L. Cavallini. "Inhibitory action of quercetin on xanthine oxidase and xanthine dehydrogenase activity." *Pharmacol Res Commun*, 1985; 17:831'39; Busse, W., D. Kopp, E. Middleton. "Flavonoid modulation of human neutrophil function." *J Allergy Clin Immunol*, 1984; 73:801'09.

HEARING LOSS

Many years ago, when we were working at a health food store, a customer complained, "You know, you see all kinds of articles on vision problems, but you never see anything on hearing problems." He was right. Despite the fact that hearing loss is one of the most common health problems amongst the elderly, you almost never see—or hear—anything about it. Well, here it is.

Ginkgo: Helping the Elderly Again

Ginkgo biloba is perhaps the most important herb for elderly people, and it is one of the best supplements for hearing. When people suffering from hearing loss due to old age were given ginkgo, 40 per cent of them improved[1].

Folic Acid And Homocysteine

Age-related hearing loss may be connected to elevations in homocysteine. Homoscysteine is better known as a risk factor for heart disease, but it means more to the elderly than that. Elevated homocysteine levels are also now known to play a role in osteoporosis and Alzheimer's. And they may play a role in age-related hearing loss as well. Researchers gave either 800 mcg of folic acid a day or a placebo to 728 people between the ages of fifty and seventy for three years. Folic acid lowers homocysteine. Those in the folic acid group suffered less loss of hearing over the three years, showing that some cases of age-related hearing loss may be preventable with folic acid[2].

Treating Tinnitus

When people suffering from hearing loss, tinnitus, vertigo, or labyrinthine syndrome were given ginkgo, 88 per cent of them improved[3]. Most cases of tinnitus can be completely treated with ginkgo, though it is probably more effective in treating recent tinnitus than it is the difficult-to-treat permanent, severe tinnitus, according to Michael Murray, N.D. Tinnitus is the perception that there is sound when there isn't. People suffering from tinnitus hear a ringing, hissing, roaring, whistling, or chirping sound. About 17 per cent of people suffer from tinnitus, but among the elderly, the number is much higher, as high as 33 per cent. So a treatment would be great, and the leading candidate is probably ginkgo.

A review of ginkgo studies found that the results on tinnitus are favourable, but made no firm conclusion[4]. Though there have been negative studies, some of them have been flawed. In one, the ridiculously low dose (29 mg) and the short length of the study (two weeks) seem to have been designed to make the ginkgo fail. The researchers, in addition, used no objective measures in their study! Several studies have found that ginkgo does help tinnitus, and the German Commission E approves this use of ginkgo. A well-designed double-blind, placebo-controlled study found that 40 mg of standardized ginkgo extract three times a day for twelve weeks worked significantly better than a placebo[5].

Zinc may also help tinnitus. When people with tinnitus were given either 50 mg of zinc or a placebo for two months, 46 per cent of them improved, which was greater than the placebo, but not significantly. However, 82 per cent of people in the zinc group reported a significant improvement in the experience of tinnitus, while those in the placebo group did not[6].

Traditional Chinese Medicine

Usually traditional Chinese medicine sees hearing loss and tinnitus as a kidney-related issue, connected to low *yin*, and uses herbs to strengthen the kidneys. Often herbs such as, schizandra, fo ti, or lycii, rehmannia, peony, or dong quai may be used. If the sound heard is high, kidney weakness is indicated. A low sound indicates gall bladder/liver problems, and so, each case is treated differently. Acupuncture is very helpful with tinnitus and hearing issues.

Hearing And Fat

Melvyn Werbach, M.D., reports that hearing loss is often associated with elevated blood levels of fat. Studies show that diets low in saturated fat protect against hearing loss and even partially restore hearing.

So there you go: Nature takes care not only of seeing, but of hearing, too. And now you've heard!

Chapter Endnotes

1. De Amicis, E. "Attivita della ginkgo biloba nelle ptopatie da arteriosclerosi." *Minera Med*, 1973; 64:4193.

2. Durga, J., *et al.* "Effects of folic acid supplementation on hearing in older adults: a randomized, controlled trial." *Ann Intern Med*, 2007; 146:1'9.

3. Montanini, R., G. Gaspari. "*Impiego di un estratto di ginkgo biloba (TEBONIN) nella terrapia delle vasculopatie cerebrali*." *Min Card*, 1969; 17:1096.

4. Ernst, E., C. Stevinson. "Ginkgo biloba for tinnitus: a review." *Clin Otolaryngol*, 1999; 24:164'67.

5. Morgenstern, C. "Ginkgo biloba extract EGb 761 in the treatment of tinnitus aurium." *Fortschr Med*, 1997; 115:7'11.

6. Arda, H.N., *et al.* "The role of zinc in the treatment of tinnitus." *Otology and Neurology*, 2003; 24:86'89.

HIGH BLOOD PRESSURE

Heart disease is the number-one killer of North Americans, and one of the most important risk factors for heart disease is high blood pressure. Blood pressure is considered to be high when it is at or above 140/90. High blood pressure is a strong risk factor for atherosclerosis, heart attack, and stroke. It can also be behind kidney failure, eye disease, headache, and dizziness.

High blood pressure will affect half of us in our later years. But it doesn't have to. There are many simple changes you can make in your diet, lifestyle, and supplements that can help you prevent, and even reverse, high blood pressure.

How to Eat for a Healthy Heart

Most cases of high blood pressure can be controlled by diet and lifestyle alone. The most important change to make is the change to a vegetarian diet. Vegetarians have lower blood pressure than people who eat meat[1]. They also have lower incidence of high blood pressure and less heart disease in general[2]. Though it is commonly thought that natural approaches to health are fine, but slow, research shows that vegetarian and vegan diets actually lower blood pressure very quickly. A twelve-day study on vegan diets revealed that blood pressure was already lowered[3]. Longer studies on vegan diets and blood pressure have also been positive[4]. Many factors in the vegetarian diet improve blood pressure, including that it is high in potassium, magnesium, calcium, complex carbohydrates, fibre, essential fatty acids, folic acid, and vitamin C, while low in saturated fat.

An important study known as DASH (Dietary Approaches to Stop Hypertension) looked at the importance of diet on high blood pressure[5] by comparing three diets. The first was the typical western diet. The second was the typical diet with extra fruits and vegetables and reduced sugar. The third was the DASH diet: high in fruit, vegetables, low-fat dairy, nuts, fibre, potassium, magnesium, and calcium, and low in cholesterol, saturated fat, total fat, sugar, and meat. Those on the typical western diet—since it is the diet that most of us are on anyway—had no significant effect. The fortified western diet had only modest effects on blood pressure. But the DASH diet caused a huge reduction in blood pressure in only two weeks. Interestingly, the study shows that the benefits of a vegetarian diet come not only from the healthy things the diet adds, but also from the elimination of meat.

Another study of diet and blood pressure found that a diet low in salt, alcohol, and protein, but rich in potassium, calcium, and magnesium is associated with lower blood pressure[6]. Similar to the DASH diet, we see the need to increase potassium, magnesium, and calcium and decrease protein. This study also points to the need to restrict salt.

Restricting salt is crucial. Salt increases blood pressure[7]. Cultures that do not add salt have virtually no high blood pressure[8]. The good news is that reducing salt usually reduces blood pressure[9].

Minerals that Lower Blood Pressure

But don't just watch your salt. The ratio of salt to potassium is important. Not only must the amount of salt be lowered, but the amount of potassium must be increased. A meta-analysis of nineteen studies shows that supplementing potassium significantly lowers blood pressure[10]. Increasing potassium is easily accomplished by switching to a vegetarian diet; plant foods are much higher in potassium, and that may be part of the reason vegetarians have lower blood pressure[11].

Another important mineral, as the dietary studies have already shown, is magnesium. Heart expert Decker Weiss, M.D., N.D., recommends magnesium supplementation for high blood pressure. Population studies show an association between high intake of magnesium and lower blood pressure. Several[12], though not all, studies have found magnesium supplements lower blood pressure.

Population studies also point to the importance of calcium, and a meta-analysis of forty-two studies found that calcium significantly lowers blood pressure[13].

Blood Pressure and the Fats You Eat

It is not surprising that the kind of fat you eat is an important determinant of blood pressure. One of the benefits of the vegetarian diet is the healthier fats it provides—it is lower in total fat and has a high ratio of polyunsaturated to saturated fat. If the ratio changes—as it does in the typical western diet—to low polyunsaturated to saturated fat, the risk of high blood pressure goes up[14]. This risk was demonstrated in a study that put people with normal blood pressure on two different diets. One group was on a high fat diet with a low ratio of polyunsaturated fats to saturated fats—their blood pressure went up; the other group was on a low fat diet with a high ratio of polyunsaturated to saturated fat—their blood pressure went down[15]. Polyunsaturated fats are the essential fatty acids and can be supplemented by taking flaxseed oil, hempseed oil, or fish oil.

Another heart healthy oil is olive oil. In a double-blind study, twenty-three people with moderately high blood pressure added three or four teaspoons of extra virgin olive oil or sunflower oil to their diet. Eight people on olive oil were able to completely stop their blood pressure medication and maintain normal blood pressure. No one in the sunflower-oil group could. In the olive-oil group, the dose of blood-pressure medication dropped by 48 per cent, while dropping only 4 per cent in the other group. Despite the 48 per cent reduction in meds, the olive oil group still had significant decreases in blood pressure[16].

Going Down! Take Your Supplements

There are several other supplements that can help control blood pressure.

Vitamin C

Ten out of fourteen population studies have found that higher vitamin C levels mean lower blood pressure, and three out four found that those with more vitamin C in their diet had lower blood pressure[17]. Double blind studies on vitamin C have had mixed results, but all show at least a trend toward lowering blood pressure, and several studies show that the vitamin can modestly lower blood pressure. A large study of elderly people found that higher levels of vitamin C meant significantly lower blood pressure[18].

Fibre

Several, but not all, double-blind studies show that increasing fibre lowers blood pressure. Clinically, I have found that taking a significant amount of fibre from flaxseeds and psyllium lowers blood pressure, in addition to getting fibre into the diet.

Coenzyme Q10

One very important heart nutrient is coenzyme Q10. Many people with high blood pressure have CoQ10 deficiencies. Several studies have shown that CoQ10 significantly lowers high blood pressure[19]. When people with high blood pressure were given either 60 mg of CoQ10 or a placebo twice a day for twelve weeks in a double-blind study, there was a significantly greater reduction of blood pressure in the CoQ10 group[20].

B Vitamins

B vitamins are proving to play an increasingly important role in heart health. One study of twenty people with high blood pressure found that B6 was able to significantly lowered their blood pressure[21]. Folic acid, B6, and B12 are crucial for controlling homocysteine. Homocysteine is a crucial risk factor for atherosclerosis, and atherosclerosis is a major cause of high blood pressure.

HERBS THAT HELP HIGH BLOOD PRESSURE

Hawthorn

The herbal star for the heart is hawthorn, and several studies have confirmed hawthorn's traditional blood-pressure-lowering ability.

Garlic

Garlic, a herb with many heart benefits, has been found by an analysis of ten double-blind studies to have a mild but significant blood-pressure-lowering effect[22]. But when a more true-to-life meta-analysis of placebo-controlled studies on garlic and blood-pressure looked only at people who actually had high blood-pressure, garlic reduced both systolic and diastolic blood-pressure significantly better than a placebo. In fact, the study's authors say that the effects of garlic are comparable to the effects of blood pressure medications[23].

That hawthorn and garlic help high blood-pressure is not surprising. But here are some blood pressure herbs that will surprise you.

Reishi

Better known as an immune booster and cancer fighter, the Chinese mushroom, reishi, is a very good heart herb and has been shown in double-blind research to significantly lower blood pressure. When people with high blood pressure who did not respond to ACE inhibitors (captopril or minodipine) added reishi to their meds, they did respond. Their blood pressure dropped significantly[24].

Pycnogenol

A double-blind, placebo-controlled study found that 200 mg a day of pycnogenol significantly lowered blood pressure in people with mild high blood pressure, and another study found that 100 mg a day allowed people to cut the dose of their blood pressure meds by half.

Hibiscus

When people with mild to moderate high blood pressure were given either a tea made from hibiscus extract, standardized for anthocyanin flavonoids, or the ACE inhibitor captopril for four weeks, the effect of the herb and of the drug were statistically similar[25].

Yarrow

Yarrow is a herb that rarely gets talked about, and, when it is talked about, it is never in relation to blood pressure. But 15 to 20 drops of yarrow extract given twice a day for six months has been shown to significantly lower blood pressure[26].

Olive Leaf

Olive leaf is another rarely discussed herb. It has a mild effect but works very quickly. In a three-month study, olive-leaf extract significantly lowered blood pressure in people with high blood pressure[27]. Decker Weiss says that a hawthorn-and-olive-leaf combination is his personal favourite for treating high blood pressure.

Mistletoe

Better known for kissing at Christmas, mistletoe has mild but real blood-pressure-lowering properties. It is an ideal herb to gently accompany a dietary treatment of mild high blood pressure. It is also remarkably good for treating the symptoms that come with high blood pressure; headache, dizziness, and low energy.

Other Herbs

Another herb with a great blood-pressure-lowering effect is *coleus forskohlii*.

Or try celery seed, or diuretics such as corn silk, bucchu, uva ursi, and perhaps the best one, dandelion leaf, that not only gets the water out, but supplies extra crucial minerals as it does so.

Lifestyle Changes

Other lifestyle changes can also help. If weight is a problem, losing weight can significantly lower blood pressure[28]. So can exercise[29]. Surprisingly, dealing with food allergies may also lower blood pressure[29]. And, if you smoke, stop[31].

If you have a juicer, don't forget to use it. Simple juices made of foods such as celery, cucumber, parsley, carrot, grapefruit, lime, and grapes can help to lower blood pressure, since they are high in the minerals that affect blood pressure.

Finally, acupuncture is also effective for treating high blood pressure.

1. Rouse, I. L., L. J. Beilin, D.P. Mahoney, *et al.* "Vegetarian diet and blood pressure." *Lancet*, 1983; ii:742'43; Margetts, B.M., *et al.* "Vegetarian diet in mild hypertension: a randomised controlled trial." *BMJ*, 1986; 293:1468-71.

2. Rouse, I. L., L. J. Beilin, D. P. Mahoney, *et al.* "Vegetarian diet and blood pressure." *Lancet*, 1983; ii:742'43.

3. McDougall, J., K. Litzaue, E. Haver, *et al.* "Rapid reduction of serum cholesterol and blood pressure by a twelve-day, very low fat, strictly vegetarian diet." *J Am Coll Nutr*, 1995; 14:491'96.

4. Lindahl, O., *et al.* "A vegan regimen with reduced medication in the treatment of hypertension." *Br J Nutr*, 1984; 52:11'20.

5. Appel, L. J., T. J. Moore, E. Boarzanek, *et al.* "A clinical trial of the effects of dietary patterns on blood pressure." *N Engl J Med*, 1997; 336:1117-24.

6. Hajjar, I. M., *et al.* "Impact of diet on blood pressure and age-related changes in blood pressure in the U.S. population: Analysis of NHANES III." *Arch Inter Med*, 2001; 161:589-93.

7. Stamler, J., G. Rose, P. Elliott, *et al.* "Findings of the international cooperative IN-TERSALT study." *Hypertension*, 1991; 17(1 Suppl):I9-15.

8. Page, L. B., A. Damon, R. C. Moellering, Jr. "Antecedents of cardiovascular disease in six Solomon Islands Societies." *Circulation*, 1974; 44:1132-46.

9. MacGregor, G. A., N. D. Markandu, G. A. Sagnella, *et al.* "Double-blind study of three sodium intakes and long-term effects of sodium restriction in essential hy-pertension." *Lancet*, 1989; 2:1244-47; Cutler, J.A., D. Follmann, P.S. Allender. "Randomized trials of sodium reduction: an overview." *Am J Clin Nutr*, 1997; 65(Suppl):643S-51S; Hajjar, I.M., C.E. Grim, V. George, T.A. Kotchen. "Impact of diet on blood pressure and age-related changes in blood pressure in the U.S. population: Analysis of NHANES III." *Arch Intern Med*, 2001; 161:589-93.

10. Cappuccio, F. P., G. A. MacGregor. "Does potassium supplementation lower blood pressure? A meta-analysis of published trials." *J Hypertens*, 1991; 9:465-73.

11. Ophir, O., *et al.* "Low blood pressure in vegetarians: the possible role of potas-sium." *Am J Clin Nurtr*, 1983; 37:755'62.

12. Motoyama, T., H. Sano, H. Fukuzaki, *et al.* "Oral magnesium supplementation in patients with essential hypertension." *Hypertension*, 1989; 13:227-32; Witte-man, J., D. E. Grobbee, F.H.M. Derkx, *et al.* "Reduction of blood pressure with oral magnesium supplementation in women with mild to moderate hypertension." *Am J Clin Nutr*, 1994; 60:129'35; Sanjuliani, A. F., V. G. de Abreu Fagundes, E. A. Francischetti. "Effects of magnesiumon blood pressure and intracellular ion levels of Brazilian hypertensive patients." *Int J Cardiol*, 1996; 56:177'83; Itoh, K., T. Kawasaki, M. Nakamura. "The effects of high oral magnesium supplemen-tation on blood pressure, serum lipids and related variables in apparently healthy Japanese subjects." *Br J Nutr*, 1997; 78:737'50.

13. Griffith, L. E., G. H. Guyatt, R. J. Cook, *et al.* "The influence of dietary and nondietary calcium supplementation on blood pressure. An updated metaanalysis of randomized controlled trials." *Am J Hypertens*, 1999; 12:84-92.

14. Zheng, H-J., A. R. Folsom, J. Ma, *et al.* "Plasma fatty acid composition and 6-year incidence of hypertension in middle-aged adults." *Am J Epidemiol*, 1999; 150:492'500.

15. Iaconon, J. M., P. Puska, R. M. Dougherty, *et al.* "Effect of dietary fat on blood pressure in a rural Finnish population." *Am J Clin Nutr*, 1983; 38:860'69.

16. Ferrara, L. A., *et al.* "Olive Oil and Reduced Need for Antihypertensive Medica-tions." *Arch Intern Med*, 2000; 160:837'842.

17. Ness, A. R., D. Chee, P. Elliott. "Viamin C and blood pressure-an overview." *J Human Hypertens*, 1998; 16:925'32.

18. Bates, C. J., *et al.* "Does vitamin C reduce blood pressure? Results of a large study of people aged 65 or older." *J Hypertens*, 1998; 16:925'32.

19. Digiesi, V., F. Cantini, B. Brodbeck. "Effect of coenzyme Q10 on essential arterial hypertension." *Curr Ther Res*, 1990; 47:841-45; Singh, R.B., M.A. Niaz, S.S. Rastogi, *et al.* "Effect of hydrosoluble coenzyme Q10 on blood pressure and in-sulin resistance in hypertensive patients with coronary artery disease." *J Hum Hy-pertens*, 1999; 13:203-08.

20. Burke, B. E., R. Neuenschwander, R. D. Olson. "Randomized, double-blind, placebo-controlled trial of coenzyme Q10 in isolated systolic hypertension." *South Med J*, 2001; 94:1112'17.

21. Ayback, M., *et al.* "Effect of oral pyridoxine hydrochloride supplementation on arterial blood pressure in patients with essential hypertension." *Arzneim Forsch*, 1995; 45:1271'73.

22. Silagy, C., A. W. Neil. "A meta-analysis of the effect of garlic on blood pressure." *J Hypertension*, 1994; 12:463-68.

23. Ried, K., *et al.* "Effect of garlic on blood pressure: a systematic review and meta-analysis." *BMC Cardiovasc Disord.*, 2008; 8:13.

24. Jin, H., G. Zhang, X. Cao, *et al.* "Treatment of hypertension by ling zhi combined with hypotensor and its effects on arterial, arteriolar and capillary pressure and microcirculation." Cited in Yarnell, E., K. Abascal, C. Hoopre. *Clinical Botanical Medicine*. Mary Ann Liebert: Larchmont NY, 2002, p.74.

25. Herrera-Arellano, A., *et al.* "Effectiveness and tolerability of a standardized ex-tract from Hibiscus sabdariffa in patients with mild to moderate hypertension: a controlled and randomized clinical trial." *Phytomedicine*, 2004; 11(5):375-82.

26. Asgary, S., G. H. Naderi, N. Sarrafzadegan, *et al.* "Antihypertensive and antihy-perlipidemic effects of Achillea wilhelmsii." *Drugs Exp Clin Res*, 2000; 26:89'93.

27. Cherif, S. "A clinical trial of a titrated Olea extract in the treatment of essential arterial hypertension." *J Pharm Belg*, 1996; 51:69'71.

28. Alderman, M. H. "Nonpharmacologic approaches to the treatment of hyperten-sion." *Lancet*, 1994; 334:307-11 [review]; Stevens, V. J., E. Obarzanek, N. R. Cook, *et al.* "Long-term weight loss and changes in blood pressure: results of the Trials of Hypertension Prevention, Phase II." *Ann Intern Med*, 2001; 134:1-11; He, J., P.K. Whelton, L.J. Appel, *et al.* "Long-term effects of weight loss and di-etary sodium reduction on incidence of hypertension." *Hypertension*, 2000; 35:544-49; McCarron, D.A., M.E. Reusser. "Body weight and blood pressure reg-ulation." *Am J Clin Nutr*, 1996; 63 (suppl):423S'425S.

29. Kukkonen, K., *et al.* "Physical training of middle-aged men with borderline hy-pertension." *Ann Clin Res*, 1982; 14(Suppl 34):139-45; Young, D.R., *et al.* "The effect of aerobic exercise and T'ai Chi on blood pressure in older people: results of a randomized trial." *J Am Geriatr Soc*, 1999; 47:277-84.

30. Grant, E. C. G. "Food Allergies and migraine." *Lancet*, 1979; 1:966-69.

31. Narkiewicz, K., G. Maraglino, T. Biasion, *et al.* "Interactive effect of cigarettes and coffee on daytime systolic blood pressure in patients with mild essential hy-pertension." *J Hypertens*, 1995; 13:965-70.

OSTEOARTHRITIS

There are many kinds of arthritis, but the most common of them all is osteoarthritis.

At the ends of our joints, there is a cushioning pillow of cartilage that protects them. In osteoarthritis, this cushioning degenerates, leading to pain and reduced motion of the joints. Osteoarthritis is the leading cause of disability in people over sixty-five.

The Disappointment of Conventional Medicine

Conventional medicine has had a tough time helping the millions of people who suffer from this painful disease. The commonly performed arthroscopic surgery has been discovered by placebo-controlled research to be no better than a placebo—the surgery doesn't work[1]. And the aspirin and other nonsteroidal anti-inflammatory drugs (NSAIDs) that are so commonly prescribed, while they do dull the pain, actually help the arthritis to progress[2]. That's because these painkilling drugs actually inhibit cartilage repair and accelerate cartilage destruction[3]. This news is not new; it's just that no one ever tells you about it.

The Promise Of Natural Medicine

The real crime is that there are natural treatments that really do work that no one ever tells you about. People who could be healing their osteoarthritis naturally, are instead having useless surgeries and taking harmful drugs. And, unlike the drugs, which only address the symptoms of osteoarthritis, the natural approach, while being every bit as good at pain control, addresses the real cause of the pain and stops the disease by stimulating the body's production of cartilage.

Glucosamine Sulfate: Putting the Brakes on Osteoarthritis

Glucosamine sulfate is a substance that occurs naturally in the body. It stimulates the production of cartilage and so is capable of repairing joints. Glucosamine does not act as a painkiller: it kills

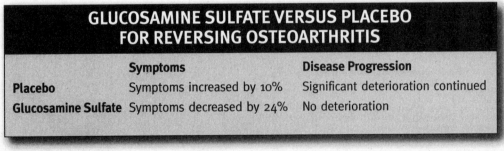

	Symptoms	Disease Progression
GLUCOSAMINE SULFATE VERSUS PLACEBO FOR REVERSING OSTEOARTHRITIS		
Placebo	Symptoms increased by 10%	Significant deterioration continued
Glucosamine Sulfate	Symptoms decreased by 24%	No deterioration

pain by stopping the disease.

Because glucosamine eases the pain by stopping the disease, and because stopping the disease takes time, glucosamine takes longer to work than aspirin does. But, surprisingly, not much! While NSAIDs may kill the pain more in the first two weeks, by the fourth week of treatment, people on glucosamine will be doing significantly better than the people on the NSAID painkillers[4].

All kinds of double-blind studies show that glucosamine sulfate works better than placebo and as well or better than NSAIDs[5]. The studies also show it to be safer and better-tolerated.

But here's the really exciting news. The studies do not only show that glucosamine matches the drugs as a painkiller. At least two studies show that glucosamine, in fact, stops the disease's destruction of cartilage. The first study[6] was both long term and very well designed. Two hundred and twelve people with osteoarthritis were given either 1,500 mg of glucosamine sulfate or a placebo once a day for three years. In the placebo group, symptoms increased by 10 per cent and X-rays showed that the disease continued to increase significantly. But in the glucosamine group, symptoms decreased by 24 per cent and—here's the important part—X-rays revealed no deterioration at all! This study was the first to show that glucosamine not only kills pain, but also prevents further joint damage—the opposite of NSAIDs, which contribute to it. This study also showed two

other things. The first is that glucosamine is not only very effective but also very safe to take long-term. The second is that you don't have to remember to take 500 mg three times a day as is always suggested; you can take all 1,500 mg at once. That you can take glucosamine once a day is important because it improves compliance.

A second study confirmed these amazing results[7]. Two hundred and two people were given either glucosamine sulfate or a placebo for three years in a double-blind study. Measurements of joint space revealed continued disease progression in the placebo group but no progression in the glucosamine group. The difference was significant. Symptoms also improved significantly more in the glucosamine group. And the glucosamine was just as safe as the placebo.

S-Adenosyl-Methionine

Another important, though much less well-known, supplement for osteoarthritis is S-adenosyl-methionine or, as it is known for short, SAMe. SAMe is important for the body to manufacture cartilage components. Unlike glucosamine, as well as addressing the causes of osteoarthritis, SAMe is also an anti-inflammatory and painkiller. Many double-blind studies have shown SAMe's ability to reduce pain, stiffness, and swelling better than a placebo and as well or better than drugs such as ibuprofen and naproxen in people with osteoarthritis. They have also proven SAMe to be safer[8]. These studies gave SAMe at a dose of 1,200 mg a day. When the clinical studies on SAMe were put together and reviewed, the results showed that SAMe's effectiveness was similar to drugs, with the advantage of being better tolerated[9].

Unlike glucosamine, which is derived from the shells of sea animals, SAMe is suitable for vegetarians.

Methylsulfonylmethane

Another nutrient that is emerging as an important supplement for osteoarthritis is methylsulfonylmethane, or MSM. MSM increases sulphur in the body, which seems to be important for osteoarthritis. It also reduces pain and inflammation. The first small study to show that MSM helps osteoarthritis found that when people were given 2,250 mg of MSM, 82 per cent of them improved by the sixth week, compared to only 18 per cent of those who were given a placebo[10]. For a few years, no one seems to have followed up this lead. But then, in 2006, researchers gave either 3 g of MSM or a placebo twice a day for twelve weeks in a double-blind study, and found that the people given the MSM had significantly more reduced pain and overall improvement in physical functioning than those given the placebo[11].

Glucosamine/MSM Combo

And it may be that taking MSM with glucosamine sulfate will help even more than taking either of them alone. When 118 people with osteoarthritis were given either 500 mg of glucosamine, 500 mg of MSM, a combination of both, or a placebo three times a day for twelve weeks, the glucosamine and the MSM both significantly improved pain and swelling. That's nothing new. What was new was that the combination of the two improved pain and swelling even more[12].

Antioxidants: Anti-arthritis

Antioxidants can also help. The two that stand out for osteoarthritis are vitamins C and E. Though it is less discussed than immunity and fighting colds, one of the main functions of vitamin C in the body is the production of collagen, the major protein in cartilage. And remember that it is the degeneration of the cartilage cushion at the ends of the joints that leads to osteoarthritis. So it is not surprising that as the level of vitamin C goes up, the degree of protection against osteoarthritis goes up, too[13]. Vitamin C significantly lowers the risk of osteoarthritis progressing and also reduces the likelihood of pain[14]. A double-blind, placebo-controlled study that gave 1 gram of vitamin C in the form of calcium ascorbate or a placebo each day to 133 people with osteoarthritis found that the vitamin C reduced the pain significantly more than the placebo[15].

Studies show that vitamin E also helps[16] because it inhibits the degeneration of the cartilage and stimulates the production of cartilage components[17]. At least two double-blind studies have proven vitamin E to be superior to a placebo at relieving the pain of osteoarthritis[18]. One study of vitamin E found no effect.

Other Cartilage-building Nutrients

The body needs several other nutrients for healthy cartilage, including vitamins A and B6 and the minerals zinc, copper and boron. You can get most of these nutrients from a good quality multivitamin. In addition to taking boron supplements you, can get boron by eating lots of fruits, nuts, and vegetables, especially green leafy vegetables. You can also get plenty of boron from the herb stinging nettle. Boron has been shown in one small double-blind study to help more people with osteoarthritis than does a placebo[19]. Nettle has also been shown to help[20].

Another nutrient that may help is niacinamide, a form of vitamin B3. In the 1940s and 1950s, Dr. William Kaufman reported that niacinamide helped people suffering from osteoarthritis. Half a century later, someone finally put his claim to the test. This double-blind, placebo-controlled study found a reduction of symptoms within twelve weeks when taking 3g a day of niacinamide[21].

Helpful Herbs for Osteoarthritis

There are also several herbs that can help people with osteoarthritis.

Devil's Claw

Devil's claw is better known for rheumatoid arthritis, but, surprisingly, it is in osteoarthritis that the real promise for this herb is showing up. Double blind research shows that it reduces pain better than a placebo. Placebos are one thing, but even more exciting research has now shown that devil's claw works better than drugs. Researchers gave 122 people with osteoarthritis either devil's claw or a drug. The herb outperformed the drug—65.3 per cent of the people using the herb got good or very good results versus 60 per cent on the drug. And the herb had significantly fewer side effects[22].

Ayurvedic Herbs

The Ayurvedic herb boswellia is anti-inflammatory and prevents decreases in cartilage production. When thirty people with osteoarthritis in their knees were given either 333 mg of boswellia extract or a placebo three times a day, there was a significant improvement in pain, swelling, and motion in those who got the boswellia[23].

Curcumin is another very powerful anti-inflammatory herb. When boswellia and curcumin were combined in a double-blind study and compared to a placebo, the herbal combination produced significant improvements in pain, swelling, and motion, while the placebo produced none[24]. A formula combining bos-wellia and curcumin with ashwagandha (another of the excellent herbs from India's Ayurvedic tradition), and zinc has also been shown to be effective[25]. And now curcumin has proven itself effective on its own. Ninety-one people with osteoarthritis in their knees were given either 400 mg of ibuprofen twice a day or turmeric extract, containing 500 mg of curcuminoids, four times a day. After six weeks, there was a significant improvement in both groups. When pain was measured on level walking, scores on turmeric dropped from 5.3 to 2.7, and scores on ibuprofen dropped from 5 to 3.1. People taking turmeric had less pain when climbing stairs and they both walked and climbed stairs faster. 91.1 per cent of people taking turmeric reported moderate to high satisfaction, compared to 80.4 per cent of those taking ibuprofen[26].

Ginger

Ginger is powerfully anti-inflammatory as well as having antioxidant effects. Evidence is mounting for ginger as an osteoarthritis herb. When 247 osteoarthritis sufferers were given either 255 mg of standardized ginger extract or a placebo twice a day for six weeks in a double-blind study, pain went down by 63 per cent in the ginger group, compared to 50 per cent in the placebo group—a

significant difference. Pain went down by 24.5 points in the ginger group but only 16.4 points in the placebo group[27]. A second double-blind, placebo-controlled study found that 250 mg of ginger extract taken four times a day significantly reduced pain and increased mobility in people with osteoarthritis of the knee[28].

Rosehips

Rosehips are the little apple-like fruits that follow the rose flower. If people know them as a herb at all, they know them as a rich source of vitamin C for fighting colds. But studies in the past few years have discovered that rosehips can reduce the pain and stiffness of osteoarthritis and improve mobility[29]. When people with osteoarthritis were given either 5 g of rosehip powder or a placebo every day in a double-blind study, there was a significant reduction in pain in the rosehip group after three weeks, but no reduction at all in the placebo group[30].

Cat's Claw

Cat's claw is a terrific anti-inflammatory herb from Peru. After four weeks on 100 mg a day of freeze-dried cat's claw, people with osteoarthritis had significantly more relief from pain and improvement in their overall condition than people given a placebo[31].

Pine Bark

The newest entry on the osteoarthritis list is pine bark extract. People with mild to moderate osteoarthritis were given either pine bark or a placebo with their regular medications for three months. Compared to the placebo group, the people in the pine bark group had significant relief from pain and stiffness. Nearly 40 per cent of pine bark users were able to reduce their pain medications and none of them needed to increase it, while in the placebo group, only 8 per cent were able to decrease their pain meds and 10 per cent had to increase them[32].

More Herbs and Nutrients

White willow bark may also offer some help[33], as could soy protein[34].

Clinically, Linda has found that bromelain, a natural anti-inflammatory and painkiller, is also extremely useful for the pain of osteoarthritis.

There is evidence that 5-HTP may also help for pain, as it increases serotonin and endorphins, two naturally occurring susbstances that help to reduce pain in the body.

Tradional herbalists would use herbs such as Oregon grape root, princes pine, sassafras, prickly ash bark, black cohosh, guaiacum, ginger, and cayenne for arthritis. Topical applications of ginger and lobelia are also helpful. Several double-blind studies show that applying a cream of cayenne extract reduces the pain and tenderness[35]. Other traditionally used herbs include burdock, butcher's broom, alfalfa, nettle, wheat grass, and barley grass.

Diet and Lifestyle

If you are overweight, achieving a healthy weight is an important step in preventing and treating osteoarthritis. Obesity increases the risk, and weight loss decreases the risk[36]. And losing weight can also reduce the pain of osteoarthritis if you already have it[37].

Since antioxidant and sulphur rich supplements are important in osteoarthritis, it is not surprising that antioxidant- and sulphur-rich foods are, too. The diet should be bursting with fruits and vegetables because they are a rich source of antioxidants. People with osteoarthritis who get a lot of antioxidants from food have slower joint deterioration[38]. Some of the best foods are the flavonoid-rich berries such as blueberries, blackberries, cranberries, cherries, and dark grapes. Grape seed, rich in flavonoids, is an excellent addition to prevent and treat arthritis.

Foods that are rich in sulphur—such as garlic, onions, broccoli, cabbage, and other foods in the cabbage family—are also important.

And finally, massage therapy can improve pain, stiffness, and physical functioning in people with osteoarthritis[39], and acupuncture can be extremely helpful[40]. In the most recent acupuncture study, osteoarthritis sufferers continued their regular care while either receiving acupuncture for three months or not getting acupuncture. Osteoarthritis severity scores improved by 17.6 points in the acupuncture group, but by only 0.9 points in the group that didn't get the acupuncture. Quality of life also improved more in the acupuncture group[41].

Chapter Endnotes

1. Mosely, J. B., et al. "A controlled trial of arthroscopic surgery for osteoarthritis of the knee." *N Engl J Med* 2002; 347:81'88.

2. Newman, N. M., R. S. M. Ling. "Acetabular bone destruction related to non-steroidal anti-inflammatory drugs." *Lancet*, 1985; ii:11'13.

3. Brooks, P. M., S. R. Potter, W.W. Buchanan. "NSAID and osteoarthritis-help or hinderance." *J Rheumatol*, 1982; 9:3'5; Shield, M. J. "Anti-inflammatory drugs and their effects on cartilage synthesis and renal function." *Eur J Rheum Inflam*, 1993; 13:7'16; Ghosh, P. "Evaluation of disease progression during nonsteroidal anti-inflammatory drug treatment: experimental models." *Osteoarthritis Cartilage*, 1999; 7:340'42; Dingle, J. T. "Cartilage maintenance in osteoarthritis: interaction of cytokines, NSAID and prostaglandins in articular cartilage damage and repair." *J Rheumatol Suppl*, 1991; 28:30'37.

4. Vaz, A. L. "Double-blind clinical evaluation of the relative efficacy of ibuprofen and glucosamine sulfate in the management of osteoarthritis of the knee in outpatients." *Curr Med Res Opin*, 1982; 8(3):145'49.

5. Drovanti, A., A. A. Bignamini, A. L. Rovati. "Therepeutic activity of oral glucosamine sulfate in osteoarthritis: a placebo controlled double-blind investigation." *Clin Ther*, 1980; 3(4):260'72; Pujalte, J. M., E. P. Llavore, F. R. Ylescupidez. "Double-blind clinical investigation of oral glucosamine sulfate in the basic treatment of osteoarthritis." *Curr Med Res Opin*, 1980; 7(2):110'14; Vaz, A.L. "Double-blind clinical evaluation of the relative efficacy of ibuprofen and glucosamine sulfate in the management of osteoarthritis of the knee in outpatients." *Curr Med Res Opin*, 1982; 8(3):145'49; Rovati, L. C. "Clinical research in osteoarthritis: design and results of short-term and long-term trials with disease-modifying drugs." *Int J Tissue React*, 1992; 14:243'51; Qiu, G.X., et al. "Efficacy and safety of glucosamine sulfate versus ibuprofen in patients with knee osteoarthritis." *Arzneimittelforschung*, 1998; 48:469'74; Poolsup, N., et al. "Glucosamine long-term treatment on the progression of knee osteoarthritis: systematic review of randomized controlled trials." *Ann Pharmacother*, 2005; 39:1080'87.

6. Reginster, J.Y., R. Deroisy, L. C. Rovatti, et al. "Long-term effects of glucosamine sulfate on osteoarthritis progression: a randomized, placebo-controlled trial." *Lancet*, 2001; 357:251'56.

7. Pavelka, K., J. Gatterova, M. Olejarova, et al. "Glucosamine sulfate use and delay of progression of knee osteoarthritis: a 3-year, randomized, placebo-controlled, double-blind study." *Arch Intern Med*, 2002; 162:2113'23.

8. Domljan, Z., et al. "A double-blind trial of ademetionine vs naproxen in activated gonarthrosis." *Int J Clin Pharmacol Ther Toxicol*, 1989; 27:329-33; Müller-Fassbender, H. "Double-blind clinical trial of S-adenosylmethionine versus ibuprofen in the treatment of osteoarthritis." *Am J Med*, 1987; 83(Suppl 5A):81-83; Vetter, G. "Double-blind comparative clinical trial with S-adenosylmethionine and indomethacin in the treatment of osteoarthritis." *Am J Med*, 1987; 83(Suppl 5A):78-80; Maccagno, A. "Double-blind controlled clinical trial of oral S-adenosylmethionine versus piroxicam in knee osteoarthritis." *Am J Med*, 1987; 83(Suppl 5A):72-77; Caruso, I., V. Pietrogrande. "Italian double-blind multicenter study comparing S-adenosylmethionine, naproxen, and placebo in the treatment of degenerative joint disease." *Am J Med*, 1987; 83(Suppl 5A):66-71; Marcolongo, R., N. Giordano, B. Colombo, et al. "Double-blind multicentre study of the activity of S-adenosyl-methionine in hip and knee osteoarthritis." *Curr Ther Res*, 1985; 37:82-94; Glorioso, S., S. Todesco, A. Mazzi, et al. "Double-blind multicentre study of the activity of S-adenosylmethionine in hip and knee osteoarthritis." *Int J Clin Pharmacol Res*, 1985; 5:39-49; Montrone, F., M. Fumagalli, P. Sarzi-Puttini, et al. "Double-blind study of S-adenosyl-methionine versus placebo in hip and knee arthrosis." *Clin Rheumatol*, 1985; 4:484-85.

9. DiPadova, C. "S-adenosylmethionine in the treatment of osteoarthritis. Review of the clinical studies." *Am J Med*, 1987; 83:60'65[review].

10. Lawrence, R. M. "Methylsulfonylmethane (MSM): a double-blind study of its use in degenerative arthritis." *International Journal of Anti-Aging Medicine*, Summer 1998; 1(1):50.

11. Kim, L. S., et al. "Efficacy of methylsulfonylmethane (MSM) in osteoarthritis pain of the knee: a pilot clinical trial." *Osteoarthritis Cartilage*, 2006; 14:286'94.

12. Usha, P. R., M. U. R. Naidu. "Randomized, double-blind, parallel, placebo-controlled study of oral glucosamine, methylsulfonylmethane and their combination in osteoarthritis." *Clin Drug Invest*, 2004; 24:353'63.

13. Krystal, G., G. M. Morris, L. Sokoloff. "Stimulation of DNA synthesis by ascorbate in cultures of articular chondrocytes." *Arthr Rheum*, 1982; 25:318'25.

14. McAllindon, T. E., et al. "Do antioxidant micronutrients protect against the development and progression of knee osteoarthritis?" *Arthritis Rheum*, 1996; 39:648'56.

15. Jensen, N. H. "Reduced pain from osteoarthritis in hip joint or knee joint during treatment with calcium ascorbate: a randomized, placebo-controlled cross-over trial in general practice." *Ugeskr Laeger*, 2003; 165:2563'66.

16. Schwartz, E. R. "The modulation of osteoarthritic development by vitamins C and E." *Int J Vit Nutr Res*, (supplement) 1984; 26:141'46; Scherak, O., et al. "Hochdosierte vitamin-E-therapie bei patienten mit aktivierter arthrose." *Z Rheumatol*, 1990; 49:369'73 (German).

17. Machtey, I., L. Ouaknine. "Tocopherol in osteoarthritis: a controlled pilot study." *J Am Geriatr Soc*, 1978; 26:328'30.

18. Machtey, I., L. Ouaknine. "Tocopherol in osteoarthritis: a controlled pilot study." *J Am Geriatr Soc*, 1978; 26:328'30; Blankenhorn, G. "Klinische wirtsamkeit von spondyvit (vitamin E) bei aktiverten arthronson." *Z Orthop*, 1986; 124:340'43 (German).

19. Travers, R. L., G. L. Rennie, R.E. Newnham. "Boron and arthritis: the results of a double-blind pilot study." *J Nutr Med*, 1990; 1:127'32.

20. Sommer, R. G., B. Sinner. "IDS 23 in the therapy of rheumatic disease. Do you know the new cytokine antagonists?" *Therapiewoche*, 1996; 46:44'49; Chrubasik, S., et al. "Evidence for antirheumatic effeciveness of Herba Urticae dioica in acute arthritis: a pilot study." *Phytomed*, 1997; 4(2):105'08.

21. Jones, W.B., C. P. Rapoza, W. F. Blair. The effect of niacinamide on osteoarthritis: a pilot study. *Inflamm Res*, 1996; 45:330'34.

22. Chantre, P., et al. "Efficacy and tolerance of Harpagophytum procumbens versus diacerhein in treatment of osteoarthritis." *Phytomedicine*, 2000; 7:177'83.

23. Kimmaticar, N., et al. "Efficacy and tolerability of Boswellia serrata extract in treatment of osteoarthritis of knee-a randomized double-blind placebo controlled trial." *Phytomedicine*, 2003; 10:3'7.

24. Badria, F., et al. "Boswellia-curcumin preparation for treating knee osteoarthritis."

Alternative & Complementary Therapies, 2002:341'48.

25. Long, L., K. Soeken, E. Ersnst. "Herbal medicine for the treatment of osteoarthritis: a systematic review." *Rheumatology*, 2001; 40:779'93.

26. Kuptniratsaikul V., *et al.* "Efficacy and safety of Curcuma domestica extracts in patients with knee osteoarthritis." *J Altern Complement Med*, 2009; 15:891-97.

27. Altman, R.D., K.C. Marcussen. "Effects of a ginger extract on knee pain in patients with osteoarthritis." *Arthritis Rheum*, 2001; 44:2531'38.

28. Wigler, I., *et al.* "The effects of Zintona EC (a ginger extract) on symptomatic gonarthritis." *Osteoarthritis Cartilage*, 2003; 11(11):783'89.

29. Larsen, C., *et al.* "An anti-inflammatory galactolipid from rose hip (Rosa canina) that inhibits chemotaxis of human peripeheral blood neutrophils in vitro." *J Nat Prod*, 2003; 66(7):994'95; Warholm, O., *et al.* "The effects of standardized herbal remedy made from a subtype of Rosa canina in patients with osteoarthritis: a double-blind, randomized, placebo-controlled clinical trial." *Curr Ther Res*, Clin & Experimental, 2003; 64(1):21'31.

30. Winther, K., K. Apel, G. Thamsborg. "A powder made from seeds and shells of rose-hip subspecies (*Rosa canina*) reduces symptoms of knee and hip osteoarthritis: a randomized, double-blind, placebo-controlled clinical trial." *Scand J Rheumatol*, 2005; 34:302'08.

31. Piscova, J., *et al.* "Efficacy and safety of freeze-dried cat's claw in osteoarthritis of the knee: mechanisms of action of the species Uncaria guianensis." *Inlamm Res*, 2001; 50:442'48.

32. Cisár P., *et al.* "Effect of pine bark extract (Pycnogenol®) on symptoms of knee osteoarthritis." *Phytother Res*, 2008; 22:1087-92.

33. Schmid, B., *et al.* "Analgesic effect of willow bark extract in osteoarthritis: results of a clinical double-blind trial." *FACT*, 1998; 3:186.

34. Argmandi, B., *et al.* "Soy protein may alleviate osteoarthritis symptoms." *Phytomed*, 2002; 11:567'75.

35. McCarthy, G. M., D. J. McCarty. "Effect of topical capsaicin in the therapy of painful osteoarthritis of the hands." *J Rheumatol*, 1992; 19:604-07; Altman, R.D., A. Aven, C.E. Holmburg, *et al.* "Capsaicin cream 0.025 per cent as monotherapy for osteoarthritis: a double-blind study." *Sem Arth Rheum*, 1994; 23(Suppl 3):25-33; Deal, C.L., T. J. Schnitzer, E. Lipstein, *et al.* "Treatment of arthritis with topical capsaicin: a double-blind trial." *Clin Ther*, 1991; 13:383-95; Schnitzer, T., C. Morton, S. Coker. "Topical capsaicin therapy for osteoarthritis pain: achieving a maintenance regimen." *Sem Arth Rheum*, 1994; 23(Suppl 3):34-40.

36. Felson, D. T., *et al.* "Risk factors for incident radiographic knee osteoarthritis in the elderly: The Framingham study." *Arthritis Rheum*, 1997; 40:728'33; Felson, D. T., *et al.* "Weight loss reduces the risk for symptomatic knee osteoarthritis in women. The Framingham study." *Ann Intern Med*, 1992; 116:535'39.

37. Altman, R. D., C. J. Lozada. "Practice guidelines in the management of osteoarthritis." *Osteoarthritis Cartilage*, 1998; 6(suppla):22'24[review].

38. McAlindon, T. E., P. Jacques, Y. Zhang. "Do antioxidant micronutrients protect against the development and progression of knee osteoarthritis?" *Arthrit Rheum*, 1996; 39:648-56.

39. Perlman, A. I., *et al.* "Massage Therapy for Osteoarthritis of the Knee: A Randomized Controlled Trial." *Arch Intern Med*, 2006; 166:2533'38.

40. Gaw, A. C., L. W. Chang, L-C. Shaw. "Efficacy of acupuncture on osteoarthritic pain. A controlled, double-blind study." *N Engl J Med*, 1975; 293:375-78; Takeda, W., J. Wessel. "Acupuncture for the treatment of pain of osteoarthritic knees." *Arthritis Care Res*, 1994; 7:118-22; Thomas, M., S.V. Eriksson, T. Lundeberg. "A comparative study of diazepam and acupuncture in patients with osteoarthritis pain: a placebo controlled study." *Am J Chin Med*, 1991; 19:95-100; Christensen, B. V., I.U. Iuhl, H. Vilbek, *et al.* "Acupuncture treatment of severe knee osteoarthrosis. A long-term study." *Acta Anaesthesiol Scand*, 1992; 36:519-25; Berman, B. M., *et al.* "A randomized trial of acupuncture as an adjunctive therapy in osteoarthritis of the knee." *Rheumatology*, 1999; 38: 346'54.

41. Witt, C. M., *et al.* "Acupuncture in patients with osteoarthritis of the knee or hip: a randomized, controlled trial with an additional nonrandomized arm." *Arthritis Rheum*, 2006; 54(11):3485'93.

OSTEOPOROSIS

It is a disease reaching epidemic proportions, despite the push for women to consume dairy products. In North America, osteoporosis continues to be the single most common bone disease, with 50 per cent of all Caucasian women, and one out of every eight men developing it in their lifetime. Yet in several other countries throughout the world, almost no one develops it. Japanese women are only half as likely as American women to suffer from spine fractures and two and a half times less likely to fracture a hip. The Chinese have one-fifth the fractures we do.

Why are the chances of getting osteoporosis so much greater in North America? Clearly something we're doing is going very wrong for our bones. So let's expose the myths and uncover the surprising facts about what really makes bones strong.

The Estrogen Push: Fact or Myth

We continue to be told that dropping estrogen levels at menopause are the cause of osteoporosis. But, although this is almost universally accepted without challenge, there are two lines of argument against it. The first is that not all bone loss happens after menopause. In 1985, the Mayo clinic found that half of all vertebral bone loss took place before menopause. The second is that osteoporosis does not seem to correlate so simply with low estrogen. Susan Brown, Ph.D., points out that if falling estrogen levels caused osteoporosis, all women would develop it, but they don't. In several cultures, post-menopausal women have less osteoporosis despite having lower estrogen levels than women in the west. And vegetarian women have lower estrogen levels than meat eaters, but higher bone density. Recent research has found that estrogen levels in women with and without osteoporosis are the same[1].

Even more interesting, not one study using estrogen alone has shown any increase in bone mass. The reason is simple: Although estrogen slows bone loss for the few years that it accelerates during menopause, the effect wears off a few years later, and estrogen cannot rebuild new bone.

A drop in estrogen levels at menopause is a nat-

THINGS THAT LEACH CALCIUM OUT OF YOUR BODY

animal protein
sugar
caffeine
phosphoric acid
salt
alcohol
tobacco
cortisone (prednisone)
antibiotics

ural—not an unnatural—thing. No longer needed for reproduction, since unnecessarily high estrogen levels increase the risk for breast cancer, the body curtails its production.

Real Risk Factors for Osteoporosis

What are the risk factors for osteoporosis? If you are thin or small-boned and have light skin and light-coloured hair, or don't lead a very active life, you are at greater risk for osteoporosis. So are those with thyroid problems, those who have never been pregnant, have bowel disease (which prevents absorption), who smoke, drink pop, eat sugar, salt, too much animal protein and refined grains. If you take drugs such as prednisone, you are also at risk, as are those with poor nutrition.

SO WHAT CAN YOU DO BOTH TO TREAT AND TO PREVENT OSTEOPOROSIS?

Calcium

Everyone knows that calcium is important to bone health, but it isn't calcium intake that is so important as much as it is calcium balance. It isn't how much calcium you take that prevents bone loss; it is how much you lose that causes bone loss. In North America, most women get loads of calcium, but they also take in so many things that leach calcium that they end up with very little calcium still in their systems. In many cultures where osteoporosis is virtually unheard of, only 175 to 540 mg of calcium a day are consumed. The difference is that not as much of the substances that leach calcium are being taken in by these women. How much calcium you need depends on how much calcium you lose. Studies show that Japanese women only need 550 mg of calcium a day, while North American women need 1,241 mg a day to offset their diets. What's wrong with our diets that we lose so much calcium? We consume way too much animal protein, sugar, phosphorus, caffeine, salt, tobacco, alcohol, cortisone, and antibiotics. Low friendly flora caused by antibiotic use can impair your body's ability to digest and absorb nutrients.

Calcium Robbers

So let's take a closer look at some of these calcium robbers that leach calcium from our bodies.

Research shows that eliminating animal protein can reduce calcium loss by 50 per cent. Increasing protein from a healthy 47g a day to a more normal North American amount of 142 g a day, doubles the amount of calcium lost by the body[2]. Summarizing several studies, Susan Brown says that at 95g of protein a day, the body is losing calcium even if you are taking in a lot. The lower amount of animal protein in the diet is one of the reasons that vegetarians have superior bone density.

Part of the reason why protein causes calcium loss is that when the body breaks down the protein it produces acid, which needs to be buffered. And calcium is what the body uses to buffer it. That calcium is drawn out of the bones. The more protein you eat, the more calcium you need. Perhaps this is one reason why a twelve-year study done at Harvard Medical School found that women who drank two or more glasses of milk a day had a 45 per cent higher risk of hip fractures than women who drank less milk[3]. Milk is high in animal protein and also contains sugar (lactose) and phosphorus, which leach calcium. Phosphorus is also found in meat and soft drinks. Soft drinks have been linked to lower levels of calcium[4] and increased incidence of bone fractures[5]. In addition to phosphorus, soft drinks are also high in sugar and caffeine. Sugar not only reduces calcium absorption, it also increases the excretion of calcium and other key bone nutrients[6], and the risk of hip fracture increases with caffeine consumption[7]. Alcohol is also like a sugar in the body. And in western cultures, where osteoporosis rates are so high, we consume plenty of meat, dairy, salt, (which causes the kidneys to excrete excess calcium) caffeine, alcohol, and sugar.

Take Calcium

How much calcium you should take is a hard question to answer, because how much you need depends on what you eat and what you are avoiding as well as your overall health and exercise levels. Some cultures only get about 175 mg of calcium a day and are fine. Again, how much you need depends a lot on how many calcium robbers are part of your diet and lifestyle.

Although just taking calcium is not enough, there is no disagreement that it is part of an effective osteoporosis program. Several studies have shown that calcium helps bone density and helps prevent fracture. Calcium supplements work best when they are divided into several small doses.

But Don't Just Take Calcium . . .

Though calcium is crucial for bone health, calcium does not work alone. Too much isolated calcium can even cause deficiencies of magnesium, manganese, zinc, phosphorus and vitamin K—all important bone-building nutrients.

Magnesium

Low magnesium levels are an important risk factor for osteoporosis[8]. Studies show that taking magnesium increases bone density[9]. Magnesium is crucial for bone density for several reasons: it increases calcium absorption; it increases the absorption of vitamin C; and it helps to convert vitamin D into its active form. Vitamins C and D are both crucial nutrients for bone health. Magnesium also stimulates hormones that preserve bone and regulates those that break it down.

Vitamin D and the Sun for Bones

Vitamin D alone can increase your bone density[10] and reduce hip fractures by 43 per cent to 60 per cent[11]. Calcium needs vitamin D to be absorbed and to be deposited in bone tissue. Taking calcium in the winter with vitamin D not only stops bone loss, but it actually increases bone density[12]. Recent evidence is suggesting that we do not get enough vitamin D because we are worried about skin cancer and either do not go out in the sun anymore or use sun screen to cover up. But rates of osteoporosis are soaring because we simply do not get enough vitamin D. Cancer rates are soaring for the same reason. Vitamin D not only protects your bones, it also protects against many types of cancer. So try to get at least some sunlight each day while you are exercising to make sure you are getting some natural vitamin D, but don't do it in the worst hours when the sun is the strongest. Also, take between 1200 to 1500 IU or more, of vitamin D a day.

Studies prove vitamin D's effectiveness even at lower dosages. In 1997, the *New England Journal of Medicine* reported a study that found when 700 IU of vitamin D was taken with 500 mg of calcium, bone-mineral density went up, while in the placebo group it went up less, or even went down[13].

Other Key Help for Bones

Vitamin C is essential for the synthesis and repair of bone. It also enhances calcium absorption and the effects of vitamin D, and stimulates cells that build bone.

Vitamin K helps to produce osteocalcin, which helps to attract calcium to bone tissue. Without vitamin K, bones would be as soft as chalk. People with osteoporosis have been reported to be low in vitamin K and to be helped by supplementing it. Since vitamin K supplementation is illegal in Canada, the best way to get it is to eat plenty of leafy green vegetables and drink green tea.

Antibiotics wipe out the friendly flora that produce vitamin K, so you may want to try taking probiotics to replenish the friendly flora. Probiotics are crucial to good digestion and it is a good idea to take at least 10 to 20 billion live cells a day to help maximize absorption of nutrients.

Boron is crucial for bone health. To get more boron, eat lots of leafy greens, apples, cherries, almonds, hazelnuts, beans, and pears. Nettle is one of the best bone herbs, partially because it contains boron. Just 3 mg a day of boron has been shown to prevent calcium and magnesium loss in post-menopausual women[14].

Other important nutrients for the bones are B6, B12, and folic acid, the trio that prevents homocysteine. Homocysteine interferes with collagen cross-linking, which causes defective bones. When elderly people who had never before fractured a hip were followed, it was found that the risk of their fracturing a hip went up as their level of homecysteine went up[15]. Similar research has found that people with high homo-cysteine can seriously lower their risk of fractures by supplementing folic acid and B12[16].

Deficiencies of manganese can also increase bone breakdown and decrease bone-mineralization. It is not surprising that women with osteoporosis have only 25 per cent as much manganese as women without osteoporosis.

Zinc helps with calcium absorption and vitamin D activity. Low levels are associated with osteoporosis[17].

Silica and copper are also important. Silica helps to supply silicon for calcium utilization and bone strength, and copper also aids in bone formation.

Beta-carotene is also important; it helps to form collagen in the bone matrix.

Strontium citrate is also key. This nutrient builds new bone, improves retention of calcium, phosphorus, and protein, and prevents the breakdown of old bone. It is found in spices, whole grains, leafy and root vegetables, and legumes.

A surprising help for osteoporosis is the essential fatty acids, such as those found in flaxseeds. It turns out that they improve bone strength by increasing calcium absorption, metabolism, and deposition in the bone, while decreasing calcium excretion in the urine. They enhance the effect of vitamin D and are needed by bone membranes.

Bones and Digestion

Anyone who is taking all of these nutrients and is still having bone trouble should look to her digestive system. Low digestive enzymes prevent the absorption and utilization of nutrients that build bone. Low stomach acid can be at fault. Taking digestive enzymes can help. As can herbs such as gentian and dandelion root, which increase the absorption of nutrients. Also, gut-sealing nutrients such as slippery elm, licorice, and the amino acid L-glutamine can help. Resealing the digestive walls and making them healthier leads to better absorption of nutrients.

As mentioned, probiotics are also important, as they increase absorption of nutrients and keep parasites that can interfere with the absorption of nutrients at bay. For the same reason, herbs that wipe out parasites are also important, such as grapefruit seed extract, black walnut, oregano oil, clove, wormwood, and bitters such as gentian. Fibres, such as psyllium and flaxseed, that keep the intestines clean and ready to absorb, are also useful. Cleaning out the bowels with fibre can help, but don't do it at the same time as you are taking your minerals because the fibre might reduce absorption of the minerals.

Soy

Thanks to the isoflavones found in soy, it too helps to build bone. When sixty-six postmenopausal women were given either 90 mg of isoflavones from soy protein or a placebo for twenty-four weeks, the soy isoflavones produced a significant increase in bone-mineral density in the lumbar spine[18]. When sixty-nine perimenopausal women were given either isoflavone-rich soy protein or whey protein for twenty-four weeks, there was significant loss in bone-mineral density and content in the whey group but not in the soy group, showing the positive effects that soy isoflavones have on bone mass[19].

Soy isoflavones are estrogenic; they may increase bone formation by stimulating bone-building cells[20]; they inhibit cells that break down bone[21]; they may improve calcium absorption[20]; and studies show that soy protein leads to less urinary loss of calcium than animal protein[22].

Finally, try drinking the following herbs as teas for bone health: nettle, which is rich in silica, calcium, magnesium, vitamins D and K, and boron; chamomile, rich in calcium; alfalfa, which is rich in minerals, vitamins D and K; and dandelion, which is rich in silica, minerals, vitamins D and K, boron, calcium, and B vitamins. Green tea also helps to prevent bone loss. Tea drinkers have significantly greater bone density[23]. Drinking not only green tea, but also black or oolong tea for ten or more years leads to significantly higher bone-mineral density[23]. Black tea has been linked to some stomach issues, so be careful. These teas are highly absorbable and taste quite pleasant. Consume three to four cups a day for strong bones. For green tea, consume eight cups a day.

Low kidney essence—yin or yang—is also linked to bone weakness. Premature greying of the hair and low back pain can be early warning signs. Take ho shou wu or schizandra to rebuild weak kidneys. Weak gums and teeth can also be early warning signs of bone problems, as can compressions, fractures, arthritis, poor nail growth, and decreased height.

Foods Rich in Calcium

Also be sure to eat foods that are rich in calcium—leafy greens, sea vegetables, whole grains, raw seeds and nuts, and legumes—for strong bones. Some particularly good sources of calcium include kelp, dulse, kale, mustard green, brewer's yeast, turnip greens, almonds, brown sesame seeds, collard greens, broccoli, figs, dandelion greens, parsley, brazil nuts, watercress, tofu, carob flour, wheat bran, and buckwheat.

Eat lots of millet, as opposed to other grains. Some believe that high acid levels in the body can cause bones to break down, and millet does not produce acid. Eat lots of vegetables, other than potato, for the same reason.

Again, don't rely on dairy. Although dairy products may be high in calcium, they are not well-absorbed. According to Michael T. Murray, N.D., kale has a better calcium absorption rate than milk. And, as mentioned, dairy is high in animal protein, sugar, and phosphorus, and both a vegetarian diet and a vegan diet (in other words, no dairy) are associated with a lower risk of osteoporosis[24].

And, of course, don't forget to exercise. Exercise helps to maintain strong and healthy bones and is one of the most important bone-building factors, especially if you do it in sunlight, which also increases bone mass. Do weight-bearing exercises for at least one hour a day.

Chapter Endnotes

1. Brown, S. *Better Bones, Better Body*. Lincolnwood IL: Keats, 2000.

2. Licata, A., *et al*. "Acute effects of dietary protein on calcium metabolism in patients with osteoporosis." *J Geron*, 1981; 36:14'19.

3. Feskanich, D., *et al*. "Milk, dietary calcium, and bone fractures in women: a 12-year prospective study." *Am J Public Health*, 1997; 87:992'97.

4. Mazariegos-Ramos, E., *et al*. "Consumption of soft drinks with phosphoric acid as a risk factor for the development of hypocalcemia in children: a case-control study." *J Pediatr*, 1995; 126:940'42.

5. Wyshak, G., R.E. Frisch. "Carbonated beverages, dietary calcium, the dietary calcium/phosphorus ratio, and bone fractures in girls and boys." *J Adolescent Health*, 1994; 15:210-15.

6. Anderson, R., A. Kozlovsky, P. Moser. "Effects of diets high in simple sugars on urinary chromium excretion of humans." *Fed Proc*, 1985; 44:251; Lemann, J., W.F. Piering, E.J. Lennon. "Possible role of carbohydrate-induced calciuria in calcium oxalate kidney-stone formation." *N Engl J Med*, 1969; 280:232'37.

7. Hernandez-Avila, M., *et al*. "Caffeine, moderate alcohol intake, and risk of fractures of the hip and forearm in middle-aged women." *Am J Clin Nutr*, 1991; 54:157'63.

8. Cohen, L., R. Kitzes. "Infrared spectroscopy and magnesium content of bone-mineral in osteoporotic women." *Isr J Med Sci*, 1981; 17:1123-25; Geinster, J.Y., *et al*. "Preliminary report of decreased serum magnesium in postmenopausal osteoporosis." *Magnesium*, 1989; 8:106-09; Stendig-Lindberg, G., R. Tepper, I. Leichter. "Tabecular bone density in a two-year controlled trial of peroral magnesium in osteoporosis." *Magnesium Res*, 1993; 6:155'63.

9. Dimai, H.P., *et al*. "Daily oral magnesium supplementation suppresses bone turnover in young adult males." *J Clin Endocrinol Metab*, 1998; 83:2742-48; Stendig-Lindberg, G., R. Tepper, I. Leichter. "Tabecular bone density in a two-year controlled trial of peroral magnesium in osteoporosis." *Magnesium Res*, 1993; 6:155'63.

10. Dawson-Hughes, B., *et al*. "Effect of vitamin D supplementation on wintertime and overall bone loss in healthy postmenopausal women." *Ann Intern Med*, 1991; 115:505-12; Ooms, M.E., *et al*. "Prevention of bone loss by viatamin D supplementation in elderly women: a randomized double-blind study." *J Clin Endocrinol Metabol*, 1995; 80:1052'58; Adams, J.S., *et al*. "Resolution of vitamin D insufficiency in osteopenic patients results in rapid recovery of bone-mineral density." *J Clin Endocrinol Metab*, 1999; 84:2729-30.

11. Dawson-Hughes, B., *et al*. "Rate of bone loss in postmenopausal women ran-domly assigned to one of two dosages of the vitamin D." *Am J Clin Nutr*, 1995 61:1140'45; Chapuy, M.C., *et al*. "Effect of calcium and cholecalfiferol treatmen for three years on hip fractures in elderly women." *Br Med J*, 1994; 308:1081'82

12. Dawson-Hughes, B., *et al*. "A controlled trial of the effect of calcium supplementation on bone density in postmenopausal women." *N Eng J Med*, 1990 323:878'83.

13. Dawson-Hughes, B., *et al*. "Effect of calcium and vitamin D supplementation or bone density in men and women 65 years of age or older." *N Eng J Med*, 1997 337:701'02.

14. Nielsen, F.H. Boron-an overlooked element of potential nutritional importance *Nutr Today* (Jan/Feb):4'7.

15. McLean, R.R., *et al*. "Homocysteine as a Predictive Factor for Hip Fracture ir Older Persons." *N Engl J Med*, 2004; 350:2047'49.

16. Sato, Y., *et al*. "Effect of folate and mecobalamin on hip fractures in patients witl stroke: a randomized controlled trial." *JAMA*, 2005; 293:1082-88.

17. Sahap, A.O. "Zinc and senile osteoporosis." *J Am Geriatr Soc*, 1983; 31:790-91

18. Potter, S.M., *et al*. "Soy protein and isoflavones: their effects on blood lipids and bone density in postmenopausal women." *Am J Clin Nutr*, 1998; 68(Suppl):1375-9S[is this correct?].

19. Alekel, D.L., *et al*. "Isoflavone-rich soy protein isolate attenuates bone loss in the lumbar spine of perimenopausal women." *Am J Clin Nutr*, 2000; 72:844'52.

20. Sugimoto, E., M. Yamaguchi. "Stimulatory effect of daidzein in osteoblastic MC3T3-E1 cells." *Biochem Pharmacol*, 2000; 59:471'75.

21. Blair, H.C., *et al*. "Variable effects of tyrosine kinase inhibitors on avian osteo-clastic activity and reduction of bone loss in ovariectomized rats." *J Cell Biochem* 1996; 61:629'37.

22. Breslau, N.A., *et al*. "Relationship of animal protein-rich diet to kidney stone formation and calcium metabolism." *J Clin Endocrinol Metab*, 1988; 66:140'46.

23. Hegarty, V.M., H.M. May, K.T. Khaw. "Tea drinking and bone-mineral density ir older women." *Am J Clin Nutr*, 2000; 71:1003-07; Wu, C-H., *et al*. "Epidemio-logical Evidence of Increased bone-mineral Density in Habitual Tea Drinkers." *Arch Intern Med*, 2002; 162:1001'06.

24. Ellis, F., S. Holesh, J. Ellis. "Incidence of osteoporosis in vegetarians and omni vores." *Am J Clin Nutr*, 1972; 25:55'58; Marsh, A., *et al*. "bone-mineral mass ir adult lacto-ovo-vegetarian and omnivorous adults." *Am J Clin Nutr*, 1983 37:453'56.

PARKINSON'S DISEASE

Parkinson's affects about 1 per cent of people over the age of fifty and most affects people after the age of sixty. It is more common in men. Parkinson's is caused by damage to nerves in the brain that make a neurotransmitter called dopamine, leading to depleted levels of that neurotransmitter, which then causes muscle tremours and rigidity, slurred speech, balance problems, loss of facial expression, depression, memory loss, and dementia. Research has pointed to many natural approaches that offer help.

Diet: Low in Protein, High in Fava Beans

A diet that is low in protein has been proven in several studies to help. It enhances the action of L-dopa, the precursor to dopamine, by reducing its competition with other amino acids to cross the blood-brain barrier. In addition to a diet that is low in protein, it is helpful to save most of the protein you eat until dinner and have almost none throughout the day[1].

Another dietary change that can help is a diet rich in beans. Eating a lot of legumes is associated with a low risk of Parkinson's[2]. One bean in particular seems most helpful. Fava beans actually contain L-dopa; in fact, L-dopa was originally discovered in fava beans. One study found that giving 250 mg of cooked fava beans substantially increased blood levels of L-dopa and substantially improved motor performance[3]. If 250 mg of fava beans a day is too much for you, then there is good news. James Duke, Ph.D., says that fava bean sprouts have ten times more L-dopa than the beans. That makes it easy.

If you use Parkinson's drugs, be careful that combining them with fava beans doesn't drive your L-dopa levels too high.

Antioxidants Prevent Parkinson's

Research shows that diets rich in antioxidants, especially vitamin E, may prevent Parkinson's[4]. One double-blind study gave 750 mg of vitamin C and 800 IU of vitamin E four times a day to people with early Parkinson's. The antioxidant group did better than the placebo group and was able to postpone the need for medicine by two and a half years, compared to the placebo group[5]. Another small double-blind study of vitamin C alone found modest improvements when people on the drug L-dopa had vitamin C added to their program[6].

Other Helpful Nutrients

The active form of B3, called NADH, significantly raises brain levels of dopamine and significantly diminishes the symptoms of Parkinson's[7]. Ten to twenty milligrams per day is the dose.

Another exciting possibility is the amino acid methionine: it seems to improve the symptoms of

Parkinson's[8]. In a tough test of this treatment, when people who had already responded to drugs were also given methionine, two-thirds of them improved even more[9].

Occasionally, something as simple as a folic acid deficiency can cause Parkinson's disease. Get your level checked, and if it is low, taking folic acid supplements should stop the progress[10].

Breaking Research: CoQ10 and Parkinson's
Recently research has focused on coenzyme Q10. In the first study, a very high dose of 1,200 mg of CoQ10 slowed down the progression of the disease. In this sixteen-month double-blind study, Parkinson's worsened by 49.8 per cent in the placebo group, but by a significantly lower 29.6 per cent in the group taking CoQ10[11].

Most recently, when twenty-eight people with Parkinson's were given a smaller 180 mg dose of CoQ10 twice a day for four weeks, some of their symptoms improved significantly more than did those of people in the placebo group[12].

Antispasmodic Passionflower
Two prominent herbalists both mention passionflower for Parkinson's. Michael Tierra says it is used for neurological disorders, including Parkinson's; David Hoffmann says it can be used as an antispasmodic for Parkinson's. Skullcap is another antispasmodic herb that is helpful for Parkinson's. Daniel Mowrey, Ph.D., and herbalist

Michael Tierra both say that pau d'arco is reported to be helpful. And ginkgo biloba can help mood and mental function, as can phosphatidylserine.

Less Animal Products, Less Parkinson's
Recent research has also taken a renewed interest in diet. One study looking at the association of food and Parkinson's found an association between dairy and Parkinson's in men, though not in women. Higher consumption of dairy may increase the risk of Parkinson's in men[13].

The finger was pointed at animal products again in a second study. In this one, while staying on their usual medication, nineteen people with Parkinson's were given 30 mg of B2 every eight hours and had all the red meat eliminated from their diet for six months. All nineteen people saw their motor capacity improve significantly[14].

Given the research on dairy and meat, it is not surprising to find that a vegan diet may be helpful for Parkinson's[15]. In their book *Medical Botany*, Walter H. Lewis and Memory P. F. Elvin-Lewis report that three case studies have found that plant fats do not increase the risk of Parkinson's disease the way that animal fat and cholesterol do.

More Help
Finally, exposure to pesticides may contribute to the development of Parkinson's disease, while exercise improves it.

Chapter Endnotes

. Pincus, J. H., K.M. Barry. "Dietary method for reducing fluctuations in Parkinson's disease." *Yale J Biol Med*, 1987; 60:133'37; Tsui, J., *et al.* "The effect of dietary protein on the efficacy of L-dopa: a double-blind study." *Neurology*, 1989; 39:549'52; Carter, J. H., *et al.* "Amount and distribution of dietary protein affects clinical response to levodopa in Parkinson's disease." *Neurology*, 1989; 39:552'56; Karstaedt, P. J., J. H. Pincus. "Protein redistribution diet remains effective in patients with fluctuating Parkinsonism." *Arch Neurol*, 1992; 49:149'51.

. Morens, D.M., *et al.* "Case-control study of idiopathic Parkinson's disease and dietary vitamin E intake." *Neurology*, 1996; 46:1270-74.

. Rabey, J.M., *et al.* "Broad bean (Vicia faba) consumption and Parkinson's disease." *Adv Neurol*, 1993;.60:681'84.

. de Pijk, M.C., *et al.* "Dietary antioxidants and Parkinson's disease. The Rotterdam Study." Arch Neurol, 1997; 54:762'65; Scheider, W.L., *et al.* "Dietary antioxidants and other dietary factors in the etiology of Parkinson's disease." *Mov Disord*, 1997; 12:190'96.

. Fahn, S. "A pilot trial of high-dose alpha-tocopherol and ascorbate in early Parkinson's disease." *Ann Neurol*, 1992; 32:S128'32.

. Reilly, D.K., *et al.* "On-off effects in Parkinson's disease: a controlled investigation of ascorbic acid therapy." *Adv Neurol*, 1983; 37:51'60.

. Birkmayer, J.G.D., *et al.* "Nicotinamide adenine dinucleotide (NAD). A new therapeutic approach to Parkinson's disease. Comparison of oral and parenteral application." *Acta Neurol Scand*, (Suppl) 1993; 146:32'35.

. Meininger, V., *et al.* "L-methionine treatment of Parkinson's disease: preliminary results." *Rev Neurol* (Paris), 1982; 297'303.

9. Smythies, J.R., J.H. Halsey. "Treatment of Parkinson's disease with L-methionine." *South Med J*, 1984; 77:1577.

10. Clayton, P., *et al.* "Subacute combined degeneration of the cord, dementia and Parkinsonism due to an inborn error of folate metabolism." J *Neurol Neurosurg Psychiatry*, 1986; 49:920'27.

11. Shults, C.W., *et al.* "Effects of coenzyme Q10 in early Parkinson's disease: evidence of slowing of the functional decline." *Archives of Neurology*, 2002; 59:1541'50.

12. *Neuroscience Letters*, 2003; 341:201-04.

13. Chen, H., *et al.* "Diet and Parkinson's disease: a potential role of dairy products in men." *Ann Neurol*, 2002; 52:793'801.

14. Coimbra, C.G., V.B.C. Junqueira. "High doses of riboflavin and the elimination of dietary red meat promote the recovery of some motor functions in Parkinson's disease patients." *Braz J Med Biol Res*, 2003; (36)409'1417.

15. McCarty, M.F. "Does a vegan diet reduce risk for Parkinson's disease?" *Med Hypotheses*, 2001; 57:318'23.

RHEUMATOID ARTHRITIS

Rheumatoid arthritis is a very common form of arthritis, that causes severe and even crippling pain. It is an autoimmune disease and a chronic inflammatory condition. The most important step in controlling the inflammation and in preventing and treating this painful disease is adapting the diet.

What to Eat and What Not to Eat

The diet should be abundant in whole foods, fibre, fruits, and vegetables; it should be low in meat, saturated fat, refined carbohydrates, and sugar. Simply put, the rheumatoid arthritis diet should be rich in plant foods and poor in animal foods.

One of the reasons for emphasizing plant foods over animal foods is that the unsaturated fats found in plant food are anti-inflammatory, while the saturated fats found in animal foods are highly inflammatory. By altering dietary fats, you can reduce inflammation. This difference in fats is one of the reasons why vegetarian diets are so helpful in inflammatory diseases.

Research shows that people with rheumatoid arthritis eat more animal fat than people without rheumatoid arthritis[1]. Research also shows that when you remove animal fats, you get better; simply adopting a vegan diet reduces the symptoms of rheumatoid arthritis[2]. Two recent studies have once again highlighted the importance of these dietary changes. When people with rheumatoid arthritis who were already on medication followed either a typical western diet or a Mediterranean diet that was high in fish, fruit, vegetables, grains, beans, and olive oil, and low in meat and dairy for three months, the Mediterranean diet group had a significant 56 per cent reduction in joint swelling, tenderness, and pain[3]. In the second study, people with rheumatoid arthritis were put on either a normal diet or on a vegan diet that was also gluten-free. While only 4 per cent of the people on the normal diet improved, a full 40.5 per cent on the vegan diet improved[4]. In addition to shifting the fats in your diet from saturated fats to unsaturated fats, supplementing with polyunsaturated omega-3 essential fatty acids can also help improve symptoms[5]

The removal of gluten in the second study also points to the importance of removing food allergens from the diet of rheumatoid arthritics. Studies show that food allergies are linked to rheumatoid arthritis. But just as rheumatoid arthritis symptoms worsen when food allergens are eaten, so they improve when the allergens are eliminated[6]. Amazingly, one-third of people with rheumatoid arthritis may be able to completely control their disease simply by eliminating the foods they are allergic to[7]. Milk, dairy products, and wheat are very common allergies in people with rheumatoid arthritis[8]. Other common offenders are beef, corn, food additives, and nightshade vegetables (peppers, eggplant, potatoes, and tomatoes). Tobacco is also a nightshade, so don't smoke.

Another helpful and—this time—delicious dietary change to make is to eat lots of flavonoid rich dark grapes and berries, such as cherries, blueberries, cranberries, and blackberries. Flavonoids are antioxidant and anti-inflammatory, two great properties for rheumatoid arthritis sufferers. You can also supplement flavonoids by taking grape seed extract and quercetin. Quercetin is a very powerful anti-inflammatory.

Adding Even More Antioxidants

In addition to increasing antioxidants in your diet, it helps to supplement them as well. Vitamin E seems especially to stand out. People with rheumatoid arthritis have low levels of vitamin E in their joint fluids[9], suggesting that supplementing vitamin E should help. And it does[10]. At least two double-blind studies have found vitamin E to be significantly more effective than a placebo for rheumatoid arthritis[11], and, even more impressively, at least two have found vitamin E to be about as effective as anti-inflammatory drugs[12].

People with rheumatoid arthritis are also low in the antioxidant mineral selenium[13]. Supple-

menting selenium has had mixed results. One double-blind study found a significant reduction in pain and joint swelling[14], but another found no benefit. Rheumatoid arthritics are also low in vitamin C and manganese.

Though not an antioxidant, another nutrient that helps is vitamin B5[15]. In a double-blind, placebo-controlled study, 2 g of B5 for two months improved morning stiffness, disability, and pain[16].

Helping Rheumatoid Arthritis with Herbs

Many herbs are powerfully anti-inflammatory and antioxidant and are enormously helpful for rheumatoid arthritis.

Bromelain

Bromelain comes from pineapples and is better known as a digestive enzyme, but when it is taken on an empty stomach instead of with the food it is meant to digest, it is one of the most powerful anti-inflammatories. In an early study done in the sixties, bromelain was shown to improve joint swelling and mobility[17]. Strangely, even though bromelain is a known anti-inflammatory that worked in its first test, we are unable to find any rheumatoid arthritis studies that have been done on it since. Clinically, Linda sees good results with it.

Curcumin

Curcumin, the active ingredient in the herb turmeric, is another remarkable anti-inflammatory. In acute inflammation, curcumin is as effective as cortisone or the nonsteroidal anti-inflammatory drug, phenylbutazone; in chronic inflammation, it is half as effective but much safer. When people with rheumatoid arthritis were given either 1,200 mg of curcumin or the powerful nonsteroidal anti-inflammatory drug phenylbutazone, the improvement in morning stiffness and joint swelling was comparable in the two groups[18].

Ginger

Ginger is both anti-inflammatory and antioxidant, a great combination for rheumatoid arthritis. So it is no surprise that studies show that it helps rheumatoid arthritis[19]. Even when medication hasn't done the job, ginger has been able to improve pain, joint mobility, swelling, and stiffness[20].

Boswellia

A less well-known anti-inflammatory herb is boswellia. Boswellia is a species of frankincense, a species of herb so valued in the ancient world that it was, according to the New Testament, one of the gifts the three Wise Men gave to Jesus. Double-blind research shows that boswellia improves pain, stiffness, and joint function. Not all, but most of the research on boswellia and rheumatoid arthritis is positive[21].

Cat's Claw

Curcumin, ginger, and boswellia all come from the Ayurvedic healing tradition of India. But South America also has something to offer—the amazing anti-inflammatory herb cat's claw. Cat's claw has been used by traditional healers in Peru to treat arthritis for thousands of years. When modern scientists put this herb to the test by adding either it or a placebo to the drugs of people with rheumatoid arthritis, joint pain went down by 53.2 per cent in the cat's claw group, but only by 24.1 per cent in the placebo group. The cat's claw group also had less morning stiffness[22].

Detox and More Herbal Help

Other herbs that may help rheumatoid arthritis include licorice, feverfew, devil's claw, and white willow bark.

A good detox can also help. Use high doses of buffered vitamin C, up to ten g, and herbs such as yellow dock, burdock, celery seed, nettle, wheat grass, barley grass, and alfalfa.

Tradional herbalists would use herbs such as Oregon grape root, prince's pine, sassafras, prickly ash bark, black cohosh, guaiacum, ginger, and cayenne for arthritis. Yucca is believed to help by gradually removing from the intestines the toxins that permeate into the bloodstream and cause joint swelling. A detox also changes the toxins in the body, helping to get rid of swelling.

Help from the Outside In

Topically, applying a cream made from cayenne has been shown in double-blind research to help[23]. Creams made from ginger or lobelia also help. And Germany's authoritative Commission E approves the topical use of the essential oils of cajeput, camphor, rosemary, eucalyptus, fir, and pine needle. Peppermint oil and topical arnica, ivy, birch, and shave grass may also help.

And one more unusual topical treatment may be worth trying. When a copper bracelet was compared to a placebo bracelet, researchers found it to be effective[24].

Lifestyle Changes

Two other things will help treat rheumatoid arthritis. The first is exercise. Several studies show that it helps[25]. The second is improving digestion and healing a leaky gut.

Clinically, Linda finds it is crucial in rheumatoid arthritis patients to take probiotics and seal up a leaky gut. She finds that 2 to 20 billion live cultures of probiotics a day and L-glutamine or licorice to seal the gut have worked very well, in combination with either cat's claw, bromelain or curcumin. MSM also helps the inflammation and the pain of rheumatoid arthritis and helps to seal the gut. MSM is an anti-inflammatory, antispasmodic and analgesic. SAMe may also help, as it detoxes the liver.

5-HTP may also help with the pain, as it increases serotonin and endorphins, two nautrally occurring susbstances that helps to reduce pain in the body.

You may also want to try immune herbs, or immune modulators, such as sterinols. Cat's claw helps partially because it is a source of sterinols.

Accupuncture is also very useful. Or try hydrotherapy.

Chapter Endnotes

1. Jacobsson, I., F. Lindgarde, R. Manthorpe, *et al.* "Correlation of fatty acid composition of adipose tissue liquids and serum phosphatidylcholine and serum concentrations of micronutrients with disease duration in rheumatoid arthritis." *Ann Rheum Dis*, 1990; 49:901'05.

2. Skoldstam, L. "Fasting and vegan diet in rheumatoid arthritis." *Scand J Rheumatol*, 1987; 15:219'21; Nenonen, M., T. Helve, O. Hanninen. "Effects of uncooked vegan food-'living food'-on rheumatoid arthritis: a three month controlled and randomized study." *Am J Clin Nutr*, 1992; 56:762[abstract #48].

3. Skoldstam, L., L. Hagfors, G. Johansson. "An experimental study of Mediterranean diet intervention for patients with rheumatoid arthritis." *Annals of Rheumatic Diseases*, 2003; 62:208'14.

4. Hafström, I. "A vegan diet free of gluten improves the signs and symptoms of rheumatoid arthritis: the effects on arthritis correlate with a reduction in antibodies to food antigens." *Rheumatology*, 2001; 40:1175'79.

5. Kremer, J. M., W. Jubiz, A. Michalek, *et al.* "Fish oil fatty acid supplementation in active rheumatoid arthritis." *Ann Int Med*, 1987; 106(4):497-503; Kremer, J. M., D. A. Lawrence, W. Jubiz, *et al.* "Dietary fish oil and olive oil supplementation in patients with rheumatoid arthritis." *Arthrit Rheum*, 1990; 33(6):810-20; Geusens, P., C. Wouters, J. Nijs, *et al.* "Longterm effect of omega-3 fatty acid supplementation in active rheumatoid arthritis." *Arthrit Rheum*, 1994; 37:824-29; Van der Tempel, H., J. E. Tulleken, P. C. Limburg, *et al.* "Effects of fish oil supplementation in rheumatoid arthritis." *Ann Rheum Dis*, 1990; 49:76-80; Cleland, L. G., J. K. French, W. H. Betts, *et al.* "Clinical and biochemical effects of dietary fish oil supplements in rheumatoid arthritis." *J Rheumatol*, 1988; 15(10):1471-75; Kremer, J. M., D. A. Lawrence, G. F. Petrillow, *et al.* "Effects of high dose fish oil on rheumatoid arthritis after stopping nonsteroidal antiinflammatory drugs." *Arthritis Rheum*, 1995; 38:1107-14.

6. Darlington, L. G., N.W. Ramsey, J. R. Mansfield. "Placebo controlled, blind study of dietary manipulation therapy in rheumatoid arthritis." *Lancet*, 1986; i:236-38; Beri, D., *et al.* "Effect of dietary restrictions on disease activity in rheumatoid arthritis." *Ann Rheum Dis*, 1988; 47:69-72; Panush, R.S. "Possible role of food sensitivity in arthritis." *Ann Allerg*, 1988; 61(part 2):31-35; Taylor, M. R. "Food allergy as an etiological factor in arthropathies: a survey." *J Internat Acad Prev Med*, 1983; 8:28-38 [review]; Hicklin, J. A., L. M. McEwen, J. E. Margan. "The effect of diet in rheumatoid arthritis." *Clin Allergy*, 1980; 10:463'67; Panush, R. S. "Delayed reactions to foods. Food allergy and rheumatic disease." *Ann Allergy*, 1986; 56:500'03; Van de Laar, M. A. F. J., J. K. Ander Korst. "Food intolerance in rheumatoid arthritis. A double-blind, controlled trial of the clinical effects of elimination of milk allergens and azo dyes." *Ann Rheum Dis*, 1992; 51:298'302

7. Darlington, L. G., N. W. Ramsey. "Diets for rheumatoid arthritis." *Lancet*, 1991; 338:1209 [letter].

8. O'Farrelly, *et al.* "IgA rheumatoid factors and IgA dietary protein antibodies are associated in rheumatoid arthritis." *Immunol Invest*, 1989; 18:753'64.

9. Fairburn, K., M. Grootveld, R.J. Ward, *et al.* "Lipids and lipoproteins in knee-joint synovial fluid and serum from patients with inflammatory joint disease." *Clin Sci*, 1992; 83:657'64.

10. Scherak, O., G. Kolarz. "Vitamin E and rheumatoid arthritis." *Arthritis Rheum*, 1991; 34:1205'06[letter].

11. Edmonds, S. E., P. G. Winyard, R. Guo, *et al.* "Putative analgesic activity of repeated oral doses of vitamin E in the treatment of rheumatoid arthritis. Results of a prospective placebo controlled double-blind trial." *Ann Rheum Dis*, 1997; 56:649-55; Miehle, W. "Vitamin E in active arthroses and chronic polyarthritis. What is the value of alpha-tocopherol in therapy?" *Fortschr Med*, 1997; 115:39-42.

12. Kolarz, G., *et al.* "High dose vitamin E for chronic arthritis." *Akt Rheumatol*, 1990; 15:233-37; Wittenborg, A., *et al.* "Effectiveness of vitamin E in comparison with diclofenac sodium in treatment of patients with chronic polyarthritis." *Z Rheumatol*, 1998; 57:215-21.

13. Aaseth, J., *et al.* "Trace elements in serum and urine of patients with rheumatoid arthritis." *Scand J Rheumatol*, 1978; 7:237'40; Munthe, E., J. Aaseth. "Treatment of rheumatoid arthritis with selenium and vitamin E." *Scand J Rheumatol*, 1984; 53(suppl):103; Tarp, U., *et al.* "Selenium treatment in rheumatoid arthritis." *Scand J Rheumatol*, 1985; 14:364'68; Tarp, U., *et al.* "Low selenium level in severe rheumatoid arthritis." *Scand J Rheumatol*, 1985; 14:97'101.

14. Peretz, A., *et al.* "Adjuvant treatment of recent onset rheumatoid arthritis by selenium supplementation: preliminary observations." *Br J Rheumatol*, 1992; 31:281'82[letter].

15. Barton-Wright, E. C., W. A. Elliot. "The pantothenic acid metabolism of rheumatoid arthritis." *Lancet*, 1963; ii:862'63.

16. General Practitioner Research Group. "Calcium pantothenate in arthritic conditions." *Practitioner*, 1980; 224:208'11.

17. Cohen, A., J. Goldman. "Bromelain therapy in rheumatoid arthritis." *Pennsylvania Med J*, 1964; 67:27'30.

18. Deodhar, S. D., R. Sethi, R. C. Srimal. "Preliminary studies on antirheumatic activity of curcumin (diferuloyl methane)." *Ind J Med Res*, 1980; 71:632'34.

19. Srivastava, K. C., T. Mustafa. "Ginger (Zingiber officianale) in rheumatism and musculoskeletal disorders." *Med Hypothesis*, 1992; 39:342'48.

20. Srivastava, K.C., T. Mustafa. "Ginger (Zingiber officianale) and rheumatic disorders." *Med Hypothesis*, 1989; 29:25'28.

21. Singh, G.B., S. Singh, S. Bani. "New phytotherapeutic agent for the treatment of arthritis and allied disorders with novel mode of action." Fourth International Congress on Phytotherapy, Munich, September 1992; Etzel, R. "Special extract of *Boswellia serrata* in the treatment of rheumatoid arthritis." *Phytomed*, 1996 3:91'94 [review].

22. Mur, E., *et al.* "Randomized double-blind trial of an extract from the pentacyclic alkaloid-chemotype of Uncaria tomentosa for the treatment of rheumatoid arthritis." *J Rheumatol*, 2002; 29:678-81.

23. Deal, C.L., T.J. Schnitzer, E. Lipstein. "Treatment of arthritis with topical capsaicin: a double-blind trial." *Clin Ther*, 1991; 13:383'95.

24. Walker, W.R., D.M. Keats. "An investigation of the therapeutic value of the 'copper bracelet'-dermal assimilation of copper in arthritic/rheumatoid conditions." *Agents Actions*, 1976; 6:454'59.

25. Kay, D.R., R.B. Weber, T.E. Drisinger, *et al.* "Aerobic exercise improves performance in arthritis patients." *Clin Res*, 1985; 33:919A[abstract]; Harcom, T.M., *et al.* "Therapeutic value of graded aerobic exercise training in rheumatoid arthritis." *Arthrit Rheum*, 1985;.28:32'38; De Jong, Z., *et al.* "Long term high intensity exercise and damage of small joints in rheumatoid arthritis." *Annals of Rheumatic Diseases*, 2004; 63:1399'1405.

FAMILY HEALTH GLOSSARY

Acetylcholine: a neurotransmitter that relays nerve impulses. It's deficiency is linked to Alzheimer's.

Adaptogen: herb that is safe, increases your resistance to things that stress the body and that normalizes body functions by bringing them up or down as necessary.

Adenosine: One of the brain's natural calming substance.

Adrenaline: A hormone secreted by the adrenal gland that prepares the body for fight or flight in times of stress. Also called epinephrine.

Amenorrhoea: Absence of period.

Amino acids: The building blocks of proteins. Those that can be synthesized by the body are nonessential amino acids; those that must be obtained by the diet are essential amino acids.

Analgesic: Herbs that relieve pain.

Angiogenesis: The formation of the new blood vessels that tumours form to get the nutrients they need to grow.

Antioxidant: A substance that prevents free radical damage.

Anthilitic: A herb that is used to prevent or remove kidney stones.

Antispasmodic: Herbs that prevent or relax muscle spasms or cramps.

Aphrodisiac: substance that increases sexual desire.

Apoptosis: Natural programmed cell death. A very safe way of killing cancer cells without killing the healthy cells around them.

Arrhythmia: An irregularity of the heart rhythm.

Astringent: Herbs that have a contracting or tightening effect on tissue and so stop the loss of body fluids like haemorrhages and other secretions.

Atherosclerosis: A hardening of the artery walls, usually caused by plaque made up of cholesterol and fatty material, that blocks the blood flow through the arteries.

Autoimmune: A kind of disease in which antibodies develop against the body's own tissue.

Balm: a topical preparation that is soothing or healing.

Carcinogen: A substance that causes cancer.

Carminative: Herbs that relieve gas and gripping.

Corpus luteum: The glandular tissue in the ovary that forms after ovulation and secretes the hormone progesterone.

Corticosteroid: Hormones produced by the adrenal glands that regulate the balanace of salt and water, act as anti-inflammatories, participate in the stress response and are needed for the utilization of carbohydrates, fats and proteins.

Cyst: An abnormal growth in the shape of a sac that is filled with fluid or semisolid matter.

Decoction: A herbal tea in which the hard parts of the plant are simmered for 20 minutes to an hour.

Demulcents: Herbs that are taken internally to soothe damaged, irritated or inflamed tissue.

Diaphoretic: Herbs that induce sweating.

Diuretic: Herbs that increase the flow of urine.

Double-blind study: A study in which neither the researcher nor the subject knows if they are taking the active substance or the placebo/control substance to protect against bias.

Dysentary: An infection of the intestine that causes severe diarrhoea with blood and mucous.

Dysmenorrhoea: Painful period.

Dyspepsia: Indigestion, the symptoms of which are heartburn, nausea and appetite loss.

Dysplasia: An abnormal growth.

Edema: An accessive accumulation of fluid in the tissue.

Elimination diet: A diet that eliminates food allergens.

Emmenogogue: A herb that helps bring on menstruation.

Enteric coated: A pill that is coated to prevent it from dissolving in the stomach to ensure that it is not destroyed before it reaches the intestines.

Enzyme: A catalyst that speeds up a biological reaction.

Epidemiological study: A study that looks at the pattern of a disease in human populations.

Essential fatty acids: Unsaturated fats that the body cannot manufacture and so must get from food, including omega-3 and omega-6 fatty acids.

Essential oil: Volatile oils that are responsible for the odour or taste of a plant and are used in aromatherapy and herbal medicine.

Expectorant: Herbs that encourage the expulsion of excess mucous from the throat and lungs.

Extract: A concentrated form of a herb that is stronger than a tincture. Liquid extracts usually contains one part herb for each part liquid solvent (1:1); solid extracts are even stronger, usually around 4:1, but sometimes as much as 50:1 or more.

Fibrinolysis: The break down of fibrin or a blood clot by an enzyme.

Flavonoid: A group of antioxidants found in many plant foods and herbs that are more powerful and work against a wider range of free radicals than the vitamin antioxidants. Flavonoids are also anti-inflammatory, antiallergic, antiviral and anticancer amongst other uses.

Free Radical: Molecules that are unstable because they have an unpaired electron. When they try to stabalize themselves they rip electrons from other molecules. The damage that results is behind many diseases.

Galactogogue: Herbs that increase the production of breast milk.

Gluten: The protein found in certain grains.

Hamilton rating scales: rating scales for clinical depression and clinical anxiety.

Hemaglobin: A substance contained in the red blood cells that carries oxygen throughout the body.

Hormone: A substance that is produced in an endocrine gland and passes through the bloodstream to distant parts of the body where it controls and regulates bodily functions.

Hyperglycemia: High blood sugar.

Hyperplasia: Excessive growth of normal tissue that grows larger but retains its normal form.

Hypertension: High blood pressure.

Hypoglycemia: Low blood sugar.

Infusion: A herbal tea in which the soft parts of the plant are steeped in a covered container for 10-20 minutes.

Insulin: A hormone produced by the beta cells of the pancreas that lowers blood sugar by stimulating the uptake of blood sugar into the body's cells.

Interferon: The human body's own immune enhancing virus and cancer fighter.

In vitro: These studies are conducted outside of a living body in laboratories, literally "in glass" or in a test tube.

In vivo: These studies are conducted in vivo, meaning in a living body.

Lactose: A sugar found in milk.

Laxative: A substance that promotes bowel movements.

Leukotrienes: Inflammatory compounds involved in many inflammatory conditions.

Lipotropic: An agent that promotes the flow of fats from the liver or accelerates the utilization of fat in the liver so the liver does not become clogged, blocking metabolism.

Menorrhagia: Exessively heavy period.

Metastasis: The spread of cancer from the primary growth to a nearby site, like the lymph nodes, or to a distant site.

Motility: The ability of a sperm cell to move spontaneously without external aid.

Myelin sheath: A substance made of proteins and fats that surrounds nerve cells and increase the speed at which nerve impulses are transmitted.

Nervine: Herbs that calm and nourish the nervous system.

Neurotransmitter: A chemical substance that transmits nerve impulses.

Phytoestrogen: Plant estrogens that have a very mild effect compared to human estrogen: they can gently lower estrogen by stealing receptor sites from your own more powerful estrogen or raise it as needed.

Placebo: An inactive substance used as a comparison in controlled studies to see if the substance being tested has more than a psychological effect.

Poultice: A thick, moist paste applied directly to the skin to relieve pain or inflammation, to promote healing and to draw out infections, like venomous bites or blood poisoning.

Prolactin: A pituitary gland hormone involved in the stimulation of breast developement and milk formation.

Qi: In Traditional Chinese Medicine, the life force or energy.

Saturated fat: A fat whose carbon molecules are bound to as many hydrogen molecules as it can carry. They are found in animal foods like meat and dairy and are bad for you.

Sedative: Herb that strongly calms the nervous system.

Serotonin: A mood enhancing neurotransmitter that plays an important role in depression and insomnia.

Tincture: A liquid form of a herb usually containing one part herb to five parts liquid solvent. Tinctures are weaker than extracts.

Tonic: Herbs that can raise or lower the activity of a system, moving it back to its optimum state.

Trans-fatty acid: The hydrogenated or partially hydrogenated oils found in margarine and so many packaged foods. These fats are bad for you even in small amounts.

Tryptophan: An essential amino acid that is the precursor to serotonin, the brain's natural anti-depressant.

Unsaturated fat: A fat which has one—monounsaturated—or more—polyunsaturated—carbon molecules not filled with hydrogen molecules. Monounsaturated fats, like olive oil, and polyunsaturated fats, like flaxseed oil, are good for you.

Vulnerary: Herbs used to heal wounds or ulcers.

INDEX

and painkillers, 148-50
and Phytodolor, 153
topical painkillers, 151-52
panic attacks *See* anxiety
Parkinson's disease, 327-29
passionflower, 131
peppermint oil, 134
period, absence of *See* amenorrhoea
period, excessively heavy *See* menorrhagia
period, painful *See* dysmenorrhoea
Phytodolor, 153
premenstrual syndrome (PMS), 231-41
    psychological toll, 239-40
    symptoms and causes, 234
    treating, 234-39
prostate cancer, 260-64
prostate, englargement of *See* prostatic hyperplasia, benign
prostatic hyperplasia, benign, 248-51
psyllium, 279

Q
quercetin, 69-70

R
raspberry leaf, 41-42
rheumatoid arthritis, 330-34
rhodiola rosea, 114-15, 164
runny nose *See* sinusitis

S
saffron, 115
SAMe, 113-14, 313-14
saw palmetto berry, 248-49
selenium, 27
seniors' health, 267
sinusitis, 156-58
sitz bath, 230
skin problems, 159-61
skullcap, 129-30
soy, 186-87, 221-22, 261, 285, 324-25
St. John's wort, 112-13, 129
statins, 286
stress, 162-65
sugar cane wax, 287
Swank Diet, 144-45

T
tea tree oil, 27-28
teas, herbal, 49, 325
teething, 58
thrush, 59-60
thyme, 43
tinnitus, 304-5
topical painkillers, 151-52, 333
turmeric, 150-51

U
ulcers, 166-69
urinary tract infection, 170-75
uva ursi, 173

V
valerian, 129
vegetarian diet, 68, 185

and blood pressure, 306, 307
and cholesterol, 283-84
and fibrocystic breast disease, 208-9
and menopause, 221
and PMS, 234-35
vitamin A, 27
vitamin B6, 93-94, 237-38
vitamin C, 35, 71, 80, 109, 314
vitamin D, 323
vitamin E, 27
vitamins, B, 27, 110, 141

W
water retention, 237-38
white willow bark, 149-50
wild indigo, 108

Z
zinc, 27, 31, 109-10, 278